Mathematical Morphology and Its Applications to Image Processing

Computational Imaging and Vision

Volume 2

Mathematical Morphology and Its Applications to Image Processing

Edited by

Jean Serra

and

Pierre Soille

Ecole des Mines de Paris,
Centre de Morphologie Mathématique,
Fontainebleau, France

SPRINGER SCIENCE+BUSINESS MEDIA, B.V.

A C.I.P. Catalogue record for this book is available from the Library of Congress.

ISBN 978-94-010-4453-0 ISBN 978-94-011-1040-2 (eBook)
DOI 10.1007/978-94-011-1040-2

Printed on acid-free paper

Originally published by Kluwer Academic Publishers in 1994
Softcover reprint of the hardcover 1st edition 1994

Contents

Sampling

Coding

Representations and slope transform

Granulometries and shape description

Random models and tessellations

Algorithmic techniques

Biological applications

Preface

The first international conference entirely devoted to Mathematical Morphology (MM) and its applications to signal and image processing took place in Barcelona in May 1993. The success of this conference and the quality of the presented papers fostered us into organizing a second international conference in September 1994 in Fontainebleau, precisely where MM was born some 30 years ago.

Among the 86 submitted extended abstracts, 45 have been selected for an oral presentation. The full papers corresponding to these presentations constitute the core of this book. They represent the latest theoretical and applied developments of MM. Over 20 poster contributions have also been selected for the conference. These contributions are published separately by the *Ecole des Mines de Paris* and listed in Appendix B. We wish to express our thanks to the scientific committee who had the difficult task of reviewing the submitted papers within a very short time frame.

The realization of this book was quite challenging since we decided to make it available to attendees at the conference. We would like to thank all contributors in their effort for providing us with high quality manuscripts in time. Special thanks are also due to Tilman Jochems (our TeXpert), Sabine Müller, Sergei Kozyrev (for converting some manuscripts to TeX format), and to Michel Hugot and Philippe Le Caer (for helping us in the printing of a high quality camera-ready copy).

JEAN SERRA
PIERRE SOILLE

Introduction

Mathematical Morphology (MM) is a theory for the analysis of spatial structures which was initiated in the late sixties by Georges Matheron and Jean Serra at the Ecole des Mines de Paris (refer to Appendix A). It is called 'Morphology' since it aims at analysing the shape and form of objects. It is mathematical in the sense that the analysis is based on set theory, topology, lattice algebra, random functions, etc.

From the very beginning, theoretical developments have been driven by actual problems such as the characterization of porous media. The resulting developments could be used outside of research environments thanks to the realization of specialized hardware or, lately, new algorithmics.

It follows that MM is not only a *theory* but also a powerful image analysis *technique*. Both the theory and the technique have diffused worldwide as is reflected by the numerous conference sessions, scientific papers, industrial applications, hardware and software dealing with MM.

The purpose of the present book is to provide the image analysis community with a snapshot of current theoretical and applied developments of MM. The book consists of 45 contributions classified by subjects. It demonstrates a wide range of topics suited to the morphological approach. Each subject is briefly introduced hereafter.

Theory. The problem of translation invariance for bounded image domains is tackled and leads to the notion of conditional translation invariance. Then, a differential characterization of morphological operators using the new mathematical framework of mutational equation is investigated. Finally, an alternative characterization of morphological operations on l–images based on thresholding and umbraic approaches is provided.

Filtering. The papers dealing with filtering issues are organized around three main subjects: adaptive filtering (for openings, weighted order statistic filters, and background normalization), the application of genetic algorithms to the design of filters, and, on a more theoretical level, the study of the minimal generator basis of a finite structural opening.

Segmentation. This is a fundamental task of most image processing chains. In this section, new segmentation techniques are proposed and existing ones are further developed.

First, a new transformation, called the waterfall, is introduced and applied to

J.Serra and P. Soille (eds.), Mathematical Morphology and Its Applications to Image Processing, 1-4

hierarchical segmentation. It is closely related to the more classical watershed-based segmentation but it is not that much subjected to oversegmentation problems. Second, the watersheds of an image are defined as a minimum spanning forest of the neighbourhood graph of the image. Next, the effectiveness of the flat zone approach to image segmentation is demonstrated for colour images.

The last two contributions concern the segmentation step of the morphological approach to image coding (refer also to the coding section). This approach is object–oriented: the image is first segmented while the contours and textural parameters of each segment are transmitted. Regarding the segmentation step, intra– and inter–frame procedures are developed and the problems of including new regions and estimating the motion is tackled.

Sampling. The search for a morphological sampling scheme better adapted to further morphological processings is addressed by two contributions.

The first sampling scheme is referred to as 'critical morphological sampling' and is defined so as to meet a prescribed reconstruction error criterion. The second is based on the equicontinuous model and allows the sampling of an image so as to preserve a given accuracy under increasing or linear transformations of the image.

Coding. As mentioned in the segmentation section, image coding is a growing activity in MM. In this section, efficient techniques for the coding contours and decomposing an object into skeletal components are presented.

The first two papers address the problem of coding the contours of segmented images (refer also the segmentation section in this volume). It is shown that geodesic skeletons can be used for coding only once each region boundary. An improved method for contour image sequence coding based on motion estimation/compensation is developed. Finally, morphological skeleton decompositions are generalized for a family of structuring–functions indexed by a generic rather than scalar index. This leads to the definition of the multi–parameter skeleton. Better compression rates are expected when combining multi– with one–parameter skeletons.

Representations and slope transform. This transform has conceptual similarities with the Fourier transform in linear signal processing in the sense that it replaces the supremum operator by the arithmetic addition. The slope transform is the anchoring point of the theoretical developments presented in the three following contributions.

First, the morphological systems theory is further investigated. Next, it is shown how to convert the parallel normal transport property for the dilation of geometrical objects. This leads to the definition of a new transform complementary to the slope transform and called the normal transform. Finally, the geometric counterpart of adjunctions called dominance and incidence structures are presented and applied to the Buffon–Sylvester problem. It is also shown that the slope transform can be viewed as the adjunction of an incidence/dominance structure.

Granulometries and shape description. 1–D sieves are constructed from alternating sequential filters and are at the basis of a multiscale morphology decomposition theorem. Then, a new shape descriptor based on a statistical extension of the pattern spectrum is presented and called the 'spectrum'.

Finally, a generalized geodesic distance is introduced and applied to shape description and interpolation of contour data.

Random models and tessellations. This section discusses methods for segmenting, simulating, or estimating tessellations of the image plane.

The computational complexity of Voronoï tessellation algorithms based on morphological dilations is first estimated. In the second contribution, an algorithm based on simulated annealing allows the authors to determine an optimal partition of the image plane into Voronoï regions.

Next, a stochastic growth model mimicing boundary characteristics of tessellations with rough boundaries (as opposed to the Voronoï polygons) is presented. Probabilistic models (two-phase Poisson mosaic, dead leaves, and Boolean) are then used for characterizing grains encountered in material sciences. Finally, the problem of estimating the discrete size distribution and size density of a random binary image by means of empirical and Monte Carlo estimators is investigated.

Algorithmic techniques. Fast implementations of morphological transformations are essential to the processing of images in both academic and industrial environments. There is a continuous effort for implementing new transformations in hardware and with the advance of powerful workstations, efficient algorithmic techniques for software implementations are also sought for as reflected by the many contributions of this section.

Algorithms based on structuring element propagations and sliding windows are proposed for speeding up morphological openings. A reduction condition is also detailed for implementing close–open filters with very little extra calculations compared to a unique erosion step. An evaluation of queue data structures for morphological transformations such as watershedding is presented next. The authors demonstrate that the hierarchical queue performs the fastest but they recommend another data structure called the SplayQ for floating point values or data items of more than 12 bits. The problem of one–pixel thick skeletons is then tackled and a solution based on the definition of osculating hexagons is presented.

Fast granulometries with linear structuring elements based on the new concept of opening tree are detailed in the following contribution. An architecture for adaptive morphological operations with a reverse window operation is proposed next. Then, the parallelization of the watershed transformation is investigated and implemented in a loosely coupled system of workstations.

The visualization of 3D objects defined as a Minkowski addition or subtraction of primitives such as points, lines, discs, and spheres is addressed and solved by using constructive solid geometry methods. Finally, algorithms to simulate the morphogenesis of aggregates are proposed. The authors show that lattice gas models are an appropriate framework.

Biological applications. Stereological estimators requiring perfectly registered serial sections such as those obtained with a confocal microscope are first presented. The following applications illustrate the performance of three important morphological concepts: the granulometries, the watershed–based segmentation, and the morphological multiresolution pyramids.

Local granulometries are first used as an input to a neural network for texture classification of Kidneys' biopsies. The advantages of this approach over several other techniques are highlighted. A method for the fusion of magnetic resonance and computed tomography images based on multiresolution morphological pyramid construction/reconstruction is then developed. Eventually, the morphological approach to image segmentation is applied to the automatic morphometric analysis of epidermal biopsy images and to the quantification of spine parameters from X–ray images.

Industrial and remote sensing applications. After a survey of image processing for industrial applications, comparative filtering and multi–dimensional classification of geophysical data are presented.

This rapid scan through the book highlights the diversity of current morphological developments. All contributions will certainly prove beneficial to people working in the area and it is hoped that they will cross–fertilize the worlds of theoreticians and practitioners.

PIERRE SOILLE

SET OPERATOR DECOMPOSITION AND CONDITIONALLY TRANSLATION INVARIANT ELEMENTARY OPERATORS

G. J. F. BANON
Instituto Nacional de Pesquisas Espaciais, Divisão de Processamento de Imagens
CP 515
12 201–970, São José dos Campos, SP, Brazil
banon@dpi.inpe.br

J. BARRERA
Instituto de Matemática e Estatística, Universidade de São Paulo
CP IME 20 570
01 498–970, São Paulo, SP, Brazil
jb@ime.usp.br

Abstract. In the first part, we recall the axiomatic definition of the elementary morphological operators (dilations, erosions, anti–dilations and anti–erosions) and their characterization in the case of Boolean lattices. This characterization is used to derive the set operator decompositions from the general decompositions of operators between complete lattices. In the second part, we define the notions of "conditionally translation invariant" (c.t.i.) and of "locally c.t.i." elementary operators. These operators are those usually implemented on digital computers. We show how any c.t.i. elementary operator can be decomposed in terms of locally ones.

Key words: set operator decomposition, conditionally translation invariant elementary operator, Boolean lattice.

1. Introduction

In Image Processing, to work with translation invariant (t.i.) operators we must assume that the image domain has a torus structure. Unfortunately, this assumption is not acceptable in many practical applications. For this reason, the linear operators or the morphological elementary operators commonly used in Image Processing, behave like t.i. operators only in the "central" area of the image domain.

In the first part of the paper, we recall the axiomatic definitions of the four classes of morphological elementary operators. When the domain or the range of these elementary operators is a Boolean lattice, we can characterize the pairs of elementary operators that form Galois connections. This characterization is useful for two reasons: on one hand, it gives the clue for the link between any operator and its left or right kernel, and, on the other hand, it can be used to characterize the elementary set operators in terms of structuring functions.

Based on theses results, we derive the set operator decompositions from the general operator decompositions introduced by Banon and Barrera (1993).

In the second part of the paper, we introduce the formal definition of the so–called conditionally translation invariant (c.t.i.) elementary operators. This definition corresponds to what is usually implemented on digital computers and it is based on the notion of c.t.i. structuring function. We present the collection of all the structuring elements that characterize the c.t.i. structuring functions.

Unfortunately, the c.t.i. elementary operators are not sufficient to represent any operator. For this reason, we introduce the notion of locally c.t.i. elementary operator and we

J.Serra and P. Soille (eds.), Mathematical Morphology and Its Applications to Image Processing, 5-12

give a constructive decomposition of any c.t.i. elementary operator. The decomposition of a c.t.i. dilation is given as an example to illustrate the theory.

2. Axiomatic Definition and Characterization of the Morphological Elementary Operators

Let $(\mathcal{L}, \leq)$, or simply $\mathcal{L}$, be a complete lattice (Birkhoff, 1967). We denote by $\bigvee$, $\bigwedge$ the union and intersection in $\mathcal{L}$. The *dual complete lattice of* $\mathcal{L}$, $(\mathcal{L}, \geq)$, is denoted $\widetilde{\mathcal{L}}$.

Let $\mathcal{L}_1$ and $\mathcal{L}_2$ be two complete lattices. The class $\mathcal{L}_2{}^{\mathcal{L}_1}$ of the mappings ψ from $\mathcal{L}_1$ to $\mathcal{L}_2$, called *operators*, equipped with the *punctual ordering* $\underset{(\mathcal{L}_2)}{\leq}$

$$\psi \underset{(\mathcal{L}_2)}{\leq} \psi' \Leftrightarrow \psi(X) \underset{\mathcal{L}_2}{\leq} \psi'(X) \ (X \in \mathcal{L}_1)$$

is a complete lattice.

We define the morphological elementary operators axiomatically. The *dilations* (resp. *erosions*) from $\mathcal{L}_1$ to $\mathcal{L}_2$ are the operators in $\mathcal{L}_2{}^{\mathcal{L}_1}$ which commute with union (resp. intersection). The *anti–dilations* (resp. *anti–erosions*) from $\mathcal{L}_1$ to $\mathcal{L}_2$ are the dilations (resp. erosion) from $\mathcal{L}_1$ to $\widetilde{\mathcal{L}}_2$ (Banon & Barrera, 1993).

We will denote by $\Delta(\mathcal{L}_1, \mathcal{L}_2)$, $\mathrm{E}(\mathcal{L}_1, \mathcal{L}_2)$, $\Delta^a(\mathcal{L}_1, \mathcal{L}_2)$ and $\mathrm{E}^a(\mathcal{L}_1, \mathcal{L}_2)$, respectively, the class of dilations, erosions, anti–dilations and anti–erosions from $\mathcal{L}_1$ to $\mathcal{L}_2$. We know (Banon & Barrera, 1993a) that these classes are complete lattices. Consequently, the Galois connections (α, β) between $\mathcal{L}_1$ and $\mathcal{L}_2$ (Birkhoff, 1967) form a complete lattice with respect the the partial ordering

$$(\alpha, \beta) \leq (\alpha', \beta') \Leftrightarrow \alpha \underset{(\mathcal{L}_2)}{\leq} \alpha' \text{ and } \beta \underset{(\mathcal{L}_1)}{\leq} \beta'.$$

If (α, β) is a Galois connection, then β is the *companion operator of* α and similarly α is the *companion operator of* β.

Let E be a non empty set, then $(\mathcal{P}(E), \subset)$, or simply $\mathcal{P}(E)$ or $\mathcal{P}$, the collection of all parts of E equipped with the inclusion $\subset$, is a complete Boolean lattice. We denote by X^c the set complement of a subset X of E.

Let $(\mathcal{L}, \leq)$ be a complete lattice. The set $\mathcal{L}^E$ of the functions a from E to $\mathcal{L}$ equipped with the punctual ordering $\underset{(\mathcal{L})}{\leq}$ is a complete lattice.

We now recall Corollary 4 of Achache (1982). A similar result (with $\mathcal{L} = \mathcal{P}(E)$) is in Serra (1988, Section 2.2).

Proposition 1 – The mapping $a \mapsto (\alpha, \beta)$ from the complete lattice $\mathcal{L}^E$ to the complete lattice of Galois connections between $\mathcal{L}$ and $(\mathcal{P}(E), \subset)$ defined by

$$\alpha(X) = \{y \in E : X \underset{\mathcal{L}}{\leq} a(y)\} \ (X \in \mathcal{L}) \quad \text{and} \quad \beta(Y) = \bigwedge_{y \in Y} a(y) \ (Y \in \mathcal{P}(E))$$

is a lattice isomorphism. Its inverse $(\alpha, \beta) \mapsto a$ is given by $a(y) = \beta(\{y\})$ $(y \in E)$. □

We know (Achache, 1982, Lemma 1) that $\alpha \in \Delta^a(\mathcal{L}, \mathcal{P})$ and $\beta \in \Delta^a(\mathcal{P}, \mathcal{L})$. From Proposition 1 we can derive the following proposition.

Proposition 2 – The mapping $a \mapsto (\alpha, \beta)$ from the complete lattice $\mathcal{L}^E$ to the complete lattice of Galois connections between $\mathcal{L}$ and $(\mathcal{P}(E), \supset)$ defined by

$$\alpha(X) = \{y \in E : X \underset{\mathcal{L}}{\leq} a(y)\}^c \ (X \in \mathcal{L}) \quad \text{and} \quad \beta(Y) = \bigwedge_{y \in Y^c} a(y) \ (Y \in \mathcal{P}(E))$$

is a lattice isomorphism. Its inverse $(\alpha,\beta) \mapsto a$ is given by $a(y) = \beta(\{y\}^c)$ $(y \in E)$. □

In this case, $\alpha \in \Delta(\mathcal{L},\mathcal{P})$ and $\beta \in \mathrm{E}(\mathcal{P},\mathcal{L})$. In Propositions 1 and 2 the function a is called the *structuring function of the elementary operators* α *and* β.

From Propositions 1 and 2 we can derive the elementary operators characterization given in Table 1 and the next corollary where $\mathcal{P}_2$ stands for $\mathcal{P}(E_2)$.

TABLE 1

Elementary operators characterization.

identifying $\mathcal{L}$ to	in Prop.	leads to	and	with
$\tilde{\mathcal{L}}_1$	1	$\alpha \in \mathrm{E}(\mathcal{L}_1,\mathcal{P}_2)$ $\beta \in \Delta(\mathcal{P}_2,\mathcal{L}_1)$	$\alpha = \varepsilon_a$ $\beta = \delta_a$	$\varepsilon_a(X) = \{y \in E_2 : a(y) \leq X\}$ $\delta_a(Y) = \bigvee_{y \in Y} a(y)$
$\mathcal{L}_1$	1	$\alpha \in \Delta^a(\mathcal{L}_1,\mathcal{P}_2)$ $\beta \in \Delta^a(\mathcal{P}_2,\mathcal{L}_1)$	$\alpha = {}_b\delta^a$ $\beta = \delta^a{}_b$	${}_b\delta^a(X) = \{y \in E_2 : X \leq b(y)\}$ $\delta^a{}_b(Y) = \bigwedge_{y \in Y} b(y)$
$\tilde{\mathcal{L}}_1$	2	$\alpha \in \mathrm{E}^a(\mathcal{L}_1,\mathcal{P}_2)$ $\beta \in \mathrm{E}^a(\mathcal{P}_2,\mathcal{L}_1)$	$\alpha = \varepsilon^a{}_a$ $\beta = {}_a\varepsilon^a$	$\varepsilon^a{}_a(X) = \{y \in E_2 : a(y) \leq X\}^c$ ${}_a\varepsilon^a(Y) = \bigvee_{y \in Y^c} a(y)$
$\mathcal{L}_1$	2	$\alpha \in \Delta(\mathcal{L}_1,\mathcal{P}_2)$ $\beta \in \mathrm{E}(\mathcal{P}_2,\mathcal{L}_1)$	$\alpha = {}_b\delta$ $\beta = {}_b\varepsilon$	${}_b\delta(X) = \{y \in E_2 : X \leq b(y)\}^c$ ${}_b\varepsilon(Y) = \bigwedge_{y \in Y^c} b(y)$

Corollary 3 – Let a and b be two functions from E_2 to $\mathcal{L}_1$. Then we have:
(1) if a is the structuring function of $\delta \in \Delta(\mathcal{P}_2,\mathcal{L}_1)$ (i.e., $a(y) = \delta(\{y\})$ $(y \in E_2)$) then its companion erosion is ε_a;
(2) if b is the structuring function of $\delta^a \in \Delta^a(\mathcal{P}_2,\mathcal{L}_1)$ (i.e., $b(y) = \delta^a(\{y\})$ $(y \in E_2)$) then its companion anti–dilation is ${}_b\delta^a$;
(3) if a is the structuring function of $\varepsilon^a \in \mathrm{E}^a(\mathcal{P}_2,\mathcal{L}_1)$ (i.e., $a(y) = \varepsilon^a(\{y\}^c)$ $(y \in E_2)$) then its companion anti–erosion is $\varepsilon^a{}_a$;
(4) if b is the structuring function of $\varepsilon \in \mathrm{E}(\mathcal{P}_2,\mathcal{L}_1)$ (i.e., $b(y) = \varepsilon(\{y\}^c)$ $(y \in E_2)$) then its companion dilation is ${}_b\delta$. □

3. Operator Decomposition in terms of Elementary Operators

In order to specialize to set operators the general decomposition theorem (Banon & Barrera, 1993) we need to derive one more corollary from Proposition 1. In this section $\mathcal{P}_1$ and $\mathcal{P}_2$ stands, respectively, for $\mathcal{P}(E_1)$ and $\mathcal{P}(E_2)$. Let ψ be an operator from $\mathcal{P}_1$ to $\mathcal{P}_2$. We recall (Banon & Barrera, 1993) that the mappings $\cdot\mathcal{K}(\psi)$ and $\mathcal{K}\cdot(\psi)$ from $\mathcal{P}_2$ to $\mathcal{P}(\mathcal{P}_1)$ given by, for any $Y \in \mathcal{P}_2$,

$$\cdot\mathcal{K}(\psi)(Y) = \{X \in \mathcal{P}_1 : Y \subset \psi(X)\} \text{ and } \mathcal{K}\cdot(\psi)(Y) = \{X \in \mathcal{P}_1 : \psi(X) \subset Y\}$$

are called, respectively, the *left* and *right kernel of* ψ.

Corollary 4 – The left and right kernel of a set operator from $\mathcal{P}_1$ to $\mathcal{P}_2$ are, respectively, an anti–dilation and an erosion from $\mathcal{P}_2$ to $\mathcal{P}(\mathcal{P}_1)$. □

Proof – For the left kernel, the result follows from Proposition 1 by identifying E, $\mathcal{L}$, a and α to, respectively, $\mathcal{P}_1$, $\mathcal{P}_2$, ψ and $\cdot\mathcal{K}(\psi)$. For the right kernel, the result follows from Proposition 1 by identifying E, $\mathcal{L}$, a and α to, respectively, $\mathcal{P}_1$, $\tilde{\mathcal{P}}_2$, ψ and $\mathcal{K}\cdot(\psi)$. □

Let $\alpha,\beta \in \mathcal{P}_1^{\mathcal{P}_2}$ and let $[\alpha,\beta]$ be the *interval function* from $\mathcal{P}_2$ to $\mathcal{P}(\mathcal{P}_1)$ *with extremities α and β* (Banon & Barrera, 1993).

Lemma 5 – Let ψ be a set operator from $\mathcal{P}_1$ to $\mathcal{P}_2$.
(1) If $\alpha \in \Delta(\mathcal{P}_2,\mathcal{P}_1)$ and $\beta \in \Delta^a(\mathcal{P}_2,\mathcal{P}_1)$ then, for any $Y \in \mathcal{P}_2$,

$$[\alpha,\beta](\{y\}) \subset \cdot\mathcal{K}(\psi)(\{y\}) \ (y \in Y) \Rightarrow [\alpha,\beta](Y) \subset \cdot\mathcal{K}(\psi)(Y).$$

(2) If $\alpha \in E^a(\mathcal{P}_2,\mathcal{P}_1)$ and $\beta \in E(\mathcal{P}_2,\mathcal{P}_1)$ then, for any $Y \in \mathcal{P}_2$,

$$[\alpha,\beta](\{y\}^c) \subset \mathcal{K}\cdot(\psi)(\{y\}^c) \ (y \in Y^c) \Rightarrow [\alpha,\beta](Y) \subset \mathcal{K}\cdot(\psi)(Y). \quad \square$$

Proof – Let us prove part (1). For any $Y \in \mathcal{P}_2$,

$$\begin{aligned}
\text{TRUE} &\Leftrightarrow [\alpha,\beta](Y) \subset [\alpha,\beta](\{y\}) \ (y \in Y) && (\alpha \text{ is isotone and } \beta \text{ is antitone})\\
&\Leftrightarrow [\alpha,\beta](Y) \subset \bigcap_{y \in Y} [\alpha,\beta](\{y\}) && (\text{property of the intersection})\\
&\Rightarrow [\alpha,\beta](Y) \subset \bigcap_{y \in Y} \cdot\mathcal{K}(\psi)(\{y\}) && ([\alpha,\beta](\{y\}) \subset \cdot\mathcal{K}(\psi)(\{y\}) \ (y \in Y))\\
&\Leftrightarrow [\alpha,\beta](Y) \subset \cdot\mathcal{K}(\psi)(\bigcup_{y \in Y} \{y\}) && (\text{by Corollary 4, } \cdot\mathcal{K}(\psi) \text{ is an anti–dilation})\\
&\Leftrightarrow [\alpha,\beta](Y) \subset \cdot\mathcal{K}(\psi)(Y). && (Y \text{ representation by singletons})
\end{aligned}$$

The proof of part (2) is similar to the proof of part (1). □

Let AB be the set defined by

$$\mathrm{AB} = \{(a,b) \in \mathcal{P}_1^{E_2} \times \mathcal{P}_1^{E_2} : \forall y \in E_2,\ (a(y) \subset b(y)) \text{ or } (a(y) = E_1 \text{ and } b(y) = \emptyset)\}$$

Let $a, b \in \mathcal{P}_1^{E_2}$. We denote by $[a,b]$ the *interval function* from E_2 to $\mathcal{P}(\mathcal{P}_1)$ *with extremities a and b*. We denote the punctual ordering $\underset{(\subset)}{\leq}$ on $\mathcal{P}(\mathcal{P}_1)^{E_2}$ simply $\leq$.

Theorem 6 – Any operator $\psi \in \mathcal{P}_2^{\mathcal{P}_1}$ can be decomposed in terms of a set of sup–generating or inf–generating operators and the constructive decompositions are

$$\psi = \bigvee_{(a,b) \in \mathrm{AB} \text{ and } [a,b] \leq \cdot\mathcal{K}(\psi)} (\varepsilon_a \wedge {}_b\delta^a)$$

where $\cdot\mathcal{K}(\psi)(y) = \{X \in \mathcal{P}_1 : y \in \psi(X)\}$, for any $y \in E_2$, and

$$\psi = \bigwedge_{(a,b) \in \mathrm{AB} \text{ and } [a,b] \leq \mathcal{K}\cdot(\psi)} (\varepsilon^a{}_a \vee {}_b\delta)$$

where $\mathcal{K}\cdot(\psi)(y) = \{X \in \mathcal{P}_1 : y \notin \psi(X)\}$, for any $y \in E_2$. □

Proof – We can make a direct proof or, as we do below, derive the result from the general decomposition theorem of Banon & Barrera (1993). For any ψ from $\mathcal{P}_1$ to $\mathcal{P}_2$,

$$\psi = \bigvee_{(\alpha,\beta) \in \Delta\Delta^* \text{ and } [\alpha,\beta] \leq \cdot \mathcal{K}(\psi)} (\overline{\alpha \mathrm{I}} \wedge \overline{\mathrm{O}\beta})$$

(Theorem 6.1 of Banon & Barrera (1993a) or Theorem 1 of Banon & Barrera (1993b))

$$= \bigvee_{(\alpha,\beta) \in \Delta\Delta^* \text{ and } ([\alpha,\beta](y) \subset \cdot \mathcal{K}(\psi)(\{y\})\ (y \in E_2))} (\overline{\alpha \mathrm{I}} \wedge \overline{\mathrm{O}\beta}) \quad \text{(Lemma 5)}$$

$$= \bigvee_{(a,b) \in \mathrm{AB} \text{ and } [a,b] \leq \cdot \mathcal{K}(\psi)} (\varepsilon_a \wedge {}_b\delta^*). \quad \text{(Corollary 3)}$$

The proof of the second decomposition is similar to the proof of the first one. □

A direct proof of a similar result is given in Banon & Barrera (1990).

The sup–generating and inf–generating operators of Theorem 6 are, respectively, the operators $\varepsilon_a \wedge {}_b\delta^*$ and $\varepsilon^*_a \vee {}_b\delta$, where a and b are functions from E_2 to $\mathcal{P}_1$.

4. Conditionally Translation Invariant Elementary Operators

Let $(\mathbf{Z}^2, +)$ be the set of ordered pairs of integers equipped with the usual addition. Let u be a point of $\mathbf{Z}^2$, we denote by $B + u$ the translate by u of a subset B of $\mathbf{Z}^2$ and by B^t its transpose (Banon & Barrera 1991). From now on, we assume that the sets E_1 and E_2 of Section 3 are subsets of $\mathbf{Z}^2$ (for example "rectangles").

A function b from E_2 to $\mathcal{P}_1$ is *conditionally translation invariant* or a *ct–function* iff

$$\exists B \in \mathcal{P}(\mathbf{Z}^2),\ \forall y \in E_2,\ b(y) = (B + y) \cap E_1.$$

Let us consider the following subcollection $\mathfrak{B}_{E_1,E_2}$, or simply $\mathfrak{B}$, of $\mathcal{P}(\mathbf{Z}^2)$

$$\mathfrak{B} = \{B \in \mathcal{P}(\mathbf{Z}^2) : \forall b \in B,\ \exists u \in E_2,\ b + u \in E_1\}.$$

Let $\oplus$ denote the Minkowski addition on $\mathcal{P}(\mathbf{Z}^2)$ (Hadwiger, 1950). We observe that $\mathfrak{B}$ is an ideal and a complete sublattice of $\mathcal{P}(\mathbf{Z}^2)$, its greatest element is $E_1 \oplus E_2^t$ and $\mathfrak{B} = \mathcal{P}(E_1 \oplus E_2^t)$. Figure 1 shows an element B of $\mathfrak{B}$ generated by two rectangles.

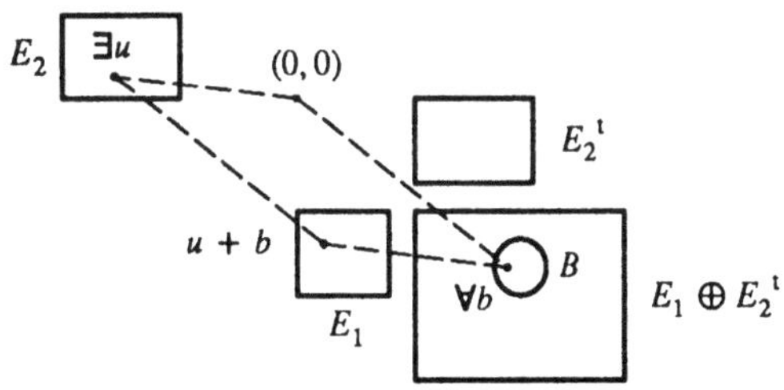

Fig. 1 – An element of an ideal generated by two rectangles.

The next proposition characterizes the ct–functions in $\mathcal{P}_1^{E_2}$ in terms of subsets of $E_1 \oplus E_2^t$.

Proposition 7 – The mapping $B \mapsto b_B$ from $\mathfrak{B}$ to the set of ct–functions in $\mathcal{P}_1^{E_2}$ given by

$$b_B(y) = (B + y) \cap E_1 \quad (y \in E_2)$$

is a bijection. Its inverse $b \mapsto B_b$ is given by $B_b = \bigcup_{y \in E_2} (b(y) - y)$. □

Proof – (1) For any $B \in \mathfrak{B}$, b_B is by construction a ct–function.

(2) For any ct–function b from E_2 to $\mathcal{P}(E_1)$

$$B_b = \bigcup_{y \in E_2} (b(y) - y) \qquad \text{(definition of } B_b\text{)}$$

$$\subset \bigcup_{y \in E_2} (E_1 - y) \qquad (b(y) \subset E_1)$$

$$= E_1 \oplus E_2^t, \qquad \text{(definition of } \oplus\text{)}$$

That is, $B_b \in \mathfrak{B}$.

(3) Let us prove that $B \mapsto b_B$ is "one to one". On one hand, for any $B \in \mathfrak{B}$,

$$\begin{aligned}
\text{TRUE} &\Leftrightarrow (B + y) \cap E_1 \subset (B + y) \quad (y \in E_2) && \text{(property of the intersection)}\\
&\Leftrightarrow ((B + y) \cap E_1) - y \subset B \quad (y \in E_2) && \text{(translation is isotone)}\\
&\Leftrightarrow \bigcup_{y \in E_2} (((B + y) \cap E_1) - y) \subset B && \text{(property of the union)}\\
&\Leftrightarrow B_{b_B} \subset B. && \text{(definitions of } b_B \text{ and } B_b\text{)}
\end{aligned}$$

On the other hand, for any $B \in \mathfrak{B}$ and $b \in \mathbf{Z}^2$,

$$\begin{aligned}
b \in B &\Rightarrow b \in B \text{ and } \exists y \in E_2,\ b + y \in E_1 && \text{(definition of } \mathfrak{B}\text{)}\\
&\Rightarrow \exists y \in E_2,\ b + y \in B + y \text{ and } y + b \in E_1 && \text{(property of the translation)}\\
&\Leftrightarrow \exists y \in E_2,\ b + y \in (B + y) \cap E_1 && \text{(definition of the intersection)}\\
&\Leftrightarrow \exists y \in E_2,\ b \in ((B + y) \cap E_1) - y && \text{(translation is isotone)}\\
&\Leftrightarrow b \in \bigcup_{y \in E_2} (((B + y) \cap E_1) - y) && \text{(definition of the union)}\\
&\Leftrightarrow b \in B_{b_B}. && \text{(definitions of } b_B \text{ and } B_b\text{)}
\end{aligned}$$

That is, for any $B \in \mathfrak{B}$, $B \subset B_{b_B}$. Therefore, $B \mapsto b_B$ is "one to one".

(4) Let us prove that $B \mapsto b_B$ is "onto". On one hand, for any ct–function b in $\mathcal{P}_1^{E_2}$ and $y \in E_2$,

$$\begin{aligned}
b_{B_b}(y) &= ((\bigcup_{v \in E_2} (b(v) - v)) + y) \cap E_1 && \text{(definitions of } B_b \text{ and } b_B\text{)}\\
&\supset b(y) \cap E_1 && (v = y \text{ e property of the union)}\\
&= b(y). && (b(y) \subset E_1)
\end{aligned}$$

On the other hand, for any ct–function b in $\mathcal{P}_1^{E_2}$ and $y \in E_2$,

$$\begin{aligned}
\text{TRUE} &\Leftrightarrow ((\bigcup_{v \in E_2} (b(v) - v)) + y) \cap E_1 \subset (\bigcup_{v \in E_2} (b(v) - v)) + y && \text{(property of } \cap\text{)}\\
&\Leftrightarrow (((\bigcup_{v \in E_2} (b(v) - v)) + y) \cap E_1 \subset (b(v) - v) + y) \ (v \in E_2) && \text{(prop. of } \bigcup\text{)}\\
&\Leftrightarrow (b_{B_b}(y) \subset (b(v) - v) + y) \ (v \in E_2) && \text{(definitions of } B_b \text{ and } b_B\text{)}\\
&\Rightarrow b_{B_b}(y) \subset b(v). && (v = y)
\end{aligned}$$

Therefore, $B \mapsto b_B$ is "onto". □

We say that an elementary operator from $\mathcal{P}(E_1)$ to $\mathcal{P}(E_2)$ is *conditionally translation invariant* (*c.t.i.*) iff its structuring function from E_2 to $\mathcal{P}(E_1)$ is a ct–function. For any $B \in \mathfrak{B}$, we denote by α_B (or ${}_B\alpha$) the c.t.i. elementary operator which has the structuring function b_B. In particular, we have $\varepsilon_B(X) = ((X \cup E_1^c) \ominus B) \cap E_2$ $(X \in \mathcal{P}(E_1))$ and $\delta_B(Y) = (Y \oplus B) \cap E_1$ $(Y \in \mathcal{P}(E_2))$ where $\ominus$ is the Minkowski subtraction on $\mathcal{P}(\mathbf{Z}^2)$ (Hadwiger, 1950).

5. Locally c.t.i. Elementary Operators

A function b from E_2 to $\mathfrak{P}_1$ is said to be a *locally ct–function* iff there exist a subset M of E_2, called *mask*, and a ct–function b' from E_2 to $\mathfrak{P}_1$, such that

$$b(y) = \begin{cases} b'(y) & \text{if } y \in M \\ \emptyset & \text{otherwise} \end{cases} \quad (y \in E_2).$$

We will now give a constructive function decomposition in terms of locally ct–function. Let b be a function from E_2 to $\mathfrak{P}_1$. We define the binary relation $\mathfrak{R}_b$ on E_2 by

$$y_1 \,\mathfrak{R}_b\, y_2 \Leftrightarrow \exists B \in \mathfrak{B},\ (B + y_1) \cap E_1 = b(y_1) \text{ and } (B + y_2) \cap E_1 = b(y_2).$$

The relation $\mathfrak{R}_b$ is an equivalence relation. We denote by $E_2/\mathfrak{R}_b$ the resulting partition of E_2.

Proposition 8 – Any function b from E_2 to $\mathfrak{P}_1$ can be decomposed in terms of locally ct–functions and the constructive decomposition is

$$b = \bigvee_{M \in E_2/\mathfrak{R}_b} b_{B_{b/M},M}$$

where, for any $M \in \mathfrak{P}(E_2)$ and $B \in \mathfrak{B}$, $b_{B,M}$ is the function from E_2 to $\mathfrak{P}_1$ given by

$$b_{B,M}(y) = \begin{cases} b_B(y) & \text{if } y \in M \\ \emptyset & \text{otherwise} \end{cases} \quad (y \in E_2)$$

and b/M denotes the restriction of b to M. □

Proof – For any $N \in E_2/\mathfrak{R}_b$ and $y \in N$,

$$\begin{aligned} (\bigvee_{M \in E_2/\mathfrak{R}_b} b_{B_{b/M},M})(y) &= b_{B_{b/N}}(y) && \text{(definition and property of } b_{B,M}) \\ &= b/N(y) && \text{(Proposition 7 applied to the ct–function } b/N) \\ &= b(y). && \text{(definition of restriction)} \end{aligned}$$

□

The locally ct–functions of Proposition 8 are the functions $b_{B,M}$.

We say that an elementary operator from $\mathfrak{P}_1$ to $\mathfrak{P}_2$ is *locally c.t.i.* iff its structuring function in $\mathfrak{P}_1^{E_2}$ is a locally ct–function. For any $M \in \mathfrak{P}_2$ and $B \in \mathfrak{B}$, we denote by $a_{B,M}$ (or ${}_{B,M}a$) the locally c.t.i. elementary operator which has the structuring function $b_{B,M}$.

6. Elementary Operator Decomposition in terms of Locally c.t.i. Elementary Operators

Theorem 9 – Any elementary operator δ (resp. ε, δ^{a} and ε^{a}) of the class $\Delta(\mathfrak{P}_1, \mathfrak{P}_2)$ (resp. $\mathrm{E}(\mathfrak{P}_1, \mathfrak{P}_2)$, $\Delta^{a}(\mathfrak{P}_1, \mathfrak{P}_2)$ and $\mathrm{E}^{a}(\mathfrak{P}_1, \mathfrak{P}_2)$) can be decomposed in terms of locally c.t.i. elementary operators of the same class and, if b is its structuring function, the constructive decomposition is $\delta = \bigwedge_M {}_{B_{b/M},M}\delta$ (respectively. $\varepsilon = \bigwedge_M \varepsilon_{B_{b/M},M}$, $\varepsilon^{a} = \bigvee_M \varepsilon^{a}{}_{B_{b/M},M}$ and

$\delta^{a} = \bigvee_M {}_{B_{b/M},M}\delta^{a}$), where the union and intersection are taken over $E_2/\mathfrak{R}_b$. □

Proof – The result is a consequence of Propositions 1, 2 and 8. The decomposition involves an union (resp. intersection) when the mapping $a \mapsto \boldsymbol{a}$ is an isomorphism (resp. a dual isomorphism). □

From Theorems 6 and 9, we see that any operator can be decomposed in terms of locally c.t.i. elementary operators.

Let E be a non empty subset of $\mathbf{Z}^2$ and $B \in \mathfrak{B}_{E,E}$. We now consider the *example* of decomposition of δ_B, the *ct–dilation by B* defined from $\mathcal{P}(E)$ to $\mathcal{P}(E)$. We know that $\delta_B(X) = (X \oplus B) \cap E$. The left kernel (as defined in Theorem 6) of δ_B is given by

$$\cdot\mathcal{K}(\delta_B)(y) = \{X \in \mathcal{P} : (B^t + y) \cap X \neq \emptyset\} \quad (y \in E).$$

For any $y \in E$, if $(B^t + y) \cap E \neq \emptyset$, then $\cdot\mathcal{K}(\delta_B)(y) \neq \emptyset$ and the pairs (a, b) of interest in the decomposition of δ_B are such that the $a(y)$ contain at least one point in $(B^t + y) \cap E$; if $(B^t + y) \cap E = \emptyset$, then $\cdot\mathcal{K}(\delta_B)(y) = \emptyset$ and by convention $a(y) = E$ and $b(y) = \emptyset$.

Let consider the following simple case where $B = \{p\}$ with $p \in E \oplus E^t$ and let $Z = E \cap (E + p)$. The pairs (a, b) of interest leading to the greatest interval functions reduce to only one defined by $a(y) = \{y - p\}$ and $b(y) = E$ if $y \in Z$, and $a(y) = E$ and $b(y) = \emptyset$ if $y \in E - Z$.

Hence, by Theorem 6, $\delta_{\{p\}} = \varepsilon_a \wedge {}_b\delta^a$ where a and b are the above ct–functions. We observe that even $\delta_{\{p\}}$ being a ct–dilation ε_a is neither a ct–erosion nor a locally ct–erosion. Just ${}_b\delta^a$ is a locally ct–anti–dilation (with $M = Z$ and $B = E$). Nevertheless, by Theorem 9, we can decompose ε_a in terms of two locally ct–erosions: $\varepsilon_a = \varepsilon_{\{-p\},Z} \wedge \varepsilon_{E,Z^c}$ Finally, we get the following decomposition of the ct–dilation $\delta_{\{p\}}$ in terms of locally ct–erosions and ct–anti–dilation:

$$\delta_{\{p\}} = (\varepsilon_{\{-p\},Z} \wedge \varepsilon_{E,Z^c}) \wedge {}_{E,Z}\delta^a.$$

7. Acknowledgements

The authors are grateful to Professor J.Serra who has suggested the present work during the previous workshop at Barcelona in May 1993 as well as the names of "conditional translation invariance" and "ct–operator".

This work has been supported by FAPESP (Fundação de Amparo à Pesquisa do Estado de São Paulo) under contract 91/3532–2.

8. References

Achache, A.: 1982, "Galois Connexion of fuzzy subset". *Fuzzy Sets and Systems*, Vol. **8**, pp. 215–218.

Banon, G. J. F. and Barrera, J.: 1990, "Set mapping decomposition by Mathematical Morphology". In R. M. Haralick ed., *Mathematical Morphology: Theory and Hardware*. To appear.

Banon, G. J. F. and Barrera, J.: 1991, "Minimal representations for translation–invariant set mappings by Mathematical Morphology". *SIAM J. Appl. Math.* Vol. **51**, pp. 1782–1798.

Banon, G. J. F. and Barrera, J.: 1993a, "Decomposition of mappings between complete lattices by Mathematical Morphology". *Signal Processing* Vol. **30**, pp. 299–327.

Banon, G. J. F. and Barrera, J.: 1993b, "A decomposition theorem in Mathematical Morphology". Proceedings of the International Worshop on Mathematical Morphology and its Application to Signal Processing, Barcelona, Spain, pp. 234–238.

Birkhoff, G.: 1967, *Lattice theory*. 3rd ed., American Mathematical Society, Providence, Rhode Island.

Hadwiger, H.: 1950, "Minkowskische Addition und Subtraktion beleibiger Punktmengen und die Theoreme von Erhard Schmidt". *Math. Zeitschrift*. Vol. **53**, pp. 210–218.

Serra, J. P. F. (edited by): 1988, *Image Analysis and Mathematical Morphology. Volume 2: Theoretical Advances*. Academic Press, London, 411 p..

MUTATIONAL EQUATIONS OF MORPHOLOGICAL DILATION TUBES

L. DOYEN
CEREMADE, Université Paris-Dauphine,
Place du Maréchal de Lattre de Tassigny, 75775 Paris Cedex 16, France

and

L. NAJMAN and J. MATTIOLI
L.C.R., Thomson-CSF, Domaine de Corbeville, 91401 Orsay, France

Abstract. The present paper provides some differential results dealing with the morphological dilation of a compact set in the nonregular case. Indeed the evolution of dilated sets with respect to time is characterized through mutational equations which are new mathematical tools extending the concept of differential equations to the metric space of all nonempty compact sets of R^n. Using the generalized gradient notion and viability theorems, we prove that a mutation of the dilation tube corresponds to the normal cone which is a generalization of the classical notion of normal.

Key words: Dilation, jauge, generalized gradient, normal cone, differential inclusions, viability tube, mutation of tube.

1. Introduction

Several works have investigated the problem of a differential characterization of the morphological operators and especially the dilation. But most of these studies have been done in a regular context [5] or through partial differential equations or inclusions ([1], [10]). We propose here to provide a geometrical point of view about this problem. To this aim, we consider it in the new mathematical framework of mutational equations ([4], [7]) which allows to extend the concept of differential equations to the metric space $\mathcal{K}(\mathbb{R}^n)$ of all non-empty compact subsets of $\mathbb{R}^n$. This means that we can characterize the evolution $K(t)$ (also called tube) of a compact geometric domain K in a differential manner, without any regularity assumptions on the shape that we deal with. Furthermore, basic theorems of classical differential systems, as the Cauchy-Lipschitz one, can be adapted to mutational equations.

In the present paper, we prove that the morphological tube $K(t) = K \oplus tS$, which corresponds to the dilation of a compact domain K by a convex compact symmetric set S with non-empty interior, satisfies some mutational equations and especially

$$\overset{\circ}{K}(t) \ni N^S_{K(t)}(\cdot) \cap S, \quad K(0) = K$$

where $N^S_K(x)$ represents the normal cone of the domain K at the point x for the norm associated with the structuring element S. This result clearly establishes, without any regularity assumptions on the compact set K, that the dilation transforms the initial domain K in the direction of the normals at any point of the set. Furthermore,

J.Serra and P. Soille (eds.), Mathematical Morphology and Its Applications to Image Processing, 13-20

when the set K is a regular manifold, the normal cone $N_K(x)$ is reduced to the half-line spanned by the outward normal $n(x)$ and we rediscover results obtained in the regular case. To state this differential characterization of the dilation, we use the notion of generalized gradient (see [6]) and viability theorems for tubes (see [3]).

2. Structuring Element, Gauge and Dilation

A basic morphological operator is the dilation. There exists several ways to define the dilation by a structuring element S. Here we propose to introduce this notion using the gauge associated with the structuring element.

The **gauge** associated to a structuring element $S \subset \mathbb{R}^n$ is defined as follows

$$j_S(x) := \inf_{\lambda \geq 0,\, x \in \lambda S} \lambda.$$

If S is equal to the Euclidean unit ball B of $\mathbb{R}^n$, the gauge appears to be the Euclidean norm. More generally, when the set S is compact, convex, with non-empty interior and symmetric with respect to the origin, then it defines a norm (see [2, Aubin]). Through the gauge, we can also define a **distance between a set K and a point x** by

$$d_K^S(x) := \inf_{y \in K} j_S(x - y),$$

and the projection of x on K associated with S as $\Pi_K^S(x) := \{z \in K \mid j_S(x - z) = d_K^S(x)\}$. When the set S has a non-empty interior, we can check that the map $x \mapsto d_K^S(x)$ is Lipschitz.

The **dilation at scale $t > 0$ of a closed set $K \subset \mathbb{R}^n$ by a structuring element S** is

$$K_S(t) := \{x \in \mathbb{R}^n \mid d_K^S(x) \leq t\} = K \oplus tS.$$

3. Generalized gradient and normal cone

In the sequel, we assume that S is a compact convex symmetric set with non-empty interior. Thus the map $x \mapsto d_K^S(x)$ is a Lipschitz map, and we can consider its generalized gradient.

3.1. Generalized gradient

A Lipschitz map is almost everywhere differentiable. But we can extend, in a set-valued way called the generalized gradient, the notion of gradient at any point of the domain of f (see [2, Aubin-Frankowska], [6, Clarke]).

Definition 3.1 *Let $f : \mathbb{R}^n \to R$ be a Lipschitz map. Let x be in $\mathbb{R}^n$.*

– *The* **circatangent epi-derivative** *of f at x in the direction v is*

$$C_\uparrow f(x)(v) := \limsup_{h \to 0+,\, x' \to x} \frac{f(x' + hv) - f(x')}{h}.$$

– *The* **generalized gradient** *of f at x is*

$$\partial f(x) := \{p \in \mathbb{R}^n \mid C_\uparrow f(x)(v) \geq \langle p, v \rangle,\ \forall v \in \mathbb{R}^n\}.$$

As described in [2, Aubin-Frankowska], the set-valued map[1] $x \rightsquigarrow \partial f(x)$ is upper semicontinuous[2] with convex compact values.

In the case of a convex map f, we obtain the following result:

Proposition 3.2 *Let $f : \mathbb{R}^n \to \mathbb{R}$ be a convex map. The generalized gradient of f at x is the set*

$$\partial f(x) = \{p \in \mathbb{R}^n \mid f(x) - f(y) \leq < p, x - y >\}.$$

3.2. Distance function and normal cone

The distance function $x \mapsto d_K^S(x)$ is a Lipschitz map and the gauge $x \mapsto j_S(x)$ is a convex map. Hence we can compare their generalized gradient. We obtain:

Proposition 3.3 *Consider a compact convex symmetric set $S \subset \mathbb{R}^n$ with non empty interior. For any $x \in \mathbb{R}^n$ and $z \in \Pi_K^S(x)$, we have*

$$\partial j_S(x - z) \subset \partial d_K^S(x)$$

Proof: Consider, for $x' \in \mathbb{R}^n$ and for any $v \in \mathbb{R}^n$ the differential quotient

$$\Delta(h, x') = \frac{d_K^S(x' + hv) - d_K^S(x')}{h}.$$

For any $z \in \Pi_K^S(x)$, we have

$$\liminf_{h \to 0+,\, x' \to x} \Delta(h, x') \leq \liminf_{h \to 0+} \Delta(h, x) \leq \liminf_{h \to 0+} \frac{j_S(x - z + hv) - j_S(x - z)}{h}.$$

Now let us take $p \in \partial j_S(x - z)$. Since j_S is a norm, it is convex and we can apply proposition (3.2) to claim that $j_S(x - z + hv) - j_S(x - z) \leq < p, hv >$. Consequently, for any v, we have $C_\uparrow d_K^S(x)(v) \geq < p, v >$. This implies that $p \in \partial d_K^S(x)$.□

The epi-derivative of the distance function allows us also to define the notions of tangent and normal spaces of a set K without any regularity assumptions on K.

Definition 3.4 *Let K be a closed subset of $\mathbb{R}^n$, S a compact convex symmetric set with non-empty interior and x an element of $\mathbb{R}^n$.*

– *The* **external circatangent cone** *of K at x associated with S is*

$$C_K^S(x) := \{v \in \mathbb{R}^n \mid C_\uparrow d_K^S(x)(v) \leq 0\}.$$

[1] A set-valued map F from a space X to a space Y is characterized by its graph Graph(F) defined as follows

$$\mathrm{Graph}(F) = \{(x, y) \in X \times Y \mid y \in F(x)\}.$$

[2] Let X be a normed space. Let F be a set valued map from X into X. The map F is said to be *upper-semicontinuous* in x_0 if

$$\forall \epsilon > 0,\ \exists \eta > 0 \text{ such that } \forall x \in \{x_0\} \oplus \eta B,\ F(x) \subset F(x_0) \oplus \epsilon B.$$

– *The* **external subnormal cone** *of K at x associated with S is the negative polar cone of $C_K^S(x)$ i.e.*

$$N_K^S(x) := C_K^S(x)^- = \{p \mid \forall v \in C_K^S(x),\ < p, v > \leq 0\}.$$

Let us precise that, when the set K is regular, this tangent cone corresponds to the classical definition of the tangent space, and when K is convex, it is the definition of convex analysis. Moreover, let us mention a link between the generalized gradient of the distance functions to K and the normal cone.

Proposition 3.5 *Let K be a compact subset of $\mathbb{R}^n$ and S a compact, convex and symmetric set with non empty interior. For any $x \in \mathbb{R}^n$, we have*

$$\partial d_K^S(x) \subset N_K^S(x) \cap S^*$$

where $S^* := \{p \in \mathbb{R}^n \mid \sup_{x \in S} < p, x > \leq 1\}$ is called **the polar set** *of S.*

Proof of the proposition: Take $p \in \partial d_K^S(x)$. Obviously, for any $v \in C_K^S(x)$, we can write $< p, v > \leq C_\uparrow d_K^S(x)(v) \leq 0$. Therefore $p \in N_K^S(x)$.
On the other hand, we have

$$C_\uparrow d_K^S(x)(v) \leq \limsup_{h \to 0^+,\ x' \to x} \frac{d_K^S(x' + hv) - d_K^S(x')}{h} \leq j_S(v).$$

Consequently, for any v, we obtain $< p, v > \leq j_S(v)$. Hence, since for any $v \in S$ we have $j_S(x) \leq 1$, this yields $\sup_{v \in S} < p, v > \leq 1$. Therefore $p \in S^*$. This completes the proof.□

4. Differential Inclusions and viability tubes

In this section, we recall briefly the main definitions and results dealing with differential inclusions, viability theory and viability tubes (see [3] for all details and proofs). We also give a characterization of the dilations in terms of viability tube.

4.1. Differential inclusions and reachable map

We consider a set-valued map $F : [0, \infty[\times \mathbb{R}^n \rightsquigarrow \mathbb{R}^n$ which associates with every (t, x) the subset $F(t, x)$ of velocities of the system at time t when its state is $x \in \mathbb{R}^n$. We now study the **differential inclusion**

$$\text{for almost all } t \in \mathbb{R}^+,\quad x'(t) \in F(t, x(t)),\quad x(0) = x_0. \tag{1}$$

We denote by $\mathcal{S}_F(x_0)$ the set of solutions to differential inclusion (1). We associate with the solution map $\mathcal{S}_F : X \rightsquigarrow \mathcal{C}(0, \infty; \mathbb{R}^n)$ of the differential inclusion (1) the **reachable map**, defined in the following way:

Definition 4.1 *For any $t \geq 0$, we denote by $\vartheta_F(t, x) := (\mathcal{S}_F(x))(t)$ the set of states $x(t)$ reached from x through differential inclusion (1) and by*

$$\vartheta_F(t, K) := (\mathcal{S}_F(K))(t)$$

the set of states $x(t)$ reached from K by solutions $x(\cdot) \in \mathcal{S}_F(x)$.

The reachable map $\vartheta_F(t,x)$ enjoys the *semigroup property*:

$$\forall\, t,s \geq 0,\;\; \vartheta_F(t+s,x) \;=\; \vartheta_F(t,(\vartheta_F(s,x))$$

4.2. Viability tubes

Viability problems deal with differential inclusions under state constraints. Viability theorem for tubes provides a geometric condition on the evolving domain of constraints represented by the tube $K(\cdot) : \mathbb{R}^+ \rightsquigarrow \mathbb{R}^n$ that guarantees the existence of a solution $x(\cdot)$ of the differential inclusion (1) starting from $x_0 \in K(0)$ that stays in $K(\cdot)$.

Definition 4.2 *We say that a tube $K(\cdot) : \mathbb{R}^+ \rightsquigarrow \mathbb{R}^n$* **is viable under** *$F$ if for any initial state $x_0 \in K(0)$, there exists a solution $x(\cdot)$ to (1) starting from x_0 which is "viable" in the sense that*

$$\forall\, t \in [0,\infty[,\;\; x(t) \;\in\; K(t)$$

Our first task is to characterize tubes enjoying the viability property thanks to its "contingent derivative".

Definition 4.3 *A tube $K : [0,\infty[\rightsquigarrow \mathbb{R}^n$ is called a* **viability tube** *of a set-valued map $F : [0,\infty[\times\mathbb{R}^n \rightsquigarrow \mathbb{R}^n$ if its graph is contained in the domain of F and if*

$$\forall\, t \in \mathbb{R}^+, \forall\, x \in K(t),\;\; F(t,x) \cap DK(t,x)(1) \neq \emptyset$$

where $DK(t,x)(1) \;=\; \left\{ v \in \mathbb{R}^n \mid \liminf_{h\to 0+} d\left(v, \frac{K(t+h)-x}{h}\right) = 0 \right\}.$

Viability Theorems for autonomous (*i.e.* time independent) systems can be easily translated in the time dependent case and yield the following summary:

Theorem 4.4 *Assume that the $F : [0,\infty[\times\mathbb{R}^n \rightsquigarrow \mathbb{R}^n$ is a Marchaud map*[3]. *A necessary and sufficient condition for a closed tube to be viable under F is that it is a viability tube.*

We shall denote by $\mathcal{S}_F(x_0)$ the set of solutions $x(\cdot)$ to the differential inclusion (1) and by Graph(K_F) its closed domain. Let $K \subset K_F(0)$ be a closed subset. We are looking for viability tubes which satisfy the initial condition $K(0) = K$, which is the Cauchy problem for tubes. The main example of a closed viability tube satisfying this initial condition is the *reachable tube* $\vartheta_F(t,K)$.

Theorem 4.5 *Assume that $F : [0,\infty[\times\mathbb{R}^n \rightsquigarrow \mathbb{R}^n$ is a Marchaud map and that a closed viability domain K of $F(0,\cdot)$ is contained $K_F(0)$. Then the reachable tube $\vartheta_F(t,K)$ is the largest closed viability tube satisfying $\vartheta_F(0,K) = K$.*

---

[3] We shall say that F is a *Marchaud map* if it is nontrivial, upper semicontinuous, has compact convex images and linear growth.

4.3. The dilation is a viability tube

We prove here that the dilation tube $K_S(t) = K \oplus tS$ is a viability tube for the set-valued map $F(x) = \frac{\partial d_K^S(x)}{j_S(S^*)}$. This result is used in the next section to give some differential (mutational) statements for this tube.

Proposition 4.6 *Let K be a compact subset of $\mathbb{R}^n$ and S a compact, convex, and symmetric set. The dilation tube $K_S(t) = K \oplus tS$ associated with the structuring element S is a viability tube for $F(x) = \frac{\partial d_K^S(x)}{j_S(S^*)}$ where $j_S(S^*) = \sup_{p\in S^*} j_S(p)$. Consequently, we have*

$$K_S(h) \subset \vartheta_F(h, K).$$

Proof: We first prove that, for any $z \in \Pi_K^S(x)$, we have $\frac{\partial j_S(x-z)}{j_S(S^*)} \in DK(t,x)(1)$. Indeed, consider $x \in K_S(t)$ and $p \in \frac{\partial j_S(x-z)}{j_S(S^*)}$. We have

$$\begin{cases} d_K^S(x+hp) & \leq j_S(x+hp-z) \leq j_S(x-z) + hj_S(p) \\ & \leq d_K^S(x) + hj_S(v)/j_S(S^*). \end{cases}$$

where $v \in \partial j_S(x-z)$. By proposition (3.3), $\partial j_S(x-z) \subset S^*$, we deduce that $j_S(v) \leq j_S(S^*)$. This yields $d_K^S(x+hp) \leq t+h$. Consequently, we obtain that for any $h > 0$, $x + hv \in K_S(t+h)$. This means that p belongs to the contingent epiderivative $DK_S(t,x)(1)$. Since, by proposition (3.3), $p \in \frac{\partial d_K^S(x)}{j_S(S^*)}$, we deduce

$$\forall t,\ \forall x \in K_S(t), F(x) \cap DK_S(t,x)(1) \neq \emptyset.$$

Consequently, by theorem (4.4), K_S is a viability tube for F. We then apply the theorem (4.5) to conclude the proof.□

5. Mutational equation of the dilation

The mathematical framework of mutational equations [4, Aubin] allows us to extend the concept of differential equations to the metric space $\mathcal{K}(\mathbb{R}^n)$ of all non-empty compact subsets of $\mathbb{R}^n$. The difficulty is due to the non-vectorial structure of this family and we have to make precise the notion of perturbation of a domain.

5.1. Mutations of tube and mutational equations

For defining mutational equations, we supply the space $\mathcal{K}(\mathbb{R}^n)$ with the **Hausdorff distance $\boldsymbol{d}$** defined by

$$\boldsymbol{d}(K_1, K_2) = \sup_{x\in\mathbb{R}^n} |d_{K_1}(x) - d_{K_2}(x)|.$$

We next associate with any domain K and with any set-valued map $F : \mathbb{R}^n \rightsquigarrow \mathbb{R}^n$, the **reachable set** $\vartheta_F(h, K)$ which plays the role of perturbed domain. The **time derivative** (mutation) of a tube $K(\cdot)$ is then characterized by:

Definition 5.1 (Mutation) *Let F be a set-valued map from $\mathbb{R}^n$ into $\mathbb{R}^n$. Consider a tube $K : \mathbb{R}^+ \leadsto \mathbb{R}^n$. If, for a given $t \in \mathbb{R}^+$, the set-valued map $K(\cdot)$ satisfies*

$$\lim_{h \to 0+} \frac{d(\vartheta_F(h, K(t)), K(t+h))}{h} = 0,$$

we shall say that F is a mutation at time t of the tube K and we shall write

$$\overset{\circ}{K}(t) \ni F.$$

Remark: Let us point out that the uniqueness of the mutation is not ensured, which justifies the notation.

We note $\mathcal{F}$ the family of set-valued maps from $\mathbb{R}^n$ to $\mathbb{R}^n$. Now, if we consider a map $f : \mathbb{R}^+ \times \mathcal{K}(\mathbb{R}^n) \mapsto \mathcal{F}(\mathbb{R}^n)$ associating with a pair (t, K) a set-valued map $x \leadsto f(t, K; x)$, we can define a **mutational equation for tubes**

$$\overset{\circ}{K}(t) \ni f(t, K(t); \cdot)\ , \ \forall t \geq 0$$

5.2. Mutational equations for the dilation tubes

As a first mutational result, dealing with the dilation, we have:

Proposition 5.2 *Let K be a compact subset of $\mathbb{R}^n$ and S a compact, convex, and symmetric set. The dilation tube $K_S(t) = K \oplus tS$ associated with the structuring element S satisfies*

$$\overset{\circ}{K_S}(t) \ni S \ \ \forall t \geq 0, \ \ K(0) = K.$$

Proof: Take $y \in \vartheta_S(h, K)$. It is clear that there exists $x \in K$ such that

$$y = x + \int_0^h x'(s)ds \in \{x\} \oplus hS.$$

Consequently $y \in K_S(h)$.

Conversely, take $y \in K_S(h)$ and consider $y(t) = z + t\frac{y-z}{h}$ where $z \in \Pi_K^S(x)$. Obviously, we have $y(h) = y$, $y' \in S$ and $y(0) = z \in K$. Therefore $y \in \vartheta_S(h, K)$ and thus $\vartheta_S(h, K) = K_S(h)$.□

But we can be more precise in the following way. Indeed we prove here that the dilation satisfies the mutational equations below which describes that the evolution of the dilation can be reduced to the evolution in the directions of the generalized gradient of the distance function or equivalently in the normal directions.

Proposition 5.3 *Let K be a compact subset of $\mathbb{R}^n$ and S a compact, convex, and symmetric set with non-empty interior. The dilation tube $K_S(t) = K \oplus tS$ satisfies*

$$\overset{\circ}{K_S}(t) \ni \frac{\partial d_K^S(\cdot)}{j_S(S^\bullet)} \ \ \forall t \geq 0, \ \ K_S(0) = K.$$

Using this proposition, we prove a theorem involving the normal cone:

Theorem 5.4 *Let K be a compact subset of $\mathbb{R}^n$ and S a compact, convex, and symmetric structuring element with non-empty interior. The dilation tube $K_S(t) = K \oplus tS$ associated with S satisfies*

$$\overset{\circ}{K_S}(t) \ni N^S_{K(t)}(\cdot) \cap S \ \forall t \geq 0, \ \ K(0) = K.$$

Proof of the theorem 5.4: It follows from the fact that

$$\frac{\partial d^S_K(\cdot)}{j_S(S^*)} \subset \frac{N^S_K(\cdot) \cap S^*}{j_S(S^*)} \subset N^S_K(\cdot) \cap S$$

since $N^S_K(x)$ is a cone. We then use the proposition 5.3.□

Proof of proposition 5.3: Let us take $h > 0$ and denote $F(x) = \frac{\partial d^S_K(x)}{j_S(S^*)}$. First, corollary (4.6) leads to $K_S(h) \subset \vartheta_F(h, K)$. Moreover, proposition (3.5) implies that $F \subset S$ and consequently that $K_S(h) \subset \vartheta_F(h, K) \subset \vartheta_S(h, K)$. But, since we also have, by proposition 5.2, $\vartheta_S(h, K) = K_S(h) = K \oplus hS$, we obtain, for any $h > 0$, $K_S(h) = \vartheta_F(h, K)$. Consequently, this gives

$$\overset{\circ}{K_S}(0) \ni \partial d^S_{K_S(0)}(\cdot)/j_S(S^*).$$

Moreover, since S is convex, we have $K_S(t + h) = K_S(t) \oplus hS$, and by the semi-group property for the reachable map, we can generalize the result for any $t > 0$. □

References

1. ALVAREZ L., GUICHARD F., LIONS P. L. & MOREL J.M.: 1992, 'Axiomatisation et nouveaux operateurs de la morphologie mathématique', *C.R.A.S. Paris*, t. 315, Série I.
2. AUBIN J.-P. & FRANKOWSKA H.: 1990, 'Set-valued analysis', *Birkhäuser*.
3. AUBIN J.-P.: 1991, 'Viability theory', *Birkhäuser*.
4. AUBIN J.-P. 1993 'Differential calculus in metric space', *Journal of Set-valued Analysis*, 1:3-46.
5. BROCKETT R. & MARAGOS P.: 1992, 'Evolution equation for continuous scale morphology', *IEEE Conference on Acoustics, Speech and Signal Processing*, San Francisco.
6. CLARKE F.H.: 1983, 'Optimization and nonsmooth analysis', *Wiley-Intersciences*.
7. DOYEN L.: 1993, 'Evolution, contrôle et optimisation de formes', *Ph-D thesis*, Université Paris-Dauphine, France.
8. DOYEN L. : 1993, 'Filippov and invariance theorems for mutational inclusions of tubes', *Journal of Set-Valued Analysis*, 1:289-303.
9. MATHERON G. : 1975, 'Random sets and integral geometry', *Wiley*, New-York.
10. MATTIOLI J.: 1993, 'Problèmes inverses et relations différentielles en morphologie mathématique', *Ph-D thesis*, Université Paris-Dauphine, France.
11. MATTIOLI J.: 1993, 'Relations différentielles d'opérations de la morphologie mathématique', *C.R.A.S. Paris*, t 316, Série I:879-884.
12. NAJMAN L.: 1994, 'Morphologie mathématique: de la segmentation d'images à l'analyse multivoque', *Ph-D thesis*, Université Paris-Dauphine, France.
13. SCHMITT M.& MATTIOLI J.: 1993, 'Morphologie mathématique', *Masson Editeur*.
14. SERRA J. : 1982, 'Image analysis and mathematical morphology', *Academic Press*, London.
15. VAN DEN BOOMGAARD R.: 1992, 'Mathematical Morphology: Extensions towards Computer Vision', *PhD Thesis*, Amsterdam University, The netherlands.

THRESHOLDINGS, UMBRAE, RESIDUALS, AND SURPLUSES OF L-IMAGES

Y.C. HSUEH*
Department of Computer and Information Science
National Chiao Tung University
Hsichu, Taiwan 300, R.O.C.

Abstract. Thresholdings and umbrae are essential in the development of mathematical morphology on numerical functions, however, they are not employed in the previous development of mathematical morphology on l-images. In the first part of this paper, we give an alternative to characterize morphological operations on l-images originated from thresholding and umbraic approaches.

In morphological image and signal processing, morphological gradients or residues, hit-or-miss transforms, and morphological skeletons are essential notions. In the second part of this paper, we propose the notions of residuals and surpluses of l-images, then we define morphological residuals and surpluses, hit-or-miss transforms and their duals, and morphological skeletons on l-images.

Key words: L-images, Thresholdings, Umbrae, Residuals, Surpluses, Morphological Skeletons

1. Introduction

In the definitions of Minkowski addition and subtraction on Euclidean space, "translation" is one of the most important operations on sets. For instance, the Minkowski addition $A \oplus B$ of two sets A and B is the union of all translated sets of A by elements of B or, equivalently, $A \oplus B$ is the set of all elements x such that the translated set of $\check{B}$ (the reflected set of B) by x hits A [15, 20]. Then, in the generalizations of matematical morphology to numerical functions and grey-level images, "thresholding" and"umbra" play essential roles [20, 22, 23]. A function f from $\Re^n$ into $\Re^*$ (the set of extended real numbers) is called a numerical function on $\Re^n$. The notion of thresholdings links numerical functions on $\Re^n$ to sets on $\Re^n$, while the notion of umbrae links numerical functions to sets on $\Re^n \times \Re$. Based on the notion of thresholdings, Serra derives morphological operations on numerical functions with

"flat" structuring elements [20, p.429] as well as Minkowski addition and subtraction on numerical functions [20, p.477]. While based on the notion of umbrae, Sternberg [23] also extends Minkowski addition and subtraction on numerical functions. However, it is pointed out by Heijmans [9] and Ronse [18] that there are some problems in umbraic approach to mathematical morphology on numerical functions from theoretical point of view. Moreover, since the grey-level overflow problem, mathematical morphology on numerical functions cannot be directly applied to grey-level images if "non-flat" structuring elements are used. Here, a grey-level image is meant a function from $\Re^n$ into the grey-scale { 0, 1, ... , m-1 } for some positive integer m.

* This work was supported by the National Science Council, Republic of China, under grant NSC82-0408-E009-437.

J.Serra and P. Soille (eds.), Mathematical Morphology and Its Applications to Image Processing, 21-28

In order to solve the grey-level overflow problem in mathematical morphology, Hsueh [12] proposes the notion of *l*-images to unify those of numerical functions and grey-level images, and then generalizes morphological operations to *l*-images. His approach is purely lattice theoretically oriented and his idea is motivated by the works of Serra [22], Heijmans and/or Ronse [9, 10, 18, 19], as well as birkhoff [4] and Goguen [6, 7, 8]. Unlike the case of numerical functions, the roles of thresholdings and umbrae are absent from the stage of derivation of morphological operations on *l*-images. Therefore, it is our first purpose in this paper to give an alternative approach to morphological operations on *l*-images based on the notions of thresholdings and umbrae.

Among morphological transformations [21], morphological residues are particularly useful in morphological high-pass filtering [14], feature detection [3, 5, 13, 17], and image segmentation [2, 16]. Given a set A and a morphological operation Ψ on sets. The Ψ-residue of A is the set difference of A and $\Psi(A)$ when Ψ is anti-extensive or the difference of $\Psi(A)$ and A when Ψ is extensive. Particularly, closing-residues and opening-residues are frequently used in corner detection while dilation-residues and erosion-residues are frequently used in edge detection. Furthermore, opening-residues of eroded sets of a compact set are used in forming the morphological skeleton [14, 20, 22] of that set.

As the second purpose of this paper, we intend to define the difference operation on *l*-images and then extend the notion of morphological residues to *l*-images. We find that a dual notion of residuals, will be called "surpluses", in a *clc*-monoid can be used to form the difference operation on *l*-images. In section 2, we review the notions of *clc*-monoids and *l*-images first. Then, the surplus of an element by another element in a *clc*-monoid is defined. In section 3, we define thresholdings, umbrae, residuals and surpluses of *l*-images. In section 4, we will derive Minkowski addition and subtraction on *l*-images based on thresholdings. In section 5, we will develop Minkowski addition and subtraction on *l*-images based on umbrae. Morphological residuals and surpluses of *l*-images are defined in section 6. Finally, conclusions are placed in section 7.

2. *Clc*-monoids and *L*-images

Conceptually, an *l*-image can be viewed as a function from a vector space V into a lattice L. However, in order to obtain most properties pertaining to mathematical morphology on Euclidean space, it has been demonstrated [12] that a better structure for the lattice L might be a complete lattice-ordered commutative monoid, or *clc*-monoid in short.

Definition 2.1 *Let* $(L, \vee, \wedge, \top, \perp)$ *be a complete lattice and* $(L, *, \iota)$ *be a commutative monoid. Then the structure* $(L, \vee, \wedge, *, \top, \perp, \iota)$ *is called [4, 12] a clc-monoid if the following infinite distributive laws are satisfied: for all* $a \in L$ *and for all* $K \subset L$*, (ID1)* $a \wedge \bigvee_{\beta \in K} \beta = \bigvee_{\beta \in K} (\alpha \wedge \beta)$*; (ID2)* $a \vee \bigwedge_{\beta \in K} \beta = \bigwedge_{\beta \in K} (\alpha \vee \beta)$*; (ID3)* $a * \bigvee_{\beta \in K} \beta = \bigvee_{\beta \in K} (\alpha * \beta)$.

Definition 2.2 *In a clc-monoids, the element $\alpha : \beta$ defined by $\alpha : \beta = \bigvee\{\gamma | \gamma * \beta \leq \alpha\}$ is called [4] the residual of α by β.*

Note that if $(L, \vee, \wedge, *, \top, \bot, \iota)$ is a *clc*-monoid, then the structure $(L, \vee, \wedge, \wedge, \top, \bot, \top)$ is also a *clc*-monoid. In general, if $(L, \vee, \wedge, \top, \bot)$ is a complete lattice satisfying the infinite distributive laws (ID1) and (ID2), then the structure $(L, \vee, \wedge, \wedge, \top, \bot, \top)$ is a *clc*-monoid. Observe that the residual of α by β in the *clc*-monoid $(L, \vee, \wedge, \wedge, \top, \bot, \top)$, will be denoted as $\alpha \sqcup \beta$, is given by

$$\alpha \sqcup \beta = \begin{cases} \alpha & \text{if } \alpha < \beta \\ -\infty & \text{otherwise.} \end{cases}$$

Definition 2.3 *A lattice L is called [4] self-dual if there exists an operation $^d : L \to L$ such that $\alpha^d \leq \beta^d$ whenever $\beta \leq \alpha$ and $(\alpha^d)^d = \alpha$ for all $\alpha, \beta \in L$.*

In a *clc*-monoid $(L, \vee, \wedge, *, \top, \bot, \iota)$, if L is self-dual, then we can define another operation $\div : L^2 \to L$ by $\alpha \div \beta = (\alpha^d * \beta)^d$. For instance, in the *clc*-monoid $([-\infty, \infty], \vee, \wedge, +, \infty, -\infty, 0)$, we have $\alpha \div \beta = \alpha - \beta$; and in the *clc*-monoid $(L, \vee, \wedge, \wedge, \top, \bot, \top)$, we have $\alpha \div \beta = \alpha \vee \beta^d$. In the case when $\alpha \div \beta = \alpha : \beta$, the *clc*-monoid $(L, \vee, \wedge, *, \top, \bot, \iota)$ is called [12] a *self-dual clc-monoid.*

Definition 2.4 *In a clc-monoid with L being self-dual, we can also define an operation $\setminus : L^2 \to L$ by $\alpha \setminus \beta = (\alpha^d : \beta^d)^d$. The element $\alpha \setminus \beta$ will be called the surplus of α by β.*

Note that in the *clc*-monoid $([-\infty, \infty], \vee, \wedge, +, \infty, -\infty, 0)$, we have $\alpha \setminus \beta = \alpha - \beta = \alpha : \beta$. However, in the *clc*-monoid $(L, \vee, \wedge, \wedge, \top, \bot, \top)$, we have $\alpha \setminus \beta = (\alpha^d \sqcup \beta^d)^d$, which is in general not equal to $\alpha \sqcup \beta$. From now on, we will write $\alpha \sqcap \beta$ to mean the surplus of α by β in stead of writing $\alpha \setminus \beta$ in the *clc*-monoid $(L, \vee, \wedge, \wedge, \top, \bot, \top)$. Note that in the *clc*-monoid $([-\infty, \infty], \vee, \wedge, \wedge, \infty, -\infty, \infty)$, we have

$$\alpha \sqcap \beta = \begin{cases} \alpha & \text{if } \alpha > \beta \\ -\infty & \text{otherwise.} \end{cases}$$

Now, let V be the underlying set of a vector space and $(L, \vee, \wedge, *, \top, \bot, \iota)$ be a *clc*-monoid.

Definition 2.5 *An $l-$image A on V is a function from V into L. For each $x \in V$, the value $A(x)$ is called the level of A at x. The set L is called the scale of A.*

For instance, numerical functions are l-images with $V = \Re^n$ and $L = \Re^*$.

3. Elementary Operations on L-images

In this section, we will define some elementary operations on l-images. Let V be the underlying set of a vector space and $(L, \vee, \wedge, *, \top, \bot, \iota)$ a *clc*-monoid.

Definition 3.1 *The translation of an element $(x,\alpha) \in V \times L$ by another element $(y,\beta) \in V \times L$, written as $(x,\alpha)\vec{+}(y,\beta)$, is defined by $(x,\alpha)\vec{+}(y,\beta) = (x+y, \alpha * \beta)$. Then, the translation of a set $Y \subset V \times L$ by an element $(x,\alpha) \in V \times L$, written as $Y_{(x,\alpha)}$, is defined by*

$$Y_{(x,\alpha)} = \{(x,\alpha)\vec{+}(y,\beta) \mid \forall\,(y,\beta) \in Y\} = \{(x+y, \alpha * \beta) \mid \forall\,(y,\beta) \in Y\}$$

Definition 3.2 *The translation of an l-image A by $(x,\alpha) \in V \times L$, also written as $A_{(x,\alpha)}$, is defined by $A_{(x,\alpha)}(y) = A(y-x) * \alpha \quad \forall y \in V$. In particular, the V-translation of an l-image A by an element $x \in V$, written as A_x, is defined by $A_x(y) = A(y-x) \quad \forall y \in V$, and the L-translation of A by an element $\alpha \in L$, written as $A * \alpha$, is defined by $(A * \alpha)(y) = A(y) * \alpha \quad \forall y \in V$.*

Definition 3.3 *The reflection $\check{Y}$ of a set $Y \subset V$ is given by $\check{Y} = \{-y \mid y \in Y\}$. Similarly, the reflection $\check{A}$ of an l-image A is given by $\check{A}(x) = A(-x)$ for all $x \in V$.*

Definition 3.4 *Given a vector space with universe V and a clc-monoid $(L, \vee, \wedge, *, \top, \bot, \iota)$ where L is self-dual. Define the difference of l-images A and B to be the surplus $A \setminus B$ of A by B. If we are working on the clc-monoid $(L, \vee, \wedge, \wedge, \top, \bot, \top)$, the difference of l-images A and B is $A \sqcap B$.*

Definition 3.5 *The thresholding of an l-image A at level τ, written as $\mathbf{X}_\tau(A)$, is a set in V defined by $\mathbf{X}_\tau(A) = \{x \in V \mid A(x) \geq \tau\}$. Another type of thresholding $\mathbf{X}^\circ_\tau(A)$ of the l-image A is defined by $\mathbf{X}^\circ_\tau(A) = \{x \in V \mid A(x) > \tau\}$.*

Note that thresholdings of an *l*-image are invariant under V-translation and reflection.

Definition 3.6 *The umbra of an l-image A, written as $\mathbf{U}(A)$, is a set in $V \times L$ defined by $\mathbf{U}(A) = \{(x,\alpha) \mid x \in V, \alpha \in L \text{ and } \alpha \leq A(x)\}$.*

Note that all operations on L in a *clc*-monoid $(L, \vee, \wedge, *, \top, \bot, \iota)$ can be extended to *l*-images point-wise. Let L^V denote the set of all *l*-images on V. Then it is shown [12] that the structure $(L^V, \vee, \wedge, *, \top, \bot, \iota)$ is also a *clc*-monoid.

Definition 3.7 *In the clc-monoid $(L^V, \vee, \wedge, *, \top, \bot, \iota)$, the residual $A : B$ and surplus $A \setminus B$ of A by B are defined point-wise by $(A : B)(x) = A(x) : B(x)$ and $(A \setminus B)(x) = A(x) \setminus B(x)$, respectively. Similarly, in the clc-monoid $(L^V, \vee, \wedge, \wedge, \top, \bot, \top)$, the residual and surplus of A by B are respectively defined by $(A \sqcup B)(x) = A(x) \sqcup B(x)$ and $(A \sqcap B)(x) = A(x) \sqcap B(x)$.*

4. Operations Based on Thresholdings

In the development of morphological operations on numerical functions, Serra [20, p.477] suggests the following definition for Minkowski addition: for any two numerical functions f and g, the Minkowski addition $f \oplus g$ is a numerical function such that $\mathbf{X}_t(f \oplus g) = \mathbf{X}_t(f) \oplus \mathbf{X}_t(g)$ for all real number t. In other words, for any $x \in \Re^n$,

$$(f \oplus g)(x) = \sup\{t \in \Re \mid x \in \mathbf{X}_t(f) \oplus \mathbf{X}_t(g)\}$$

By following the same approach, we can define the Minkowski addition $A \oplus B$ of any two l-images A, B on a vector space V with values from a clc-monoid L by

$$(A \oplus B)(x) = \bigvee \{\tau \in L \mid x \in \mathbf{X}_\tau(A) \oplus \mathbf{X}_\tau(B)\}$$

Theorem 4.1 *For any two l-images A and B on V with values from L, let the Minkowski addition $A \oplus B$ be defined by equation (1). Then, we have $(A \oplus B)(x) = \bigvee_{y \in V} \{A(x - y) \wedge B(y)\}$ and $\mathbf{X}_t(f \oplus g) = \mathbf{X}_t(f) \oplus \mathbf{X}_t(g)$.*

Denote the set of all l-images on V with values from L by L^V. It has been shown [7] that if the structure $(L, \vee, \wedge, \wedge, \top, \bot, \top)$ is a clc-monoid, then the structure $(L^V, \vee, \wedge, \oplus, I, O, U)$ is also a clc-monoid, where

$$I(x) = \top, \quad O(x) = \bot \quad \forall x \in V, \quad U(x) = \begin{cases} \top & \text{if } x = \vec{0}, \text{ the origin of } V, \\ \bot & \text{otherwise.} \end{cases}$$

The residual of A by B in the clc-monoid $(L^V, \vee, \wedge, \oplus, I, O, U)$, written as $A \ominus B$, is given [12] by $A \ominus B = \bigvee \{C \mid C \oplus B \le A\}$ and $(A \ominus B)(x) = \bigwedge_{y \in V} \{A(x + y) \sqcup B(y)\}$ for all $x \in V$. The following theorem shows that $A \ominus B$ can also be defined in terms of the Minkowski subtraction of thresholdings of A and B.

Theorem 4.2 *For any l-images A and B in the clc-monoid $(L^V, \vee, \wedge, \oplus, I, O, U)$, we have $\mathbf{X}_\tau(A \ominus B) = \bigcap_{\alpha \le \tau} \mathbf{X}_\alpha(A) \ominus \mathbf{X}_\alpha(B)$. In other words,*

$$(A \ominus B)(x) = \bigvee \{\tau \in L \mid x \in \bigcap_{\alpha \le \tau} \mathbf{X}_\alpha(A) \ominus \mathbf{X}_\alpha(B)\}$$

If L is self-dual, we can consider the complementary dual [20] $\bar{\ominus}$ of $\ominus$ defined by $A \bar{\ominus} B = (A^d \oplus \check{B})^d$. It can be easily shown that $(A \bar{\ominus} B)(x) = \bigwedge_{y \in V} \{A(x + y) \vee B^d(y)\}$.

Theorem 4.3 *Suppose the lattice L is self-dual. Then for any l-images A, B in L^V, we have $\mathbf{X}_\tau(A \bar{\ominus} B) = \{x \in V \mid A^d \le \tau^d \sqcup B_x\}$.*

Note that $A \bar{\ominus} B \ne A \ominus B$ in general. Moreover, if L is a chain, then $\mathbf{X}_{\tau^d}(A^d) = [\mathbf{X}^\circ_\tau(A)]^c$ for any l-image A and any element $\tau \in L$. In this case, we have

$$\begin{aligned} \mathbf{X}_\tau(A \bar{\ominus} B) &= \mathbf{X}_\tau(A^d \oplus \check{B})^d = [\mathbf{X}^\circ_{\tau^d}(A^d \oplus \check{B})]^c \\ &= [\mathbf{X}^\circ_{\tau^d}(A^d) \oplus \mathbf{X}^\circ_{\tau^d}(\check{B})]^c = [(\mathbf{x}_\tau(A))^c \oplus \check{\mathbf{X}}^\circ_{\tau^d}(B)]^c = \mathbf{X}_\tau(A) \ominus \mathbf{X}^\circ_{\tau^d}(B) \end{aligned}$$

It should be noted that, in general, $\mathbf{X}_\tau(A) \ominus \mathbf{X}^\circ_{\tau^d}(B) \ne \mathbf{X}_\tau(A) \ominus \mathbf{X}_{\tau^d}(B)$.

5. Operations Based on Umbrae

In the development of Minkowski operations on l-images discussed in the previous section, the operation "$*$" in the clc-monoid $(L, \vee, \wedge, *, \top, \bot, \iota)$ is not used. The reason for this is that thresholdings are sets on V, operations on thresholdings mainly dependent on the operations of subsets of V. In this section, we will give alternative approach to Minkowski addition on l-images based on umbrae, which are subsets of $V \times L$.

First of all, we should define Minkowski addition on subsets of $V \times L$. In terms of translations, the Minkowski addition of two sets A and B in $V \times L$, will be written as $A \times B$ in order to distinguish it from the Minkowski addition on sets in V, can be define by

$$A \otimes B = \{(x + y, \alpha * \beta) \mid (x, \alpha) \in A, (y, \beta) \in B\} = \bigcup_{(y,\beta)\in B} A_{(y,\beta)}$$

Similarly, the Minkowski subtraction of A from B, will be written as $A \oslash B$, can be defined by $A \oslash B = \{(z, \gamma) \in V \times L \mid B_{(z,\gamma)} \subset A\}$. It can be easily shown that $A \oslash B = \bigcup\{C \mid C \otimes B \subset A\}$. Then, analogous to the case of numerical functions, the Minkowski addition and subtraction of two l-images A and B can also be defined in terms of umbrae. That is,

$$(A \otimes B)(x) = \bigvee\{\tau \mid (x, \tau) \in \mathbf{U}(A) \otimes \mathbf{U}(B)\} \tag{1}$$

and

$$(A \oslash B)(x) = \bigvee\{\tau \mid (x, \tau) \in \mathbf{U}(A) \oslash \mathbf{U}(B)\} \tag{2}$$

Theorem 5.1 *For any two l-images A and B in L^V, if the Minkowski addition $A \otimes B$ is defined by equation (1), then we have* $(A \otimes B)(x) = \bigvee_{y\in V} \{A(x - y) * B(y)\}$.

Theorem 5.2 *For any two l-images A and B in L^V, if the Minkowski addition $A \oslash B$ is defined by equation (2), then we have* $(A \oslash B)(x) = \bigwedge_{y\in V} \{A(x - y) : B(y)\}$.

The following theorem provides another alternative to evaluate $A \oslash B$.

Theorem 5.3 *For any two l-images A and B,* $(A \oslash B)(x) = \bigvee\{\tau \in L \mid B_x * \tau \leq A\}$.

Note that if we define an l-image N by

$$N(x) = \begin{cases} \iota & \text{if } x = 0^n \\ \bot & \text{otherwise.} \end{cases}$$

then the structure $(L^V, \vee, \wedge, \oplus, I, O, N)$ is shown [12] to be a *clc*-monoid. In this *clc*-monoid, the residual of A by B is precisely $A \oslash B$.

Now consider the complementary dual $\bar{\oslash}$ of $\otimes$ if the lattice L is self-dual. It can be easily shown that

$$(A \bar{\oslash} B)(x) = (A^d \otimes \check{B})^d(x) = \bigwedge_{y\in V} \{(A^d(x + y) * B(y))^d\}$$

Moreover, if the *clc*-monoid $(L, \vee, \wedge, *, \top, \bot, \iota)$ is self-dual, i.e., if $\alpha^d * \beta = (\alpha : \beta)^d$, then

$$\begin{aligned}(A\bar{\oslash}B)(x) &= \bigwedge_{y\in V} \{(A^d(x+y) * B(y))^d\} \\ &= \bigwedge_{y\in V} \{A(x+y) : B(y)\} = (A \oslash B)(x)\end{aligned}$$

That is, if the *clc*-monoid $(L, \vee, \wedge, *, \top, \bot, \iota)$ is self-dual, then the complementary dual $A\bar{\oslash}B$ of the Minkowski addition $A \otimes B$ coincides with the residual $A \oslash B$ for all l-images A, B.

6. Morphological Residuals and Surpluses

In this section, we assume that Ψ is a morphological operation on l-images.

Definition 6.1 *The Ψ-residuals of an l-image A, written as $R^*_\Psi(A)$ and $R^\wedge_\Psi(A)$, are respectively defined by $R^*_\Psi(A) = A : \Psi(A)$ and $R^\wedge_\Psi(A) = A \sqcup \Psi(A)$. Similarly, the Ψ-surpluses of an l-image A, written as $S^*_\Psi(A)$ and $S^\wedge_\Psi(A)$, are respectively defined by $S^*_\Psi(A) = A \setminus \Psi(A)$ and $S^\wedge_\Psi(A) = A \sqcap \Psi(A)$.*

Consider the case of grey-level images defined on a vector space V with values from the *clc*-monoid $([0, m], \vee, \wedge, *, m, 0, m)$, where $a * b = 0 \vee (a + b - m)$, we have

$$(f : g)(x) = m \wedge (f(x) - g(x) + m), \qquad (f \setminus g)(x) = 0 \vee (f(x) - g(x)),$$

$$(f \sqcup g)(x) = \begin{cases} f(x) & \text{if } f(x) < g(x) \\ m & \text{otherwise,} \end{cases}$$

and

$$(f \sqcap g)(x) = \begin{cases} f(x) & \text{if } f(x) > g(x) \\ 0 & \text{otherwise.} \end{cases}$$

for all $x \in V$. Thus, for any structuring element g, let $\mathcal{C}_g$ and $\mathcal{O}_g$ respectively denote the closing and opening with respect to g, then the $\mathcal{C}_g$-residuals and $\mathcal{O}_g$-surpluses of an image f are given as follows:

$$R^*_{\mathcal{C}_g}(f)(x) = f(x) - \mathcal{C}_g(f)(x) + m, \qquad S^*_{\mathcal{O}_g}(f)(x) = f(x) - \mathcal{O}_g(f)(x),$$

$$R^\wedge_{\mathcal{C}_g}(f)(x) = \begin{cases} f(x) & \text{if } f(x) < \mathcal{C}_g(f)(x) \\ m & \text{if } f(x) = \mathcal{C}_g(f)(x), \end{cases}$$

and

$$S^\wedge_{\mathcal{O}_g}(f)(x) = \begin{cases} f(x) & \text{if } f(x) > \mathcal{O}_g(f)(x) \\ 0 & \text{if } f(x) = \mathcal{O}_g(f)(x). \end{cases}$$

7. Conclusion

In this paper, we first propose an alternative approach to characterize Minkowski addition and subtraction on l-images. Based on thresholdings, we obtain the Minkowski addition $\oplus$ and its duals $\ominus$ and $\bar{\ominus}$. While based on umbrae, we obtain the Minkowski addition $\otimes$ and its duals $\oslash$ and $\bar{\oslash}$. It should be noted that if we are working on the *clc*-monoid $(L, \vee, \wedge, \wedge, \top, \bot, \top)$, then thresholding and umbraic approaches give the same results.

Next, we propose the notions of image residuals and surpluses. Conventional morphological residues are represented by morphological residuals when the underlying morphological operations are extensive and by morphological surpluses when the underlying morphological operations are anti-extensive.

References

1. Banon, G.J.F. and Barrera, J., 'Minimal representation of translation invariant set mappings by mathematical morphology', *SIAM J. Appl. Math.* Vol. **51**, No. 6, 1991, pp. 1782-1798.
2. Beucher, S., 'Watersheds of functions and picture segmentation', *Proceedings IEEE International Conference on Acoustic, Speech and Signal Processing*, Paris, 1982, pp. 1928-1931.
3. Beucher, S. and Lantuéjoul, J., 'Use of watersheds in contour detection', *International Workshop on Image Processing: Real-Time Edge and Motion detection/estimation*, Rennes, 1979.
4. Birkhoff, G., *Lattice Theory*, American Mathematical Society, Providence, RI, 1979.
5. Fechs, R.J. and Arce, G.R., 'Multidimensional morphological edge detection', *Proc. SPIE*, Vol. **845**, 1987, pp. 285-292.
6. Goguen, J.A., 'L-fuzzy sets', *J. Mathematical Analysis and Applications*, Vol. **18**, 1967, pp. 145-174.
7. Goguen, J.A., 'The logic of inexact concepts', *Syntheses*, Vol. **19**, 1969, pp. 325-373.
8. Goguen, J.A., 'Concept representation in natural and artificial languages: Axioms, extensions and applications for fuzzy sets', in: E.H. Mamdani and B.R. Gaines, Ed., *Fuzzy Reasoning and its Applications*, Academic Press, London, 1981, pp. 67-115.
9. Heijmans, H.J.A.M., 'Theoretical aspects of gray-level morphology', *IEEE Trans. PAMI*, Vol. **13**, 1991, pp. 568-582.
10. Heijmans, H.J.A.M. and Ronse, C., 'The algebraic basis of mathematical morphology; Part I: Dilations and erosions', *Comput. Vision Graphics Image Process.*, Vol. **50**, No. 3, 1990, pp. 245-295.
11. Heijmans, H.J.A.M. and Serra, J., 'Convergence, continuity, and iteration in mathematical morphology', *Journal of Visual Communication and Image Representation*, Vol. **3**, No. 1, 1992, pp. 84-102.
12. Hsueh, Y.C., 'Mathematical morphology on *l*-images', *Signal Processing*, Vol. **26**, 1992, pp. 221-241.
13. Lee, J.S.J., Haralick, R.M. and Sharpiro, L.G., 'Morphologic edge detection', *IEEE J. Robotics and Automation*, Vol. **RA-3**, No. 2, 1987, pp. 142-156.
14. Maragos, P.A., *A Unified Theory of Translation-Invariant Systems with Application to Morphological Analysis and Coding of Images*, Ph.D. Thesis, Georgia Institute of Technology, 1985.
15. Matheron, G., *Random Sets and Integral Geometry*, Wiley, New York, 1975.
16. Meyer, F. and Beucher, S., 'Morphological segmentation', *J. Visual Communication and Image Representation*, Vol. **1**, No. 1, 1990, pp. 21-46.
17. Noble, J.A., 'Morphological feature detectors', *Proceedings of the Second International Conference on Computer Vision*, Tarpon Springs, FL, 1988, pp. 112-116.
18. Ronse, C., 'Why mathematical morphology needs complete lattices', *Signal Processing*, Vol. **21**, No. 2, 1990, pp. 129-154.
19. Ronse, C. and Heijmans, H.J.A.M., 'The algebraic basis of mathematical morphology; Part II: Openings and Closings', *CVGIP: Image Understanding*, Vol. **54**, 1991, pp. 74-97.
20. Serra, J., *Image Analysis and Mathematical Morphology*, Academic Press, London, 1982.
21. Serra, J., 'Introduction to mathematical morphology', *CVGIP*, Vol. **35**, 1986, pp. 283-305.
22. Serra, J., ed., *Image Analysis and Mathematical Morphology, Vol.2: Theoretical Advances*, Academic Press, London, 1988.
23. Sternberg, S.R., 'Grayscale morphology', *Comput. Vision Graphics Image Process.*, Vol. **35**, No. 3, 1986, pp. 333-355.

ADAPTIVE PARAMETERIZED OPENINGS

Y. CHEN and E. R. DOUGHERTY
Center for Imaging Science
Rochester Institute of Technology
Rochester, N.Y. USA

Abstract. Adaptive reconstructive τ-openings are to employed to recover signal from noise in the binary union-noise model. Openings are parameterized in accordance with Euclidean granulometric representation, the parameter being restricted to nonnegative integers. The filter-parameter space is treated as the countably infinite state space in a Markov chain whose transitions occur at each encounter with a grain when scanning the image. An upward or downward transition occurs when a noise or signal grain, respectively, is misrecognised.

Key words: Markov chain, adaptive filter, optimal filter, opening, granulometry.

1. INTRODUCTION

Optimization of binary nonlinear filters in the context of mathematical morphology can roughly be divided into three design paradigms involving three kinds of translation-invariant operators: increasing [1, 2, 3, 4], nonincreasing [5], and τ-openings (reconstructive or ordinary) [6, 7, 8, 9]. Optimization of increasing and nonincreasing filters has focused on search procedures to find optimal erosion expansions. Generally, full searches are intractable and constrained search methods are employed. The search problem can be mitigated by applying adaptive methods to find good, if not optimal, structuring elements for increasing filters [10].

τ-opening optimization has been more analytic and optimal parameterized structuring elements have been derived from probabilistic image models. The mathematical problems inherent in such analysis can be very difficult if the image models are geometrically complex, which is typical for segmentation models employing the watershed transformation [7, 8]. The present paper, which is an abbreviated version of Ref. [11], circumvents the full optimization problem by employing adaptive reconstructive parameterized τ-openings. The parameter space is treated as the state space in a Markov chain having a countably infinite number of states. The chain is itself discretely parameterized by allowing transitions at each grain encounter during a scanning process. When a signal grain is recognized as a noise grain, there is a parameter transition $r \rightarrow r - 1$; when a noise grain is recognized as a signal grain, $r \rightarrow r + 1$; when there is correct recognition, $r \rightarrow r$. Filter convergence is interpreted via existence and representation of a steady-state distribution. We defer to Ref. [11] for theoretical details, Markov chain models arising from various discrete scanning methodologies, continuously parameterized Markov processes arising from time scanning, transient analysis, and further applications to specific probability models.

J.Serra and P. Soille (eds.), Mathematical Morphology and Its Applications to Image Processing, 29-36

2. EUCLIDEAN GRANULOMETRIES

In binary mathematical morphology, opening with structuring element E is defined by $S \circ E = \cup\{E + x : E + x \subset S\}$, where $E + x = \{e + x : e \in E\}$ is the translation of E by x. A binary operator Ψ is called an algebraic opening if it is increasing [$S \subset T$ implies $\Psi(S) \subset \Psi(T)$], antiextensive [$\Psi(S) \subset S$], and idempotent [$\Psi\Psi = \Psi$]. If Ψ is also translation-invariant [$\Psi(S) + x = \Psi(S + x)$], then it is called a τ-opening. The invariant class, Inv[Ψ], of a τ-opening Ψ is composed of all sets for which $\Psi(S) = S$. Subset $\mathbf{B}$ of Inv[Ψ] is called a base for Inv[Ψ] if Inv[Ψ] is the closure of $\mathbf{B}$ under translations and unions. There is a representation for τ-openings [12]: Ψ is a τ-opening if and only if there exists a class of sets $\mathbf{B}$ such that

$$\Psi(S) = \bigcup_{B \in \mathbf{B}} S \circ B \tag{1}$$

$\mathbf{B}$ is a base for Inv[Ψ].

A granulometry is a family $\{\Psi_t\}$, $t > 0$, of mappings such that (i) Ψ_t is increasing, (ii) Ψ_t is antiextensive, and (iii) $\Psi_r\Psi_s = \Psi_s\Psi_r = \Psi_{max(r,s)}$. For $t = 0$, Ψ_0 is defined by $\Psi_0(S) = S$. If Ψ_t is translation invariant, $\{\Psi_t\}$ is a τ-granulometry and if Ψ_t satisfies the Euclidean condition $\Psi_t(S) = t\Psi_1(S/t)$, $\{\Psi_t\}$ is a Euclidean granulometry. A key type of Euclidean granulometry is defined by

$$\Psi_t(S) = \bigcup_{B \in \mathbf{B}} S \circ tB \tag{2}$$

where the sets in $\mathbf{B}$ are compact and convex. $\mathbf{B}$ is called the generator of the granulometry. This union represents a parameterized τ-opening. Some key properties of Euclidean granulometries: $r \geq s$ implies $\Psi_r(S) \subset \Psi_s(S)$; $r \geq s$ implies Inv[Ψ_r] $\subset$ Inv[Ψ_s]; Ψ_t is a τ-opening; if the generator consists of connected sets and S_1, S_2,... are mutually disjoint compact sets, then

$$\Psi_t\Big(\bigcup_{i=1}^{\infty} S_i\Big) = \bigcup_{i=1}^{\infty} \Psi_t(S_i) \tag{3}$$

A granulometry that distributes over disjoint unions will be called *distributive.* The present paper concerns distributive granulometries with convex generators; that is, it concerns parameterized τ-openings whose unions form a granulometry.

3. OPTIMAL τ-OPENINGS

The fundamental τ-opening optimization problem for random Boolean images degraded by random Boolean union noise can be phrased in the following manner. Let A and B be independent random variables whose ranges are the natural numbers. Then the pure signal is modeled as a union of A independent translates of a random compact, connected primitive set X, and the noise (clutter) is modeled as a union of B independent translates of a random compact, connected primitive set Y that is independent of X. Signal and noise take the forms

$$\begin{aligned} S &= \textstyle\bigcup_{i=1}^{A} X_i + x_i \\ N &= \textstyle\bigcup_{j=1}^{B} Y_j + y_j \end{aligned} \tag{4}$$

where X_1, X_2,..., X_A are independent and identically distributed with X, Y_1, Y_2,..., Y_B are independent and identically distributed with Y, and x_1, x_2,..., x_A, y_1, y_2,..., y_B are random locations. The observed image is $S \cup N$. Given a distributive, finite-generator Euclidean granulometry $\{\Psi_t\}$ according to Eq. 3, the optimization problem is to find a value of t for which $\{\Psi_t\}$ best estimates S from $S \cup N$. Estimation is optimized relative to the symmetric difference of signal and estimate: t must be found that minizimizes the expectation $E[m[\Psi_t(S \cup N)\Delta S]]$, where m denotes area (measure). Because τ-openings are increasing, it is assumed that X and Y are distributed so that X tends to be larger than Y relative to the base of the τ-opening.

Of special interest is the case where X and Y are randomly sized homothetics of fixed compact, convex primitives C and D, respectively. Then

$$\begin{aligned} S &= \textstyle\bigcup_{i=1}^{A} s_i C + x_i \\ N &= \textstyle\bigcup_{j=1}^{B} n_j D + y_j \end{aligned} \tag{5}$$

where the sizing parameters s_i and n_j come from known sizing distributions Π_S and Π_N, respectively, and all sizings are independent. It is assumed that Π_N lies to the left of Π_S in the sense that $\mu_{\Pi_N} < \mu_{\Pi_S}$. Two important special cases are when all grains are assumed to be mutually disjoint and when $C = D$. An analytic solution relative to Eq. 5 was given in Ref. [6], where it was assumed that $C = D$, $\Psi_t(S \cup N) = (S \cup N) \circ tC$, and all grains are mutually disjoint.

As so far stated, τ-opening optimization involves filtering the observed image by some selected filter from a Euclidean granulometry. In order to achieve a geometric, model-based approach, Refs. [7] and [8] employ τ-openings by reconstruction. If Ψ_t is distributive, then its action on any connected component in an image is independent of its action on the rest of the image. The classical reconstructive approach in morphology is to let the output image consist of all connected components that do not vanish entirely under an opening operation. Not only does the reconstructive optimization paradigm allow nonsimilar generators for image and opening in the nonoverlapping model, it also facilitates optimal opening filtering in the overlapping model by interpreting Ψ_t reconstructively following a watershed segmentation.

The present paper uses adaptive reconstructive parameterized τ-openings to find a good, if not necessarily the best, filter.

4. ADAPTIVE RECONSTRUCTIVE τ-OPENINGS

Consider the image-noise model $S \cup N$ according to Eq. 4 under the assumption that the grains are nonoverlapping. Let Ψ_t be a distributive granulometry defined according to Eq. 3 and let Λ_t be the filter derived from Ψ_t via reconstruction. Application of Λ_t to $S \cup N$ produces an output image $\Lambda_t(S \cup N)$ composed of a subset of the grains (connected components) forming $S \cup N$. Error results from signal grains erroneously not passed and noise grains erroneously passed. We desire a filter that removes noise grains while passing signal grains.

Error can be expressed in terms of the granulometric measure (sizes) of X and Y. Since Λ_t arises by reconstruction from Ψ_t, $\Lambda_t(X) = X$ if and only if there exists

$B \in \mathbf{B}$ and a point x such that $tB + x \subset X$. The $\{\Psi_t\}$-*measure* of X is defined by

$$\begin{aligned} M_X &= \max\{s : \text{ there exists } B \in \mathbf{B} \text{ and } x \text{ such that } sB + x \subset X\} \\ &= \max\{s : \Psi_s(X) \neq \emptyset\} \\ &= \max\{s : \Lambda_s(X) = X\} \end{aligned} \tag{6}$$

The maximum is attained for each realization because X is compact and B contains a finite number of compact sets. Thus, M_X is a random variable depending on X. The $\{\Psi_t\}$-measure of Y is defined similarly. If $\Psi_t(X) = X \circ tB$, where B is a ball of radius 1, then M_X is the radius of the maximum ball fitting inside X. Because signal S and noise N are generated by the random grains X and Y, we may write M_S and M_N in place of M_X and M_Y.

For filter Λ_r, error is given by

$$e[r] = E[A]E[U] + E[B]E[V] \tag{7}$$

where $U = m[X]$ if $M_X < r$, $U = 0$ if $M_X \geq r$, $V = m[Y]$ if $M_Y \geq r$, and $V = 0$ if $M_Y < r$ [8]. Optimization is achieved by finding r to minimize $e[r]$, which can be a difficult task involving random geometry and expectation integrals having complicated domains of integration depending on M_X^{-1} and M_Y^{-1}.

To adaptively obtain a good filter, we shall initialize the filter Λ_r and scan the image in such a manner as to successively encounter grains. In fact, this procedure will be applied to realizations of $S \cup N$. The adaptive filter will be of the form $\Psi_{r(n)}$, where n corresponds to the nth grain encountered and $r = r(n)$ is the size of the filter at step n. When a grain G is encountered (arrives) there are a number of possibilities: a. G is a noise grain and $\Psi_{r(n)}(G) = G$; b. G is a signal grain and $\Psi_{r(n)}(G) = \emptyset$; c. G is a noise grain and $\Psi_{r(n)}(G) = \emptyset$; d. G is a signal grain and $\Psi_{r(n)}(G) = G$.In the latter two cases, the filter has acted as desired; in either of the first two it has not. Consequently, we employ the following adaptation rule:

$$\begin{aligned} &i.\ r \to r + 1 \text{ if condition a occurs} \\ &ii.\ r \to r - 1 \text{ if condition b occurs} \\ &iii.\ r \to r \text{ if conditions c or d occur} \end{aligned} \tag{8}$$

We treat $r(n)$ as the state of the system at step n, where each arriving grain determines a step. Since S and N are independent, as are their grains, and there is no grain overlapping, $r(n)$ determines a discrete-state-space Markov chain over a discrete parameter space. There are three positive homogeneous transition probabilities associated with each state r:

$$\begin{aligned} &i.\quad p_{r,r+1} &&= P(N)P(M_N \geq r) \\ &ii.\quad p_{r,r-1} &&= P(S)P(M_S < r) \\ &iii.\quad p_{r,r} &&= P(S)P(M_S \geq r) + P(N)P(M_N < r) \end{aligned} \tag{9}$$

where $P(S)$ and $P(N)$ are the probabilities of a signal and noise grain arriving.

The equivalence classes of the length chain are determined by the distributions of M_S and M_N. To avoid trivial anomalies, we shall assume that the supports of distributions are connected (intervals) with endpoints $a_S < b_S$ and $a_N < b_N$, where

$0 \leq a_S$, $0 \leq a_N$, and it is possible to have $b_S = \infty$ or $b_N = \infty$. We also assume that $a_N \leq a_S < b_N \leq b_S$. There are four cases regarding state communication.

Suppose $a_S < 1$ and $b_N = \infty$: then the length chain is irreducible since each state can be reached from every other state in a finite number of steps. Suppose $1 \leq a_S$ and $b_N = \infty$: then, for each state $r < a_S$, r is accessible from state s if $s < r$, but s is not accessible from r; on the other hand, all states $r \geq a_S$ communicate and form a single equivalence class. Suppose $a_S < 1$ and $b_N < \infty$: then, for each state $r > b_N$, r is accessible from state s if $s > r$, but s is not accessible from r; on the other hand, all states $r \leq b_N$ communicate and form a single equivalence class. Suppose $1 \leq a_S < b_N < \infty$: then states below a_S are accessible from states below themselves, but not conversely, states above b_N are accessible from states above themselves, but not conversely, and all states r such that $a_S \leq r \leq b_N$ communicate and form a single equivalence class. In sum, the states between a_S and b_N form an irreducible equivalence class C of the length chain's state space and each state outside this class is transient. With certainty, the chain will eventually enter C and once inside C will not leave. Thus, we focus our attention on C. Within C, the chain is irreducible and aperiodic. If it is also positive recurrent, then it will be ergodic and possess a stationary (steady-state) distribution.

5. STEADY-STATE DISTRIBUTION

If $b_N < \infty$, then the state space is finite and the Markov chain must be positive recurrent and possess a stationary distribution. For $b_N = \infty$, existence of the stationary distribution and the form of the distribution have been demonstrated rigorously in Ref. [11] via a basic theorem on countably infinite Markov chains. For engineering intuition, here we apply the heuristic approach taken in queueing theory. Let $p_r(n)$ denote the probability that the system is in state r at step n. According to the Chapman-Kolmogorov equation and the transition probabilities of Eq. 9,

$$\begin{aligned} p_r(n+1) &= p_{r-1,r}p_{r-1}(n) + p_{r+1,r}p_{r+1}(n) + p_{r,r}p_r(n) \\ &= P(N)P(M_N \geq r-1)p_{r-1}(n) + P(S)P(M_S < r+1)p_{r+1}(n) \\ &+ (P(S)P(M_S \geq r) + P(N)P(M_N < r))p_r(n). \end{aligned} \tag{10}$$

Using the probability relations $P(S) + P(N) = 1$, $P(M_S \geq r) = 1 - P(M_S < r)$, and $P(M_N < r) = 1 - P(M_N \geq r)$ yields

$$\begin{aligned} p_r(n+1) - p_r(n) &= P(N)P(M_N \geq r-1)p_{r-1}(n) + P(S)P(M_S < r+1)p_{r+1}(n) \\ &\quad -(P(S)P(M_S < r) + P(N)P(M_N \geq r))p_r(n) \\ &= \lambda_{r-1}p_{r-1}(n) + \mu_{r+1}p_{r+1}(n) - (\lambda_r + \mu_r)p_r(n) \end{aligned} \tag{11}$$

for $r \geq 1$. For $r = 0$, $p_{-1}(n) = 0$ and $\mu_0 = 0$ yield the initial state equation

$$p_0(n+1) - p_0(n) = \mu_1 p_1 + \lambda_0 p_0 \tag{12}$$

Equations 11 and 12 are the forward Kolmogorov equations for the system. In the steady state, the left-hand sides become 0, so that these equations form the system

$$\begin{cases} 0 = \mu_1 p_1 - \lambda_0 p_0 \\ 0 = \lambda_{r-1}p_{r-1} + \mu_{r+1}p_{r+1} - (\lambda_r + \mu_r)p_r \quad (r \geq 1) \end{cases} \tag{13}$$

Solving iteratively yields

$$\begin{cases} p_1 = \frac{\lambda_0}{\mu_1} p_0 \\ p_r = p_0 \prod_{k=1}^{r} \frac{\lambda_{k-1}}{\mu_k} \quad (r \geq 1) \end{cases} \tag{14}$$

Using the boundary condition $\sum_{k=0}^{\infty} p_k = 1$, gives

$$p_0 = \frac{1}{\sum_{r=1}^{\infty} \prod_{k=1}^{r} \frac{\lambda_{k-1}}{\mu_k} + 1} \tag{15}$$

Thus, $(p_0, p_1, \ldots)$ gives steady-states distribution if the infinite sum in the denominator of Eq. 15 converges. Convergence is proved in Ref. [11].

Having established convergence of the adaptive filter, in the sense that it reaches a steady state, key characteristics of the filter are its size mean and variance in the steady state. In the steady state, r is a random variable. To indicate it randomness, we will sometimes write R. Its mean and variance are

$$\mu_R = \sum_{r=0}^{\infty} r p_r = \sum_{r=1}^{\infty} \left[r p_0 \prod_{k=1}^{r} \frac{\lambda_{k-1}}{\mu_k} \right] \tag{16}$$

$$\sigma_R^2 = \sum_{r=1}^{\infty} \left[r^2 p_0 \prod_{k=1}^{r} \frac{\lambda_{k-1}}{\mu_k} \right] - \mu_R^2 \tag{17}$$

Both mean and variance exist. In fact, R has finite moments of all orders.

Transition probabilities depend on the arrival probabilities $P(S)$ and $P(N)$, which in turn depend on the grain-selection protocol. Various protocols are discussed in Ref. [11]. Here we assume a protocol that is probabilistically straightforward and leads to relatively simple expressions: each grain in the image is labeled and the labels are uniformly randomly chosen with replacement. For this protocol, $P(S) = E[A]/E[T]$ and $P(N) = E[B]/E[T]$, where T is the total number of grains in the image and $E[T] = E[A] + E[B]$.

If X and Y are governed by the random variables Z and W respectively, and both M_X and M_Y are strictly increasing functions of Z and W, respectively, then Eq. 7 takes the tractable form

$$e[r] = E[T] \left[P(S) \int_0^{M_X^{-1}(r)} m[X](z) f_Z(z) dz + P(N) \int_{M_Y^{-1}(r)}^{\infty} m[Y](w) f_W(w) dw \right] \tag{18}$$

Averaging over r in the steady state yields

$$E\left[e[r]\right] = \sum_{r=0}^{\infty} e[r] p_r \tag{19}$$

The otpimal value of r, say $\hat{r}$, is found by minimizing Eq. 18 [8]. The expected cost of adaptivity can be measured by $E[e[r]] - e[\hat{r}]$, which must be nonnegative. Even if the cost is very small, actual filtering is done with some choice of r, so actual cost, $e[r] - e[\hat{r}]$, is a random variable and filter goodness is therefore dependent on both expected cost and state variance.

6. A SINGLE-GENERATOR HOMOTHETIC MODEL

Closed-form expression of $E[e[r]]$ is rarely possible but it can be achieved when signal and noise take the forms given in Eq. 5 with $C = D = B$, nonoverlapping grains, and sizing distributions Π_S and Π_N both uniform. For general discrete Π_S and Π_N (not necessarily uniform),

$$e[r] = E[T]m[B]\left[P(S)\sum_{k=0}^{r-1} k^2 P(M_S = k) + P(N)\sum_{k=r}^{\infty} k^2 P(M_N = k)\right] \qquad (20)$$

where, in this model, $f_Z(k) = P(M_S = k)$ and $f_W(k) = P(M_N = k)$. Let Π_S and Π_N be discrete uniform densities over $[a, b)$ and $[c, d)$ for signal and noise, respectively, with $c < b$. Let $m_S = (d - c)^{-1}$ and $m_N = (b - a)^{-1}$. The effective state space for the parameter r is $[c, b]$ because all other states are transient and r will move into $[c, b]$ and remain there. According to Ref. [11] p_0 is found from

$$\sum_{r=c+1}^{b} \prod_{k=c+1}^{r} \frac{\lambda_{k-1}}{\mu_k} + 1 = \left(1 + \frac{m_N P(N)}{m_S P(S)}\right)^{b-c} \qquad (21)$$

the steady-state (structuring-element size) probabilities are

$$p_{c+i} = \begin{cases} \left[\sum_{r=c+1}^{b} \prod_{k=c+1}^{r} \frac{\lambda_{k-1}}{\mu_k} + 1\right]^{-1} = \left(\frac{m_S P(S)}{m_S P(S) + m_N P(N)}\right)^{b-c}, & i = 0 \\ p_c \binom{b-c}{i} \left[\frac{m_N P(N)}{m_S P(S)}\right]^i, & 1 < i \leq b - c \end{cases} \qquad (22)$$

and the mean size and size variance are

$$\mu_R = \frac{c m_S P(S) + b m_N P(N)}{m_S P(S) + m_N P(N)} \qquad (23)$$

$$\sigma_r^2 = \frac{m_S m_N P(S) P(N)(b - c)}{(m_S P(S) + m_N P(N))^2} \qquad (24)$$

Mean size is a weighted mean of c and b by the weights $m_S P(S)$ and $m_N P(N)$.

Applying the error expression of Eq. 20 in the present case yields the optimization

$$\min_r\{e[r]\} = \begin{cases} E[T]m[B]P(S)m_S \sum_{k=c}^{b-1} k^2, & \text{at } r = b, & \text{if } P(S)m_S < P(N)m_N, \\ E[T]m[B]P(N)m_N \sum_{k=c}^{b-1} k^2, & \text{at } r = c, & \text{if } P(S)m_S > P(N)m_N, \\ E[T]m[B]P(N)m_N \sum_{k=c}^{b-1} k^2, & \text{at } r \in [c, b], & \text{if } P(S)m_S = P(N)m_N. \end{cases} \qquad (25)$$

For $P(S)m_S < P(N)m_N$, the optimum occurs at the upper endpoint b of the discrete interval over which the states can vary; for $P(S)m_S < P(N)m_N$, the optimum occurs at the lower endpoint c; for $P(S)m_S = P(N)m_N$, all states in $[c, b]$ are equivalent, and hence optimal. These results can be compared with the weighted average giving the mean size of the adaptive filter (Eq. 23). For $P(S)m_S < P(N)m_N$, the mean size tends towards b; for $P(S)m_S > P(N)m_N$, the mean tends towards c; for $P(S)m_S = P(N)m_N$, the mean is $(c + b)/2$.

Taking the expectation in Eq. 20 yields the expected error in the steady state:

$$E[e[r]] = E[T]m[B]\left[\sum_{i=c}^{b-1} p_i \sum_{k=i}^{b-1} k^2 P(N)P(M_N = k) + \sum_{i=c+1}^{b} p_i \sum_{k=c}^{i-1} k^2 P(S)P(M_S = k)\right] \tag{26}$$

We have the following error bound for the adaptive filter [11]:

$$\begin{aligned} \min\{m_S P(S), m_N P(N)\} E[T]m[B] \textstyle\sum_{k=c}^{b-1} k^2 &\leq E[e[r]] \\ \leq \max\{m_S P(S), m_N P(N)\} E[T]m[B] \textstyle\sum_{k=c}^{b-1} k^2 & \end{aligned} \tag{27}$$

The optimal filter possesses an error no larger than the expected steady-state error for the adpative filter. For the special case $P(S)m_S = P(N)m_N$ in the uniform model, the two errors agree because all filters whose parameter lies in the single recurrent class of the Markov chain have the same error.

References

1. Dougherty, E. R., 'Optimal Mean-Square N-Observation Digital Morphological Filters – Part I: Optimal Binary Filters,' *Computer Vision, Graphics, and Image Processing - Image Understanding*, Vol. 55, No. 1, January, 1992.
2. Loce, R. P., and E. R. Dougherty, 'Facilitation of Optimal Binary Morphological Filter Design Via Structuring-Element Libraries and Observation Constraints,' *Optical Engineering*, Vol. 31, No. 5, May, 1992.
3. Loce, R. P., and E. R. Dougherty, 'Optimal Morphological Restoration: The Morphological Filter Mean-Absolute-Error Theorem,' *Visual Communication and Image Representation*, Vol. 3, No. 4, December, 1992.
4. Dougherty, E. R., and R. P. Loce, 'Efficient Design Strategies for the Optimal Binary Digital Morphological Filter: Probabilities, Constraints, and Structuring-Element Libraries,' *Mathematical Morphology in Image Processing*, ed. E. R. Dougherty, Marcel Dekker, New York, 1993.
5. Dougherty, E. R., and R. P. Loce, 'Optimal Mean-Absolute-Error Hit-or-Miss Filters: Morphological Representation and Estimation of the Binary Conditional Expectation,' *Optical Engineering*, Vol. 32, No. 4, April, 1993.
6. Dougherty, E. R., Haralick, R. M., Chen, Y., Agerskov, C., Jacobi, U., and P. H. Sloth, 'Estimation of Optimal T-Opening Parameters Based on Independent Observation of Signal and Noise Pattern Spectra,' *Signal Processing*, Vol. 29, December, 1992.
7. Cuciurean-Zapan, C. and E. R. Dougherty, 'Optimal Openings for Overlapping Signal and Noise Grains,' *Proc. SPIE Image Algebra and Morphological Image Processing*, Vol. 2300 July 1994.
8. Cuciurean-Zapan, C. and E. R. Dougherty, 'Optimal Reconstructive τ-Openings for Disjoint and Statistically Modeled Nondisjoint Grains,' *Morphological Imaging Laboratory Report*, MIL-04-94, Rochester Institute of Technology, Rochester, N.Y. April 1994.
9. Schonfeld, D., and Goutsias, J., 'Optimal Morphological Pattern Restoration from Noisy Binary Images,' *IEEE Transactions on Pattern Analysis and Machine Intelligence*, Vol. 13, No. 1, January, 1991.
10. Salembier, P., 'Structuring Element Adaptation for Morphological Filters,' *Visual Communication and Image Representation*, Vol. 3, No. 2, June, 1992.
11. Chen, Y., and E. R. Dougherty, 'Adaptive Reconstructive τ-Openings,' *Morphological Imaging Laboratory Report*, MIL-05-94, Rochester Institute of Technology, Rochester, N.Y. May 1994.
12. Matheron, G., *Random Sets and Integral Geometry*, John Wiley, New York, 1975.

SYNTHESIS OF ADAPTIVE WEIGHTED ORDER STATISTIC FILTERS WITH GRADIENT ALGORITHMS

MICHAËL ROPERT and DANIELLE PELÉ
C.C.E.T.T., 4 rue du Clos Courtel, BP 59, 35512 Cesson-Sévigné, France, tel: 33-99-12-41-84, fax: 33-99-12-40-98, e-mail: pele@ccett.fr, ropert@ccett.fr.

Abstract. This paper deals with adaptive optimization of the non linear Weighted Order Statistic Filters (WOSF). We propose two gradient based approaches to adapt the filter weights and rank in order to minimize mean square and mean absolute error criteria. One solution uses an explicit formulation of the filter output while the second one is derived from an implicit formulation yet introduced to optimize rank order based filters. Some practical examples illustrate the ability of the adaptive solutions to cope with texture and noise in image processing.

Key words: Adaptive filtering, weighted order statistic filters.

1. Introduction

Non linear filters based on sorting operation have been of growing interest since the introduction of the standard median filter by Tukey for smoothing statistical data [6]. Famous non linear filters are multistage FIR hybrid median filters, rank order based filters such as morphological filters and more generally stack filters. In [1], relations and intersections that exist between these classes are emphasized. All these non linear filters find many applications in image processing. Their most famous property is their ability to remove noise without blurring. Image segmentation, texture prediction and multiresolution decomposition seem also promising areas of applications [4].

Our paper addresses the problem of synthesis of Weighted Order Statistic Filters (WOSF), which are part of rank order based filters, for image applications. Most of the methods developed for designing rank order based filters are either based on structural or estimation approaches. The structural approach consists in finding a filter that preserves relevant structures of the signal and removes noise. In the estimation approach, the filter is designed to best estimate the desired signal in sense of some error criterion, given a corrupted observation of the signal. Mean square error (MSE) and mean absolute error (MAE) are the most used criteria. The first method proposed within this approach had been derived from the theory of optimal stack filtering [1], but this method suffers on the one hand from the fact that some knowledge about the noise characteristics is required, and on the other hand from the computational complexity inherent to the use of the involved linear programming method.

In order to avoid these problems and to allow to cope with non stationary signals such as images, many adaptive algorithms have been developed to solve the optimization problem for designing rank order based filters such as morphological filters

J.Serra and P. Soille (eds.), Mathematical Morphology and Its Applications to Image Processing, 37-44

with flat or gray valued structuring elements and WOSF [3, 5, 7].

We propose two gradient based adaptive approaches to design WOSF. The first one is an original approach while the second one results from an adaptation of an existing theory. Some comparisons with a neural based approach and practical examples on images are provided.

2. Statement of the optimization problem

Let $\underline{x}$ be the vector composed of the N discrete values x_j contained in a mask M ($|M| = N$), j is the index location in the mask ($1 \leq j \leq N$):

$$\underline{x} = [x_1, \ldots, x_N]^T$$

Let $\underline{w}$ be a weighting vector defined by:

$$\underline{w} = [w_1, \ldots, w_N]^T$$

Where w_j is a weight associated with the mask's location j. The weighting of x_j by w_j is defined as the repetition of x_j, w_j times. $\diamond$ is the weighting operator:

$$w_j \diamond x_j = \underbrace{x_j, \ldots, x_j}_{w_j \text{ times}}$$

and

$$\underline{v} = \underline{w} \diamond \underline{x} = [w_1 \diamond x_1, \ldots, w_N \diamond x_N]^T$$

The output y of the WOSF is given by:

$$y = \text{Rank}(r, \underline{w} \diamond \underline{x})$$

Where $\text{Rank}(r, \underline{v})$ is the operator which selects the r-ordered value of the vector $\underline{v}$. The goal of the optimization approach is to get optimal w_j ($1 \leq j \leq N$) and r, realizing the minimum of the MSE quantity:

$$J(\underline{w}, r) = E[(d - y)^2]$$

E is the mathematical expectation, y the filter output, and d the desired output. Adaptive solutions can be derived from the gradient algorithm which leads to the formulas:

$$w_j^{n+1} = w_j^n + 2\mu(d - y)\frac{\partial y}{\partial w_j} \tag{1}$$

$$r^{n+1} = r^n + 2\lambda(d - y)\frac{\partial y}{\partial r} \tag{2}$$

where n is the iteration number, μ and λ two fixed stepsizes controlling the convergence. When the MAE criterion is used, $2(d - y)$ is replaced by $sgn(d - y)$ in Eqs. 1 and 2.

The problem is to get the expression of the derivatives of the filter output with respect to the variables. One way is to express an analytical (if possible derivable)

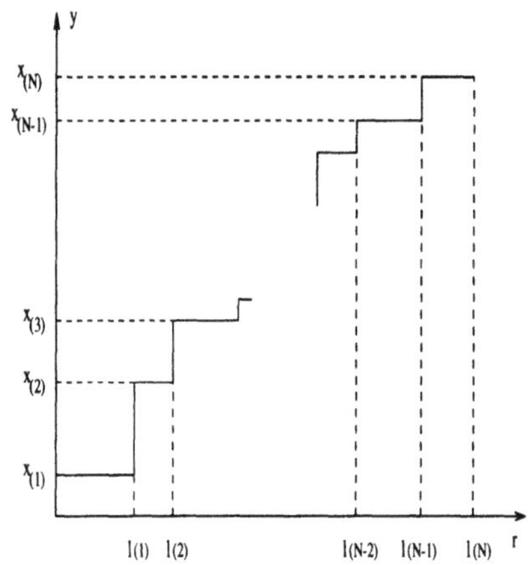

Fig. 1. Output with respect to the rank.

expression of the output as a function of the input parameters. Another approach is to propose an alternative solution where expressions of the derivatives can be obtained with no need of an explicit formulation of y. We propose a new solution resulting from an analytical expression of y and a solution relevant of the second approach with an adaptation of the implicit formulation of Salembier [3].

3. Adaptive solutions

3.1. One adaptive solution from an analytical approach

The idea which governs the analytical approach is to order the input samples and to perform the same permutation on weights so that the correct associations (inputs/weights) are preserved. The output is then chosen on the resulting ordered weighted data. We can say that weighting is controlled by ordering.

Let $\underline{x_{()}} = [x_{(1)}, \ldots, x_{(N)}]^T$ be the vector of the ordered data x_j belonging to $\underline{x}$ and $\underline{w_{()}} = [w_{(1)}, \ldots, w_{(N)}]^T$ the associated vector of the permuted weights. Define $l(k) = \sum_{i=1}^{k} w_{(i)}$, $k = 1, \ldots, N$ and $l(0) = 0$. Then the output y can be defined as a function of r by:

$$y = \sum_{k=1}^{N} x_{(k)} P_k(r)$$

$$\text{with } P_k(t) = \begin{cases} 1 & \text{if } l(k-1) \leq t < l(k) \\ 0 & \text{otherwise} \end{cases}$$

The Fig. 1 shows the shape of y with respect to the parameters. So we can derive:

$$\frac{\partial y}{\partial r} = \sum_{k=1}^{N-1} [x_{(k+1)} - x_{(k)}]\delta[r - l(k)]$$

$$\frac{\partial y}{\partial w_{(m)}} = \sum_{k=m}^{N-1} [x_{(k)} - x_{(k+1)}]\delta[r - l(k)]$$

The $\frac{\partial y}{\partial w_j}$ can be obtained from the known permutation to get from $\underline{x}$ to $\underline{x_{()}}$. As many authors do, linear piecewise approximation is chosen for the δ distribution.

3.2. A SECOND ADAPTIVE SOLUTION FROM AN IMPLICIT FORMULATION

The solution that requires no analytical expression for y is just an adaptation of Salembier's approach. In [3], Salembier proposes an implicit formulation using only sign functions to design rank order based filters where both the filter mask and the normalized rank can be optimized. A continuous variable m_k is assigned to each possible location k in a maximum search area A. This approach can easily be derived for the synthesis of WOSF of fixed size where continuous w_k replace the m_k. The output y of the WOSF is the value $y = x_{j_0}$ belonging to the set A such that:

$$F = [\sum_{j \in A} P(w_j)(sgn(x_j - y) + 2r - 1)] + P(w_{j_0})(1 - 2r) = 0$$

$$\text{with } sgn(x) = \begin{cases} -1 & \text{if } x < 0 \\ 0 & \text{if } x = 0 \\ 1 & \text{if } x > 0 \end{cases}$$

$$\text{and } P(x) = \begin{cases} 0 & \text{if } x < 0 \\ x & \text{if } x \geq 0 \end{cases}$$

Adaptation of the theory developed by Salembier yields then to:

$$\frac{\partial y}{\partial r} = \frac{\sum_{j \in A} P(w_j)}{P(w_{j_0})} - 1$$

$$\frac{\partial y}{\partial w_k} = \frac{sgn(x_k - y) + 2r - 1}{2P(w_{j_0})}$$

with j_0 such that $x_{j_0} = y$. A lower bound is imposed on $P(w_{j_0})$ to eliminate numerical instabilities.

3.3. COMPARISONS

In order to compare the performances of the different algorithms, one simulation result is presented in this section. Consider the preset periodic signal X=(1,2,4,3,2,1, 3). Its filtering with a four weights WOSF produces the output signal Y=(2,4,3,3,3, 3,2). In this experiment, initial weights are set to 1, the normalized rank r is set to 0.5, and the stepsizes μ and λ are set to 0.001. After 1000 times training, we get the results of the table I. In [8], Yin *et al.* propose another adaptive solution for the synthesis of WOSF which is based on their deterministic properties and the backpropagation algorithm of neural networks. To obtain the same rate of convergence, the stepsizes μ and λ are set to 0.8333. Figure 2 shows the evolution of rank and weights with respect to the iteration number n. Only w_4 is presented as the convergence rate is the same for the four weights. The weights derived from the optimal adaptive optimization algorithms are positive real valued. We use the conversion algorithm proposed in [10] to provide the equivalent set of integer weights and rank representing the equivalent WOSF. The conversion is done by finding the positive boolean function (PBF) corresponding to the WOSF with real weights.

TABLE I
solutions

Algorihms	w_1	w_2	w_3	w_4	r
Algo 1	0.215	0.215	0.266	w_4=0.304	r=0.696
Algo 2	0.252	0.244	0.245	w_4'=0.260	r'=0.747
Yin's Algo	0.210	0.199	0.199	w_4''=0.392	r''=0.695

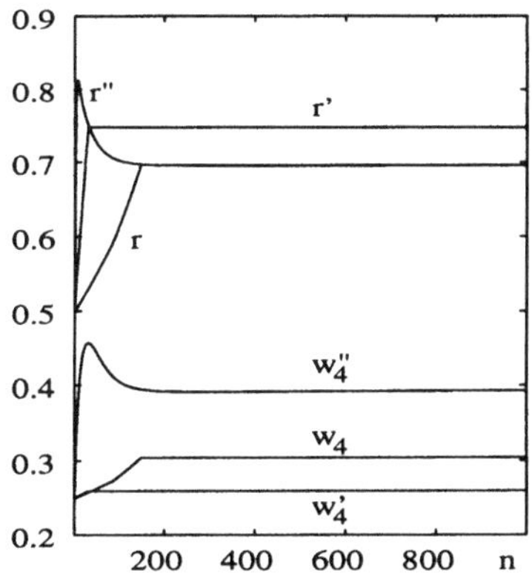

Fig. 2. Rank and weights convergence.

Then integer linear programming is performed to obtain integer weights. The three solutions lead to the same filter: $<w_1, w_2, w_3, w_4; r> = <1, 1, 1, 2; 4>$.

4. Application to image processing

4.1. Texture prediction

In this sub-section, results concerning texture prediction are presented. Figures 3 and 5 are the original textures. Figures 4 and 6 are the predicted textures. In these figures, each pixel is replaced by its predictor calculated by a WOSF of size 5×5 centered on it. The weights and rank are optimized with the approach described in section 3.1. The image is scanned line by line from top to bottom. The stepsizes λ and μ are set to 10^{-3}. Only three image lines are necessary to reach convergence. The quality of the results make the adaptive WOSF well suited for restoration of missing points or detection of texture defects in images.

5. Noise cancellation

We refer there to suppression of randomly distributed noise. In Fig. 7, the original image is corrupted by an impulsive "salt and pepper" noise (33% level of noise). The WOSF is constrained to be a weighted median filter. In a preliminary step, the

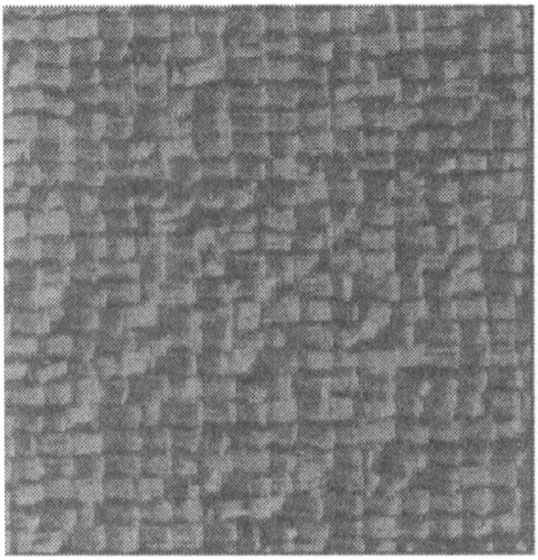

Fig. 3. Original texture 1.

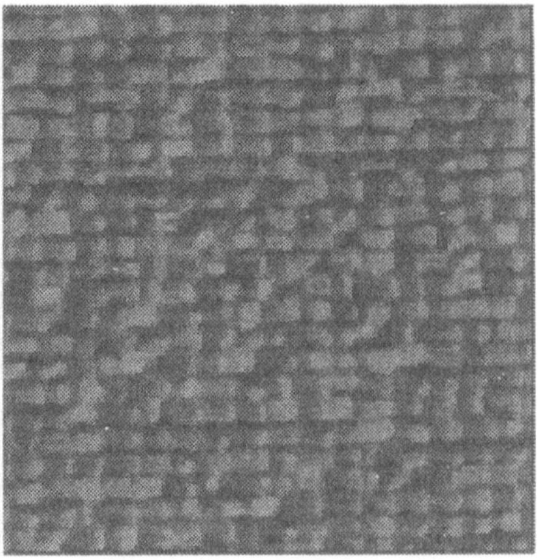

Fig. 4. Predicted texture 1.

Fig. 5. Original texture 2.

Fig. 6. Predicted texture 2.

adaptive filter is used as a predictor but the optimization is done on the noisy image. The filter is optimized with the approach of section 3.1. In order to emphasize the quality of the prediction, the predicted part of the filtering process (without taking the central pixel into account) is presented in Fig. 8. Then, provided the amount of noise is known, a weight can be assigned to the central pixel in order to accept it when it has chance to be an original point. The filtered image is presented in Fig. 9. Referring to Fig. 10, the absolute difference between Figs. 7 and 9, one can see the very good noise suppression capability of the filter while preserving the original texture.

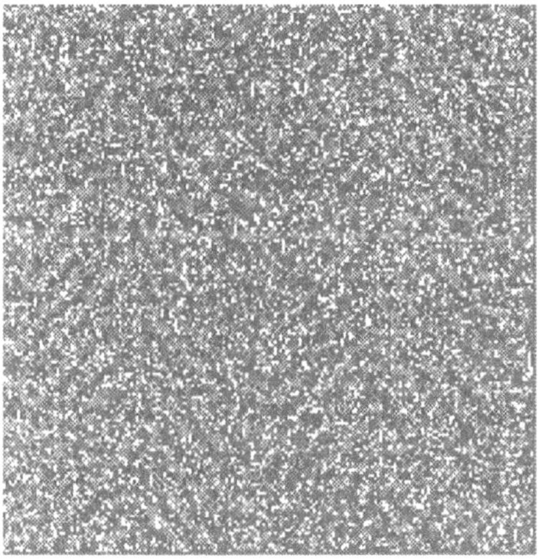

Fig. 7. Noisy texture.

Fig. 8. Predicted part.

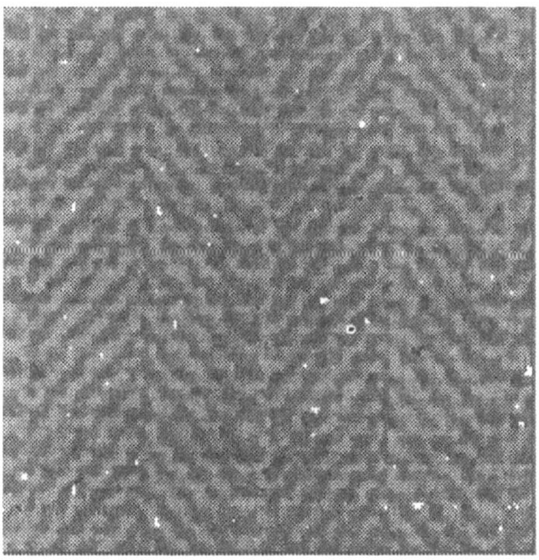

Fig. 9. Filtered noisy texture.

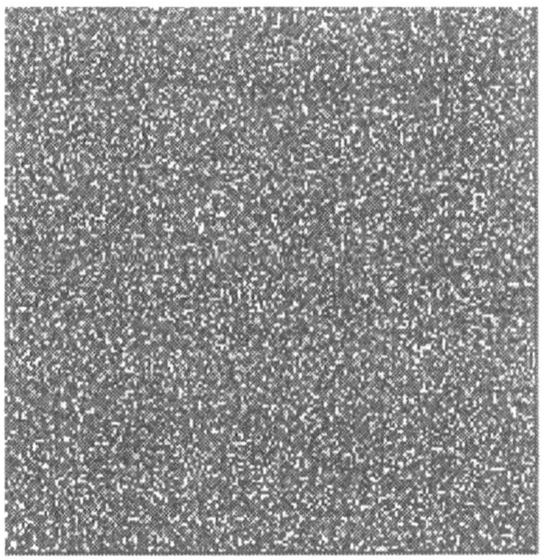

Fig. 10. Absolute difference between the filtered and the noisy texture.

6. Conclusion

In this paper, two gradient based solutions to derive adaptive Weighted Order Statistic Filters were described. Comparisons between these algorithms and a neural network approach were performed. Applications to image processing were also presented. The quality of results shows the ability of these adaptive non linear filters to cope with texture and noise in images.

7. Acknowledgment

The authors thank the reviewers for their useful comments. They also acknowledge Pierre Soille for his advices for improving the readability of this paper.

References

1. Coyle, E. J., Lin, J. H. and Gabbouj, M.: 1989, 'Optimal Stack Filtering and the Estimation and Structural Approaches to Image Processing', *IEEE Trans. Acoust. Speech Signal Processing*, Vol. 37 no. **12**, pp. 2037–2066.
2. Gabbouj, M. and Coyle, E. J.: 1990, 'Minimum Mean Absolute Error Filtering with Structural Constraints and Goals', *IEEE Trans. Acoust. Speech Signal Processing*, Vol. 38 no. **6**, pp. 955–968.
3. Salembier, P.: 1992, 'Adaptive Rank Order Based Filters', *Signal Processing*, Vol. 27 no. **1**, pp. 1–25.
4. Salembier, P. and Kunt, M.: 1992, 'Size-sensitive Multiresolution Decomposition of Images with Rank Order Based Filters', *Signal Processing*, Vol. 27 no. **2**, pp. 205–241.
5. Serra, J.: 1982, 'Image Analysis and Mathematical morphology', *Academic Press*, New York.
6. Tukey, J. W.: 1982, 'Nonlinear (nonsuperposable) methods for smoothing data', *Cong. Rec. EASCON'74*, pp. 673.
7. Wang, Q. and Neuvo, Y.: 1992, 'Adaptive Grayscale Morphological Filters for Image Noise Smoothing', *Proc. IEEE Int. Conf. Systems Engineering*, Japan, pp. 588–591.
8. Yin, L., Astola, J. T. and Neuvo, Y.: 1990, 'Adaptive Weighted Order Statistic Filters Using Backpropagation Algorithm', *Proc. IEEE Int. Symp. Circuits and Systems*, New Orlean, pp. 499–502.
9. Yin, L., Astola, J. T. and Neuvo, Y.: 1993, 'Adaptive Stack Filtering with Application to Image Processing', *IEEE Trans. Acoust. Speech Signal Processing*, Vol. 41 no. **1**, pp. 162–184.
10. Nieweglowski, J., Gabbouj , M. and Neuvo, Y.: 1993, 'Weighted medians - Positive Boolean Function Conversion Algorithms', *Signal Processing*, Vol. 34 no. **2**, pp. 149–161.

A SPATIALLY VARIANT, LOCALLY ADAPTIVE, BACKGROUND NORMALIZATION OPERATOR

ROBERT C. VOGT
Environmental Research Institute of Michigan
P. O. Box 134001, Ann Arbor, MI 48113-4001, U.S.A.

Abstract.
This paper describes a spatially variant, locally adaptive, background normalization operator that is defined in terms of morphological openings and closings. The *variable opening (and closing) residue* operators address the problems that can occur when one attempts to choose a single structuring element size for background normalization purposes, in cases where the objects of interest have multiple or unknown widths. The operators attempt to assign a natural width to each pixel in an image, based on the opening or closing size that causes the largest change in its value. This size then also determines a local contrast value for that pixel. The size, local contrast and original grey values of pixels in an image can be used to cluster pixels as an aid to performing image segmentation, or foreground-background discrimination. This paper describes and illustrates the algorithm, and discusses how its outputs may be used for image analysis and parameter selection.

Key words: mathematical morphology, background normalization, morphological top-hat, image segmentation, image analysis, object recognition

1. Introduction

The opening residue and threshold, or 'top-hat' operator [1] [2], is a well-known and commonly used morphological technique for extracting locally bright (positive contrast) objects from a grey-level image, based on size and relative brightness. The analogously defined closing residue is likewise used to extract negative contrasts. While in principle one only has to choose a structuring element for these operations that is wider than the largest possible object to be extracted, in actual practice the need to choose a single element size for them can present difficulties. If the element is chosen too small, portions of the spatial extent or contrast of some objects may be missed. If the element is too large, interference may occur with nearby image structures, causing the extraction of some objects to be imprecise.

In particular, when the exact sizes of the objects of interest are not known in advance, or when the objects vary in width over the same image or over a large population of images to be processed, the selection of a single element size for performing background normalization and foreground extraction can be problematic. Examples of such situations include the extraction of vessel networks from digital angiography images, extraction of waterways from overhead terrain images, and the extraction of text from images of documents, particularly when multiple fonts are present. In these cases, the edges and sizes of the objects to be extracted are generally quite obvious to the human eye, even if variable. One wishes for a more sophisticated morphological operator that would effectively use a different opening or closing residue at different locations in an image, based on a self-selection process

J.Serra and P. Soille (eds.), Mathematical Morphology and Its Applications to Image Processing, 45-52

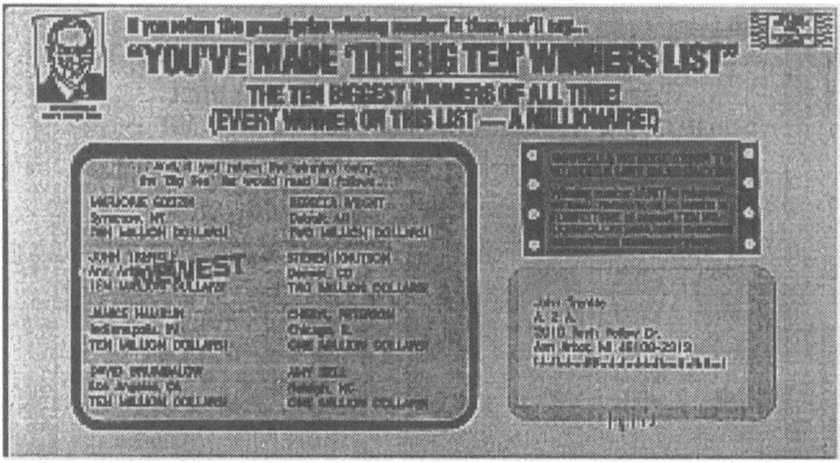

Fig. 1. Mailpiece image with mutiple fonts and inks

that would choose the 'best' size by some reasonable criterion for cleanly extracting the contrast present.

This paper describes such an operator, and compares its effects to the more common opening residue and 'rolling-ball' algorithms, as well as to other segmentation and foreground extraction operations such as simple thresholding, the top-hat, and the watershed algorithm. Illustrations are performed on grey-level images of letter mail, where the object has been to find the text that makes up the destination address block. The technique described here, which is called the *variable opening (or closing) residue*, was developed precisely for this purpose. Because the nature of a printing or writing process typically assumes a 'pen' having a reasonably constant width, as well as fairly constant color or pressure on the paper, this operator is particularly well-suited for extraction and clustering of multi-font text from images of documents that have variable backgrounds and inks, as illustrated in Figure 1. A further motivation for its development was to devise a means of segmenting images that *simultaneously* uses grey-level, intrinsic size, and local contrast criteria to cluster pixels, in much the same way that the human visual system does virtually automatically.

Because the variable opening residue operator is based on a notion of using maximum contrast differences to decide the appropriate size to use at every location in an image, it is best suited to problems where the objects of interest are expected to have fairly sharp edges and limited interior noise, but different or variable widths, grey-level values, and contrasts or backgrounds. It should therefore be viewed as practical tool that may have great utility in certain situations, but may not be applicable or most efficient in every case. For example, it would not be expected to work as well where objects are blurred or very noisy internally, or where grey values of edges fall off gradually. Likewise, it would not be necessary where simple thresholding or a fixed top-hat operator was sufficient.

In most of the discussion that follows, we will assume we are extracting positive

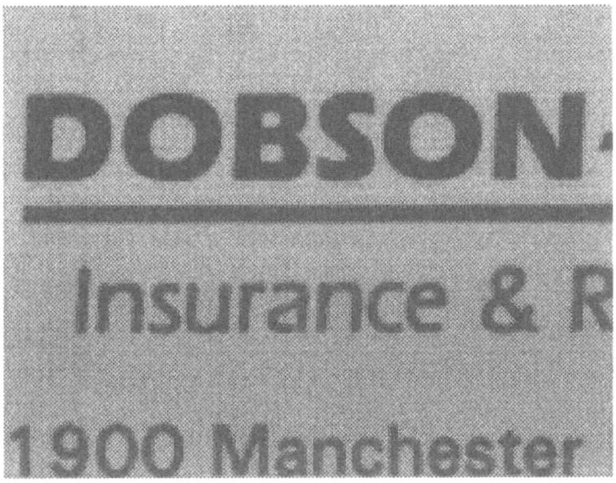

Fig. 3. Coded Size image generated by variable closing residue

contrast and speak in terms of a *variable opening residue* operator, for the sake of clarity. The corresponding *variable closing residue* is easily defined symmetrically, and is indeed the basis of the example letter mail images (dark text on light paper) that appear in the following sections.

2. Operator Description and Illustrations

Given a grey-level image as a starting point (Figure 2), the essence of the variable opening residue operator is to perform a series of successively larger openings (or closings), up to the maximum size of interest, and compute the paired differences between these. Each point in the image is then assigned a *size* classification, based on the opening pair that produced the maximum difference at that spot (Figure 3). For example, if the maximum difference occurred between sizes *k-1* and *k*, then that point would be assigned a *size class* of *k* .

At the same time, the *local contrast* assigned to the same point would be the difference between its original grey-level image value, and its value after the opening

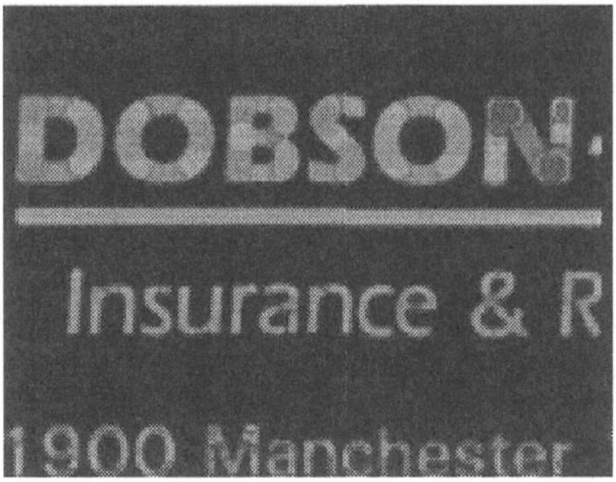

Fig. 4. LocalContrast image generated by variable closing residue

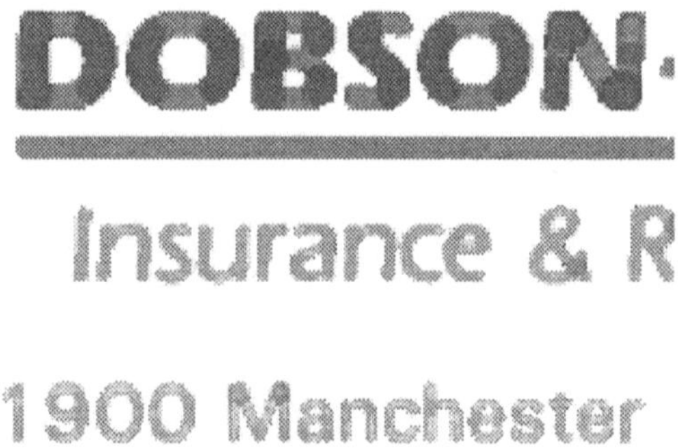

Fig. 5. Coded Size image with low contrast pixels suppressed

by size k. Note that the size and contrast values assigned to each pixel are linked in this way, but are nevertheless independent, because they come from orthogonal dimensions. The 'LocalContrast' image defined in this manner is the primary output of the variable opening residue operator (Figure 4). It represents, for each point, the total contrast present at that point based on the opening that produced the largest *change* in grey value there. Assuming reasonably well-behaved images, and strong edges, this should extract the width and contrast of the object that the human eye would typically choose, and do a somewhat better job than a fixed-size opening residue, particularly over diverse image sets containing variable-width objects.

While the LocalContrast image is the primary output of this operation, the corresponding 'Size' image is also of interest, by itself and in conjunction with the others. Since the size assigned by this algorithm for pure noise areas may be random and not of interest, it is customary to assign a 'null' size state to flat, background areas that have very little local contrast. Individual size classes can then be colored with different values to make it easier to see them. The result, for letter images, is typically a fairly clean segmented image, with most of the pixels along strokes from the same font having the same value, as shown in Figure 5.

More formally, the variable opening residue operator is defined algorithmically below (without regard to optimization issues). We assume here that grey-level images are represented as unsigned byte data (0-255). The parameter *MaxSize* designates the largest structuring element size to consider in performing the successive openings. The parameter *MinContrast* is used to suppress regions of the Size output image that are not of interest due to low contrast.

```
-- VARIABLE OPENING RESIDUE ALGORITHM --

Given original image, X, and image buffers:

Size             =  0
LocalContrast    =  0
MaxDiff          =  0
Previous         =  X
Current
Difference
UpdateMask

FOR k = 1 THRU MaxSize
    BEGIN
       Current = X OPEN DISK[k]
       Difference = Previous - Current
       UpdateMask = IF (Difference > MaxDiff)
                    THEN 255, ELSE 0
       MaxDiff = MaxDiff MAX Difference
       Size = Size MAX (UpdateMask MIN k)
       LocalContrast = LocalContrast MAX
                       (UpdateMask MIN (X - Current))
       Previous = Current
    END

UpdateMask = IF (LocalContrast >= MinContrast)
             THEN 255, ELSE 0
Size = Size MIN UpdateMask

RETURN X, LocalContrast, Size
```

By way of explanation, the Size image is initialized to zero. (Zero is reserved as a special state for areas whose contrast is very low, and thus whose 'true' size may be somewhat indeterminate). LocalContrast and MaxDiff are also initialized to zero. Previous and Current keep track of two successive openings (or closings in the case of negative contrast), with Current using a larger element than Previous.

Previous is initialized to the original image, which is equivalent to an opening by a structuring element of size 0.

The algorithm proceeds by calculating the next larger opening into Current, after which the (binary) UpdateMask is determined by finding those locations where the difference between Previous and Current is greater than the previously stored MaxDiff value. These are the locations where the MaxDiff, Size, and LocalContrast images will be modified. MaxDiff will get the new difference maxima, the Size image will have the value of the current '*k*' written into these pixels, and the LocalContrast image will have written the value of the original image X, minus the Current opening image. (The use of MAX to perform the overwriting is predicated on the fact that '*k*' and 'X - Current' increase monotonically with each loop pass).

At the end of the loop, UpdateMask is used to select those portions of the image that have significant local contrast as determined by the MinContrast parameter, and all other areas within the Size image are set to zero. The algorithm then returns the original image X, along with the LocalContrast and Size images (and possibly MaxDiff as well). Thresholding the LocalContrast image can be used to perform foreground/background discrimination, producing a result analogous to a morphological top-hat. Modification of the above algorithm for negative contrast extraction via closings is straightforward and will not be presented here.

3. Operator Comparisons and Analysis

The variable opening residue operator described above can be compared to a traditional opening residue by either a single flat disk, or by a true grey-level element such as a half-sphere ('rolling-ball') or paraboloid. While the paraboloid is constructed from flat disks spaced at fixed distances in the grey dimension, the variable opening residue is more flexible in some sense because it has no fixed distances between successively applied disk elements; it lets them slide in trying to determine when the maximum opening value change occurs for each pixel.

While the differences between these alternative means of calculating local contrast may be difficult to see in a grey-level contrast image, following a thresholding operation the differences may be more apparent. By thresholding the LocalContrast output of the variable opening residue, one obtains a result that can be compared to a simple global threshold, a traditional top-hat operation, or an opening residue threshold based on a non-flat structuring element. In cases where background variation prevents the use of a simple global threshold, and where the objects of interest have different sizes, both on the same image, and over the population of images to be processed (as is the case in our postal address block location problem), we have found the variable closing residue to provide cleaner extraction of printed text, though admittedly at somewhat greater cost.

As a segmentation method, the variable closing residue can also be compared to the traditional morphological watershed algorithm [3] [4]. Our experience with this on mailpiece and address block images is that image quality and sensor noise often lead to over-segmented images coming out of the watershed, at times creating extra segments within the text strokes. Because the variable opening or closing residue looks for the maximum opening or closing change in order to determine the size and

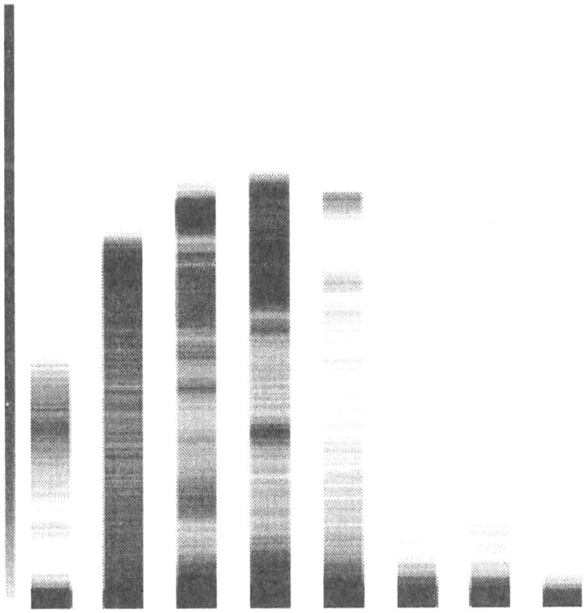

Fig. 6. Joint distribution plot of size(x) vs. local contrast(y)

local contrast of a pixel, it is somewhat immune to small levels of noise inside a character stroke, as long as the edges are relatively stronger.

As described earlier, one of the reasons for creating this algorithm was to devise a means of segmenting images that simultaneously uses grey-level, intrinsic size, and local contrast criteria to cluster pixels, in situations where more detailed analysis is required. At the end of the variable residue calculation, each pixel has been assigned a size and local contrast value, in addition to its original grey-level value. These three dimensions can be used to create joint distributions of pixels, for the purpose of clustering them into groups that have similar sizes, contrasts, and/or grey values. The clusters so-defined can be used to extract text of the same type or font. Even in cases where clean distinctions cannot be made in the distributions between all of the pixels in two different types of text, by concentrating on the central portions of the clusters, we can obtain excellent marker sets, which can then be used to reconstruct and extract the desired text via conditional dilation, possibly with other filtering operations. This can be of great help in cases where multiple fonts and colors exist on a mailpiece, and a detailed analysis is required to decide which text really represents the address block, and which is irrelevant.

The joint distribution of size vs. local contrast is especially interesting, because it displays the contrast that each pixel has, after an opening or closing residue by the disk element size that 'best extracts' the bright portion of that pixel, in the sense described earlier. Figure 6 illustrates such a plot for the images shown previously. Size, based on octagons with even radii from 2 through 16, is plotted on the x-axis. These eight columns correspond to the values of the Size coded image. Local contrast (0-255) is plotted along the y-axis. Frequencies are plotted using a reversed grey scale (shown at the left) from white (0) to black (saturated at 255 counts). Strong clusters for the top line of the address text appear at size 8, for the second line at size 6, for the third and fourth lines at size 4, and for the fourth or bottom line at size 2. Determination of the correspondence of clusters to portions of the image can be aided by watching the plot fill in as the Size and LocalContrast images are scanned.

This size vs. local contrast distribution can be used to decide what typical contrast and size combinations are present in an image, as a potential analysis aid for selecting a specific top-hat operation. If training data are available in which foreground and background pixels have been explicitly identified, then their separate distributions generated from the variable opening or closing residue outputs can be used to choose operators and parameters to best discriminate them over a population of images. More detail on how this is done may be found in [5] and [6]. Using the size vs. local contrast distribution, one can additionally define a granulometry that simultaneously makes use of both dimensions, simply by choosing a series of bracketing rectangles defined on the plot space, that satisfy a containment relation.

4. Conclusion

This paper has defined a spatially variant, locally adaptive background normalization operator for the purpose of more precisely extracting positive or negative contrast objects in grey-level images via openings and closings. The variable opening and closing residue operators described here are designed for situations where background normalization is required prior to thresholding, and where the objects to be extracted are complex, and vary in width, both in an individual image and across the population of images to be processed. They work best when the objects to be extracted have fairly clear boundaries, and they return a Size image and LocalContrast image that can be used, in conjunction with the original grey-level image, to cluster pixels along three different dimensions as a means of discriminating groups of them. The LocalContrast image can also be used separately as a spatially variant background normalization result that can be thresholded to extract high-contrast objects.

References

1. F. Meyer, 'Automatic screening of cytological specimens', *Computer Vision, Graphics, and Image Processing*, v. 35, pp. 356–369, 1986.
2. J. Serra, *Image Analysis and Mathematical Morphology*, Academic Press, London, 1982.
3. S. Beucher and C. Lantuéjoul, 'Use of watersheds in contour detection', *Intl. Workshop on Image Processing*, Rennes, France, September 1978.
4. S. Beucher and F. Meyer, 'The morphological approach to image segmentation: the watershed transformation', in E. Dougherty (ed.), *Mathematical Morphology in Image Processing*, ch. 12, Marcel-Dekker, New York, 1993.
5. R. Vogt, *Automatic Generation of Morphological Set Recognition Algorithms*, Springer-Verlag, New York, 1989.
6. R. Vogt, 'Set discrimination analysis tools for grey level morphological operators', *SPIE Proc. on Image Algebra and Morphological Image Processing II*, v. 1568, San Diego, CA, July 1991.

USING GENETIC ALGORITHMS IN THE DESIGN OF MORPHOLOGICAL FILTERS

NEAL R. HARVEY and STEPHEN MARSHALL
Signal Processing Division, Dept. of Electronic & Electrical Engineering
University of Strathclyde
204 George Street, Glasgow, G1 1XW
Scotland, U.K.

Abstract. Morphological filters are an important class of non-linear digital signal processing and analysis filters, which have found a range of applications, giving excellent results in areas such as noise reduction, edge detection and object recognition. However, few design methods exist for these morphological filters, with selection of filter type and sequence of application tending to be both ad-hoc and application specific. This paper demonstrates how simple genetic algorithms can be employed in the search for optimum morphological filters for specific signal/image processing tasks.

Key words: Genetic Algorithms, Morphological Filters, Design, Optimisation

1. Introduction

Morphological filters are non-linear transformations, locally modifying geometric features of signals/images. Structures of an image can be analysed by selecting a filter able to interact properly with these structures. A structuring element is a set or function describing a simple shape that probes the image, providing various types of information about the image. The number of possible structuring elements from which to choose is very large and this, combined with the possible choices of morphological operator sequence, indicates the complexity of the morphological filter design problem.

Genetic Algorithms are a relatively new paradigm for search, based on the principles of evolution. Problem areas which may benefit from the use of GAs are optimisation problems which are made difficult by substantial complexity and uncertainty. Genetic algorithms have been established as a valid approach to problems requiring efficient, effective and robust search in complex spaces.

This paper demonstrates how simple genetic algorithms can be employed in the search for morphological filters realising optimum performance in a given image processing task.

2. Genetic Algorithms

A Genetic Algorithm (GA) is an implementation of an adaptive plan, employing specific structural modifiers (operators) in the search for optimally performing structures in a particular environment. Genetic algorithms are computationally quite simple, yet they are powerful in their search for improvement, and are not funda-

J.Serra and P. Soille (eds.), Mathematical Morphology and Its Applications to Image Processing, 53-59

mentally limited by restrictive assumptions about their search space.

A population of individuals is successively modified from one generation to another. Individuals in the population are known as chromosomes and are made up of strings of genes. Each gene can have several different forms, knowns as alleles, producing differences in the set of characteristics associated with that gene.

The metaphor underlying genetic algorithms is that of evolution. In evolution, the problem each species faces is one of searching for beneficial adaptations to a complicated and changing environment. The knowledge that each species has gained is embodied in the makeup of the chromosomes of its members. Operators that alter this chromosomal makeup are applied when parents reproduce. Among these genetic operators are mutation and crossover, the most commonly used operators in genetic algorithms.

Crossover is basically the exchange of genetic material between two parents' chromosomes, exchanging corresponding genetic material from the parent chromosomes, allowing beneficial material from the two parent chromosomes to be combined in their offspring. Mutation provides background variation and occasionally introduces beneficial material into a species' chromosomes.

For a genetic algorithm to perform its adaptive task, there has to be some means of assigning an observable performance to each individual. A fitness function is employed, which attributes some objective measure of how well an individual performs in an environment, i.e. the fitness of an individual. Formation of the next generation proceeds in two phases: During phase one, the population is modified to produce an intermediate population, by copying each individual in the population in proportion to the individual's observed performance. The number of copies made is determined stochastically, so that the expected number of copies increases in proportion to its observed performance. During phase two, genetic operators are applied to the intermediate population, interchanging and modifying sets of alleles, to produce the new generation.

3. Using Genetic Algorithms in the Design of Morphological Filters

In order for a GA to be used in the design for morphological filters, the problem has to be encoded for genetic search, i.e. the parameters of the optimisation problem have to be mapped to a finite length string, over some alphabet. As a rule, when coding a problem for genetic search, one should select the smallest possible alphabet which permits a natural expression of the problem, this being known as the principle of minimal alphabets, [5]. This leads almost automatically to consider the use of the binary digits $\{0, 1\}$ as the alphabet. How then should the parameters of the morphological filter design problem be coded?

In the case of morphological filters there are two basic parameters: the structuring element and the sequence of morphological operations. Thus, it is necessary to code these parameters and map them to positions in the chromosome.

3.1. Coding the Structuring Element

A binary structuring element is relatively simple to code, by simply mapping the 0s and 1s to their appropriate positions in the structuring element portion of the chromosome. For grey-scale structuring elements, if the range of possible values for each position within the structuring element's region of support is $0 - I_{max}$, these integer values can be coded to binary strings, the length of which is $|log_2(I_{max})| + 1$ binary digits. Each of these binary strings, representing an integer value for each position within the structuring element's region of support, can then be mapped to their appropriate positions in the structuring element portion of the chromosome.

If the overall dimensions of the structuring element are fixed, it may be that not all positions are in the region of support. In order to take this into account in the GA optimisation, it is necessary for positions outside the structuring element's region of support, but within the overall dimensions of the structuring element to be distinguishable. A suitable code, therefore, would be one which includes a unique representation for those "null" positions. An example of such a code is illustrated in Table I. Here the asterisk represents a position outside the structuring element's region of support.

TABLE I
Example of a code suitable for encoding positions both within and outside the structuring element's region of support

Binary Code	Corresponding value in position within structuring element's overall dimensions
0 0 0	*
0 0 1	0
0 1 0	1
0 1 1	2
1 0 0	3
1 0 1	4
1 1 0	5
1 1 1	6

A function-processing dilation or erosion, with a structuring element having zero values at all positions within its region of support is equivalent to function-set processing dilation or erosion with a structuring element having the same region of support. Thus, using a coding method for structuring elements, similar to that described, the possible search space of structuring elements includes all shapes of function-set processing and function-processing structuring elements, governed by the overall dimensions of the structuring element and the value of I_{max}.

In most cases, structuring elements used in morphological filters are symmetric. It was possible to reduce the search space of the optimisation by ensuring that only structuring elements symmetrical about two orthogonal axes (horizontal and vertical) were searched for. Thus, it was only necessary for one quadrant of the structuring element to be coded into the chromosome. This quadrant could then be mapped onto the full sized equivalent structuring element.

3.2. Coding the Sequence of Morphological Operators

When considering the sequence of morphological operations in the context of design of morphological filters, there are two basic decisions to be made:

1. The set of individual morphological operators from which to choose.
2. The number of morphological operations in the sequence.

For example, for the close-open morphological filter, the set of morphological operators necessary is {dilation, erosion} and the sequence length required is four (i.e. four separate fundamental morphological operations: dilate-erode-erode-dilate).

It is necessary to include the do-nothing operation to the set of morphological operations, as this ensures that simple one or two stage morphological filters may be searched for, e.g. the basic erosion and dilation filters, the close and open filters and the close-open and open-close filters.

Each member of the set of morphological operations to be considered in the GA optimisation can be coded to a binary string and these strings can then be mapped to their appropriate positions in the morphological sequence portion of the chromosome. Table II shows an example of coding, for the set {erosion, dilation, do-nothing}.

TABLE II
Example of a code for morphological operations, if choice is from {erosion, dilation, do-nothing}

Binary Code	Morphological Operator
0 0	Do-Nothing
0 1	Do-Nothing
1 0	Erosion
1 1	Dilation

3.3. Combining the Coded Structuring Element and Sequence of Morphological Operations

To form the complete chromosome, it is simply a matter of concatenating the two separate coded binary strings for the structuring element and the sequence of morphological operations.

4. The Genetic Algorithm

4.1. Fitness Function

For each chromosome, the morphological filter configuration represented by that particular chromosome is obtained by a decoding process, i.e. the reverse of the coding processing described previously. Then, a corrupted image is filtered using

*	2	2	2	*
2	1	0	1	2
2	0	0	0	2
2	1	0	1	2
*	2	2	2	*

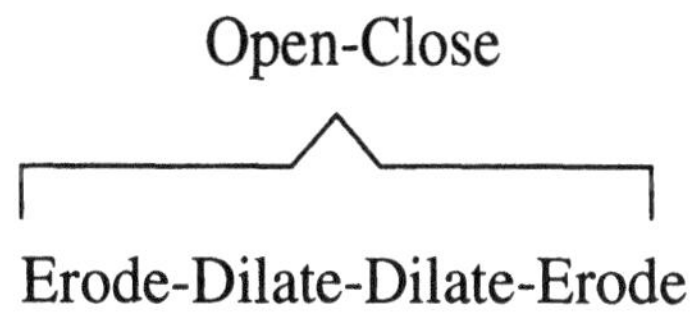

Structuring Element Sequence of Morphological Operations

Fig. 1. Morphologhical Filter used to test GA

this filter configuration. The fitness function is based on the MAE criterion. If the MAE of the filtered image is worse than that of the corrupted image, then the fitness value of the chromosome is set to zero, otherwise, the fitness value of the chromosome is set as the improvement gained in MAE by filtering using the morphological filter configuration corresponding to that particular chromosome.

5. Application of the GA

In order to determine whether or not the GA described was capable of finding/ searching for the optimum morphological filter for a particular application, and to observe the convergence characteristics, the GA was tested using a set of training images for which the optimum filter was known. An image which had been previously filtered with a known morphological filter, together with the original unfiltered image were therefore used as the training set.

The morphological filter used to "clean" the noisy test image was an open-close operation using a 5×5 spheroid structuring element. Fig. 1 shows the structuring element and sequence of morphological operations used.

To further test the GA's ability to discover the optimum morphological filter, the region of support of the structuring element in the GA was set at 7×7. Thus, if the GA performed correctly, it would still find the optimum 5×5 structuring element, within its overall dimensions of 7×7.

After running the GA for 1000 generations the GA had determined the correct sequence of morphological operations as well as the correct overall size and shape of structuring element.

The GA was then used to determine the optimum morphological filter for a second training set, shown in Fig. 2. Fig. 2a shows an uncorrupted image and Fig. 2b shows the same image, corrupted with salt and pepper noise.

After running for 750 generations, the best filter found by the GA was that shown in Fig. 3. This is a close-open operation, which is what could be expected for the type of corruption present. The result of applying this filter to the corrupted image is shown in Fig. 4. It can be seen that the filter performs well in this situation.

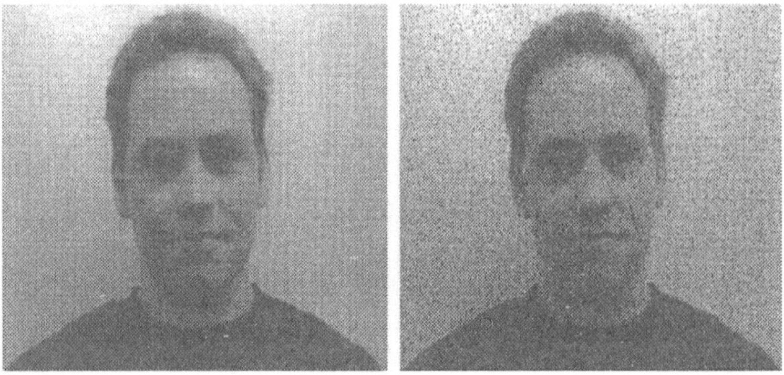

(a) (b)

Fig. 2. Images used as training set for GA

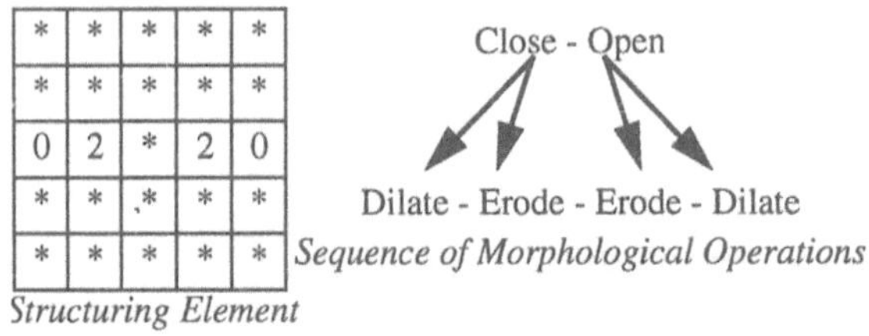

Fig. 3. Morphological Filter found using training set shown in Fig. 1

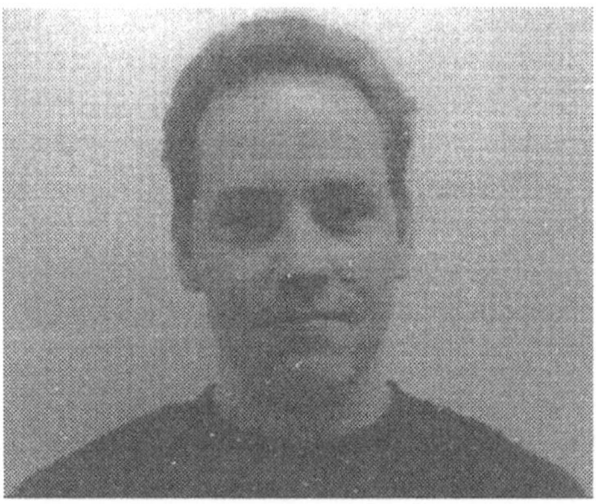

Fig. 4. Corrupted image filtered using filter shown in Fig. 3

6. Conclusions

In this paper, a method of designing morphological filters for specific noise-reduction tasks using Genetic Algorithms has been presented. An example, showing results of employing the GA in the search for the optimum filter in a particular situation has been shown. This shows that the GA is capable of being employed in the search for optimum morphological filters for particular applications, such as noise-reduction in images. The technique so far has searched for a single global optimum filtering sequence and structuring element. Another area of future work could be the investigation of locally adaptive morphological filters which use different sequences of operations and structuring elements in different areas of the image. A new objective function and thus fitness function will have to be derived for this approach. Additional areas to be investigated include the possibility of using a GA, similar to that described, in the design of soft morphological filters. Also, the current design method only makes use of a simple genetic algorithm. Investigations into improving the genetic algorithm's performance will be carried out.

References

1. Maragos, P., Schafer R.W.: 1987, 'Morphological Filters - Part I and II', *IEEE Trans. Acoust. Speech, Signal Processing* ASSP-35 **8**, pp. 1153–1184.
2. Sternberg, S.R.: 1986, 'Grayscale Morphology', *Computer Vision, Graphics and Image Processing*, [Academic Press, 1986], pp. 333–355.
3. Pitas, I., Venetsanopoulos, A.N.: 1991, *Nonlinear Digital Filters*, [Kluwer Academic Publishers, 1991].
4. Holland, J.H.: 1992, *Adaptation in Natural and Artificial Systems*, [MIT Press/Bradford Books, 1992].
5. Goldberg, D.E.: 1989, *Genetic Algorithms in Search, Optimization and Machine Learning*, [Addison-Wesley, 1989].
6. Goldberg, D.E.: 'Zen and the Art of Genetic Algorithms', *Proc. Third Int. Conf. Genetic Algorithms, ICGA'89, Fairfax, VA, June 1989*, pp. 80–85.
7. De Jong, K.A.: 1975, *An Analysis of the Behaviour of a Class of Genetic Adaptive Systems*, [Doctoral Dissertation, University of Michigan, 1975].
8. Chu, C.H.: 1989, 'A Genetic Algorithm Approach to the Configuration of Stack-Filters', *Proc. Third Int. Conf. Genetic Algorithms, ICGA'89, Fairfax, VA, June 1989*, pp. 219–224.

MINIMAL GENERATOR BASIS OF A FINITE STRUCTURAL OPENING

JULIETTE MATTIOLI
L.C.R., Thomson-CSF,
Domaine de Corbeville, 91401 Orsay, France
Email: mattioli@lcr.thomson.fr

Abstract.
In a pseudo-ring structure of the power space where the "max" plays the role of the addition and the Minkowski sum the role of the multiplication, all idealoids are invariance domain of an algebraic opening which is translation invariant. Since a finite structural opening is completely characterized by its invariance domain, the purpose of this paper is to find a "*minimal generator basis*" of a subset which is closed under union and translation, and which is the invariance domain of a finite structural opening, *i.e.* a minimal generator basis of the associated idealoid.

Key words: Dioid, idealoid, algebraic opening, structural opening, invariance domain, generator basis, prime set.

1. Finite Structural Opening

1.1. Algebraic structure for the power space

The power space $\mathcal{P}(\mathbb{R}^n)$ (*i.e.* the set of all subsets of $\mathbb{R}^n$), supplied with an order relation $\subseteq$, a complementary operation, union, intersection and Minkowski sum, enjoys many algebraic structures. We shall not emphasize here the Boolean structure of the power set, which makes it a Boolean ring for the *addition* $K \Delta L = (K \backslash L) \cup (L \backslash K)$ (symmetric difference) and the *multiplication* $K \cap L$.

Morphological operations lead rather to single out the "max-plus" structure of what is called a dioid, which is a "pseudo-ring" where the union plays the role of the addition and the Minkowski sum the role of the multiplication.

Definition 1.1 [6, 7, 2] *A* semi-ring *is a set $\mathcal{D}$ supplied with:*

1. *one associative and commutative operation $+$, whose neutral element is denoted by $\emptyset$*
2. *one associative operation $\times$, whose neutral element is denoted by $\mathbb{1}$*

satisfying the distributivity conditions

$$\forall a, b, c \in \mathcal{D}, \quad (a+b) \times c = (a \times c) + (b \times c) \tag{1}$$

$$\forall a, b, c \in \mathcal{D}, \quad c \times (a+b) = (c \times a) + (c \times b) \tag{2}$$

$$\forall a \in \mathcal{D}, \quad a \times \emptyset = \emptyset \times a = \emptyset \tag{3}$$

It is said to be idempotent *if* $\forall a \in \mathcal{D}, \quad a + a = a$. *An idempotent semi-ring is called*

J.Serra and P. Soille (eds.), Mathematical Morphology and Its Applications to Image Processing, 61-68

a dioid[1]. *It is said to be* commutative *when the operation* $\times$ *is commutative, and to be* entire *if* $(a \times b = \emptyset \Rightarrow b = \emptyset$ *or* $a = \emptyset)$. *An element* u *is a* unit *of the dioid if there exists* v *such that* $u \times v = \mathbb{1}$, v *is called the* inverse *of* u. *Two elements* x *and* y *are* associated *if there exists a unit* u *such that* $x = y \times u$.

Naturally, the power set $\mathcal{P}(\mathbb{R}^n))$ is a commutative dioid for the union and the Minkowski sum, since the distributivity condition $(K \cup L) \oplus M = (K \oplus M) \cup (L \oplus M)$ is satisfied. In the dioid $(\mathcal{P}(\mathbb{R}^n), \cup, \oplus)$, $\emptyset$ is the empty set and $\mathbb{1}$ is $\{O\}$ where O is the origin of $\mathbb{R}^n$. This dioid is also entire but in general the simplification rule $A \oplus B = A \oplus C \Rightarrow B = C$ is not true. The units are singletons and two subsets are associated if and only if they are translated.

Definition 1.2 *Let* $(\mathcal{D}, +, \times)$ *be a commutative dioid. An* idealoid $\mathcal{I} \subset \mathcal{D}$ *is a subset of the dioid* $\mathcal{D}$ *satisfying*

$$\begin{cases} i) \ \forall x, y \in \mathcal{I}, \ x + y \in \mathcal{I} \\ ii) \ \forall x \in \mathcal{I}, \ \forall z \in \mathcal{I}, \ x \times z \in \mathcal{I} \end{cases}$$

The set $\mathcal{I} = a\mathcal{D} = \{a \times x \mid x \in \mathcal{D}\}$ for $a \in \mathcal{D}$, is an idealoid, called principal. We say that a is a generator of $\mathcal{I}$ and we write $\mathcal{I} =< \{a\} >$. In particular $\mathcal{D}$ is a principal idealoid whose generator is $\mathbb{1}$.

According to the definition, every principal idealoid of $(\mathcal{P}(\mathbb{R}^n), \cup, \oplus)$ admits the representation: $A \oplus \mathcal{P}(\mathbb{R}^n) = \{A \oplus K | K \in \mathcal{P}(\mathbb{R}^n)\}$ for an element $A \in \mathcal{P}(\mathbb{R}^n)$. It means that a principal idealoid generated by A is the set of all dilated [2] subsets by the structuring element $\check{A} = -A$.

Let $\mathbf{T}$ be the group of translations of $\mathbb{R}^n$. Given $\mathcal{B} \subset \mathcal{P}(\mathbb{R}^n)$, let us put $< \mathcal{B} >^{\mathbf{T}}_{\text{sup}}$ the smallest subset of $\mathcal{P}(\mathbb{R}^n)$ closed under the union $\cup$ and translation, containing $\mathcal{B}$. Each element of $< \mathcal{B} >^{\mathbf{T}}_{\text{sup}}$ is a union of translated sets of $\mathcal{B}$.

<u>EXAMPLE 1:</u> If $\mathcal{B}$ is the set of all open balls of the Euclidean space $\mathbb{R}^n$, centered at the origin, then $< \mathcal{B} >^{\mathbf{T}}_{\text{sup}}$ is the set $\mathcal{G}(\mathbb{R}^n)$ of all topological open subsets of $\mathbb{R}^n$.

Proposition 1.3 [20] *Let* $\mathcal{B}$ *an arbitrary subset of* $\mathcal{P}(\mathbb{R}^n)$. *The set* $< \mathcal{B} >^{\mathbf{T}}_{\text{sup}}$ *is the idealoid generated by* $\mathcal{B}$ *of the commutative dioid* $(\mathcal{P}(\mathbb{R}^n), \cup, \oplus)$.

In any dioid $(\mathcal{D}, +, \times)$, we can associate an order relation with the operation $+$ by setting $x \preceq y$ if and only if $x + y = y$. This relation is consistent with the two operations on the dioid in the sense that

$$\begin{cases} i) \ x \preceq y \text{ implies } x + z \preceq y + z \\ ii) \ x \preceq y \text{ implies } x \times z \preceq y \times z \end{cases}$$

It follows that in the power space $\mathcal{P}(\mathbb{R}^n)$, the natural order relationship is the inclusion order $\subseteq$. The supremum and the infimum are given by:

$$\forall \mathcal{H} \subset \mathcal{P}(\mathbb{R}^n), \ \vee \mathcal{H} = \bigcup_{K \in \mathcal{H}} K \text{ and } \wedge \mathcal{H} = \bigcap_{K \in \mathcal{H}} K$$

[1] The usual example of dioid [2] is $(\mathbb{R} \cup \{-\infty\}, \max, +)$ which has been popularized by its applications to Discrete Event Dynamics sytems.

[2] We recall that the dilation of $K \in \mathcal{P}(\mathbb{R}^n)$ by a structuring element B is the operator $K \mapsto K \oplus \check{B} := \{x \mid K \cap B_x \neq \emptyset\}$ where B_x is the translation of B by x.

1.2. Structural opening

For all $X, K \in \mathcal{P}(\mathbb{R}^n)$, the structural opening [22, 26] of the set X by K is defined as:

$$X_K = \{K_x \mid x \in \mathbb{R}^n \text{ and } K_x \subset X\}$$

where K_x is the translated of K along the vector x, *i.e.* $K_x = \{k+x \mid k \in K\}$. The set K is called the structuring element. In fact the structural open set X_K consists of all translated sets of K which are contained within X.

We recall that an operator $\psi : \mathcal{P}(\mathbb{R}^n) \mapsto \mathcal{P}(\mathbb{R}^n)$ is called a τ-operator (or translation invariant operator) if $\forall x \in \mathbb{R}^n$, $\forall X \in \mathcal{P}(\mathbb{R}^n)$, we have $\psi(X_x) = (\psi(X))_x$.

Definition 1.4 [16, 25] *An operator ψ on $\mathcal{P}(\mathbb{R}^n)$ is an* algebraic opening *if: ψ is increasing, $(X \subset Y \Rightarrow \psi(X) \subset \psi(Y))$, anti-extensive $(\psi(X) \subset X)$, and idempotent $(\psi \circ \psi = \psi)$.*

A structural opening is an algebraic opening which is translation invariant.

Definition 1.5 [9] *The* invariance domain *of an operator ψ on $\mathcal{P}(\mathbb{R}^n)$ is defined as the set of fixpoints, i.e.:* $\mathrm{Inv}(\psi) = \{X \subset \mathbb{R}^n \mid \psi(X) = X\}$.

Let us recall an important result on the invariance domain:

Theorem 1.6 (Tarski fixpoint theorem) [17, 18, 21]
Let ψ be an increasing idempotent operator on a complete[3] *lattice $\mathcal{L}$. Then* $\mathrm{Inv}(\psi)$ *is a non empty complete lattice included in $\mathcal{L}$.*

It is obvious that for all operator ψ, the set $\mathrm{Inv}(\psi)$ is ψ-closed, because $\forall X \in \mathrm{Inv}(\psi)$ we have $\psi(X) = X$, and $\psi(\psi(X)) = \psi(X)$ implies that $\psi(X) \in \mathrm{Inv}(\psi)$. Then, for any algebraic opening ψ on $\mathcal{P}(\mathbb{R}^n)$, there is an associated subset of invariants points. Since ψ is idempotent, $\mathrm{Inv}(\psi)$ is nothing but the image of $\mathcal{P}(\mathbb{R}^n)$ under ψ, *i.e.* $\mathrm{Inv}(\psi) = \psi(\mathcal{P}(\mathbb{R}^n))$. Since ψ is anti-extensive, $\mathrm{Inv}(\psi)$ is closed under the union, that is if $X_i \in \mathrm{Inv}(\psi)$ for $i \in I$ then $\cup_{i\in I} X_i \in \mathrm{Inv}(\psi)$. Furthermore, if ψ is a τ-operator then $\mathrm{Inv}(\psi)$ is closed under translation. It follows:

Proposition 1.7 [20] *Let ψ be an algebraic opening on $\mathcal{P}(\mathbb{R}^n)$ which is translation invariant. Then* $\mathrm{Inv}(\psi)$ *is an idealoid of* $(\mathcal{P}(\mathbb{R}^n), \cup, \oplus)$.

Conversely, every subset $\mathcal{B} \subset \mathcal{P}(\mathbb{R}^n)$ which is closed under union is the invariance domain of a unique algebraic opening ψ given by: $\psi(X) = \{B \in \mathcal{B} \mid B \subset X\}$. It means that every idealoid in $(\mathcal{P}(\mathbb{R}^n), \cup, \oplus)$ is the invariance domain of a unique algebraic opening which is translation invariant. Since the family of all opens by a structuring element K is equal [25] to the set of all subsets $Y \oplus K$ for $Y \in \mathcal{P}(\mathbb{R}^n)$,

[3] A complete lattice $(\mathcal{L}, \leq)$ is a partial ordered set such that every subset $\mathcal{H}$ of $\mathcal{L}$ has a supremum and and infimum denoted by $\vee\mathcal{H}$ and $\wedge\mathcal{H}$. The power space $\mathcal{P}(\mathbb{R}^n)$ supplied with the union $\cup$ and the intersection $\cap$ is an example of complete lattice.

If ψ is an increasing idempotent operator in $(\mathcal{L}, \leq)$, then the supremum (resp. the infimum) of any family $(x_i)_{i\in I}$ of $\mathrm{Inv}(\psi)$ is given by $\psi(\vee_{i\in I} x_i)$ (resp. $\psi(\wedge_{i\in I} x_i)$.)

it follows that if Inv(ψ) is a principal idealoid of $(\mathcal{P}(\mathbb{R}^n), \cup, \oplus)$ then there exists a subset $B \in \mathcal{P}(\mathbb{R}^n)$ such that ψ is the structural opening by B. Conversely, the invariance domain of an opening by a structuring element is a principal idealoid.

The following theorem due to Matheron [16, chapter 7] is very important:

Theorem 1.8 [16, 18] *Let $\psi : \mathcal{P}(\mathbb{R}^n) \mapsto \mathcal{P}(\mathbb{R}^n)$ be an algebraic opening which is translation invariant. Then ψ can be written as $\psi(X) = \cup_{K \in \mathcal{B}} X_K$ for some family of structuring elements $\mathcal{B}$.*

In this previous theorem, we can take for $\mathcal{B}$ any family of K such that Inv(ψ) is the smallest subset of $\mathcal{P}(\mathbb{R}^n)$ generated by $\mathcal{B}$ and which is closed under translation and union. Since an algebraic τ-opening ψ is the supremum of structural openings, we say that ψ is also a structural opening. The set $\mathcal{B}$ is a generator basis[4] of the invariance domain of ψ if $<\mathcal{B}>_{\cup}^{\mathbf{T}} = \text{Inv}(\psi)$.

For example [22], the topological opening $K \mapsto Int(K)$ where $Int(K)$ denotes the interior of K, is an algebraic opening on $\mathcal{P}(\mathbb{R}^n)$ which is translation invariant. Its invariance domain is $\mathcal{G}(\mathbb{R}^n)$ the set of all topological open subsets of $\mathbb{R}^n$. It is obvious that $\mathcal{G}(\mathbb{R}^n)$ is closed under union and invariant under translation. The set $\{B(O, 1/n) \mid n \in \mathbb{N}^*\}$ of all open balls centered about the origin and of radius $1/n$ will be a generator basis of its invariance domain.

Definition 1.9 *We say that ψ is a* finite structural opening *if there exists a finite compact generator basis $\mathcal{B}$ of its invariance domain, i.e. $\exists p \in \mathbb{N}$ such that $\exists K_1, K_2, ..., K_p$ compact (non necessarily convex) subsets of $\mathbb{R}^n$ and*

$$\psi(X) = \bigcup_{i=1}^{p} X_{K_i} \iff <\{K_1, K_2, ..., K_p\}>_{\cup}^{\mathbf{T}} = \text{Inv}(\psi).$$

Since a finite structural opening is completely characterized by its invariance domain, we aim to find a "*minimal generator basis*" of a finite idealoid $\mathcal{I}$ which is the invariance domain of a finite structural opening. Here, we mean by minimal generator basis, a subset Θ of $\mathcal{P}(\mathbb{R}^n)$ such that for any $\mathcal{B}$ satisfying $< \Theta >_{\cup}^{\mathbf{T}} = < \mathcal{B} >_{\cup}^{\mathbf{T}} = \mathcal{I}$, we have $Card(\Theta) \leq Card(\mathcal{B})$ where $Card(.)$ represents the number of elements.

2. Minimal generator basis of a finite structural opening

Let $\mathcal{R}$ be the following equivalence relationship:

$$\forall X, Y \in \mathcal{P}(\mathbb{R}^n),\ X \,\mathcal{R}\, Y \iff \exists x \in \mathbb{R}^n \text{ such that } X_x = Y.$$

It means that $X \,\mathcal{R}\, Y$ if and only if there exists a translated of X which is equal to Y. In the sequel, we consider that ψ is a finite structural opening. We denote

[4] By proposition 1.7 Inv(ψ) is an idealoid. Since $< \mathcal{B} >_{\cup}^{\mathbf{T}} = \text{Inv}(\psi)$, it is obvious that $\mathcal{B}$ is a generator of Inv(ψ). Conversely, every idealoid of $(\mathcal{P}(\mathbb{R}^n), \cup, \oplus)$ is the invariance domain of a structural opening.

by $\mathcal{Q}$ the quotient set $\text{Inv}(\psi)_{|\mathcal{R}}$, *i.e.* the set of all equivalence classes $\dot{X}$ for $\mathcal{R}$: $X\ \mathcal{R}\ Y \Leftrightarrow \dot{X} = \dot{Y}$. We supply $\mathcal{Q}$ by a distance $\tilde{d}$ defined by:

$$\tilde{d}(\dot{X}, \dot{Y}) = \inf_{x \in \mathbb{R}^n} d(X_x, Y)$$

where $d(X, Y)$ is a distance between X and Y.

Remark: Let K_1, K_2 be two compact subsets of $\mathbb{R}^n$ and let ϕ_i be the opening by the structuring element K_i for $i = 1, 2$. Then $\tilde{d}(\dot{K}_1, \dot{K}_2) = 0$ if and only if $\phi_1 = \phi_2$.

2.1. First order relationship on the quotient set

We first consider the order relationship $\leq$ defined on the quotient set $\text{Inv}(\psi)_{|\mathcal{R}}$ (the set of the equivalence classes of $\mathcal{R}$) as:

$$\forall \dot{X}, \dot{Y} \in \text{Inv}(\psi)_{|\mathcal{R}}, \qquad \dot{X} \leq \dot{Y} \Longleftrightarrow \exists x \in \mathbb{R}^n \text{ such that } X_x \subseteq Y$$

Proposition 2.1 [20] *Let ψ be a finite structural opening defined such that a generator basis of the invariant domain is the finite set family $\mathcal{B} = \{B_1, ..., B_p\}$. Let $\mathcal{M}_{\leq}$ the set of all minimal elements of $(\text{Inv}(\psi)_{|\mathcal{R}}, \leq)$. Then we unfortunately only have:*

$$<\mathcal{M}_{\leq}>^{\mathbf{T}}_{\text{sup}} \subset \text{Inv}(\psi).$$

EXAMPLE 2: Let ψ be an opening defined on the plane $\mathbb{R}^2$ by: $\psi = \phi_1 \vee \phi_2$, where $\phi_1(X) = X_{K_1}$ and $\phi_2(X) = X_{K_2}$, and where K_1 is the unit square $\{x|\ \|x\|_\infty \leq 1\}$ and K_2 is the unit disk $\{x|\ \|x\|_2 \leq 1\}$. It follows that $\text{Inv}(\psi) = <\{K_1, K_2\}>^{\mathbf{T}}_{\text{sup}}$. Since $K_2 \subset K_1$, we only have $\mathcal{M}_{\leq} = \{\dot{K}_2\}$. Furthermore K_1 is not open by K_2, then $<\mathcal{M}_{\leq}>^{\mathbf{T}}_{\text{sup}} \neq \text{Inv}(\psi)$.

2.2. Second order relationship on the quotient set

We can supply the quotient set $\text{Inv}(\psi)_{|\mathcal{R}}$ with a second order relationship defined by:

$$\dot{X} \ll \dot{Y} \Longleftrightarrow Y_X = Y.$$

This relation means that $\dot{X}$ is smaller than $\dot{Y}$ under $\ll$ if and only if the compact set Y (and all of its translated) is open by X. Let $\mathcal{M}_{\ll}$ be the set of all minimal elements of $(\Theta_{|\mathcal{R}}, \leq)$ then we have: $<\mathcal{M}_{\ll}>^{\mathbf{T}}_{\cup} = \Theta$, but $\mathcal{M}_{\ll}$ is not necessarily a minimal basis of Θ (see example 2 again).

2.3. Prime set of a family of the power space

Definition 2.2 *Let $\mathcal{A}$ be a set of compact connected subsets of $\mathbb{R}^n$. We say that $A \in \mathcal{A}$ can not be split up in $\mathcal{A}$ if for every finite family $(A_i)_i$ of $\mathcal{A} \setminus \{A\}$ we have $\cup_i (A)_{A_i} \neq A$. The set A is called an prime set in $\mathcal{A}$. We say that A can be split up in $\mathcal{A}$ if there exists a finite family $(A_i)_i$ of $\mathcal{A} \setminus \{A\}$ such that $\cup_i (A)_{A_i} = A$.*

In fact, if A is not a prime set in $\mathcal{A}$, then A can be written as a union of translated elements of $\mathcal{A}$ distinct to A. It means that, there exists a finite structural opening ψ whose generator basis is a subset of $\mathcal{A} \setminus \{A\}$ such that A is invariant by ψ.

Theorem 2.3 [20] *Let ψ be a finite structural opening. Let Θ_ψ be the set of all prime set of the quotient set $Inv(\psi)_{|\mathcal{R}}$. Then Θ_ψ is a non empty set which is a minimal generator basis of $Inv(\psi)$, i.e. :*

$$<\Theta_\psi>_{\cup}^{\mathbf{T}} = \mathrm{Inv}(\psi) \text{ and } \forall \mathcal{B} \text{ generator basis of } \mathrm{Inv}(\psi),\ Card(\mathcal{B}) \geq Card(\Theta_\psi)$$

We have the following implications:

$$\begin{pmatrix} B \text{ minimal in } (\mathrm{Inv}(\psi)_{|\mathcal{R}}, \leq) \\ \Downarrow \\ B \text{ prime in } \mathrm{Inv}(\psi)_{|\mathcal{R}} \\ \Downarrow \\ B \text{ minimal in } (\mathrm{Inv}(\psi)_{|\mathcal{R}}, \ll) \end{pmatrix}$$

Unfortunately, the converse relations are in general false.

3. Algorithm for the construction of a minimal generator basis of an invariance domain of a finite structural opening

Let $\mathcal{A}$ be a finite subset of $\mathcal{K}(\mathbb{R}^n)$ (the set of all compact subsets of $\mathbb{R}^n$). Assume that $\mathcal{A}$ is a (not necessarily minimal) generator basis of a finite structural opening ψ. The following algorithm allows us to find a minimal generator basis Θ_ψ of ψ included in $\mathcal{A}$. We denote by $V^{(n)}(X)$ the Lebesgue measure of $X \in \mathcal{K}(\mathbb{R}^n)$.

$k := 0$;
Labeling every $K \in \mathcal{A}$ with the value of $V^{(n)}(K)$;
$\mathcal{A}_0 := \mathcal{A}$;
$\Theta_\psi := \emptyset$;

Repeat until $\mathcal{A}_0 = \emptyset$
> $k := k + 1$;
> Choose a set $K \in \mathcal{A}_0$, denoted by K_k with minimum Lebesgue measure;
> Compute the structural opening of elements of $\mathcal{A}_0$ by Φ_k, where Φ_k is the supremum of structural opening by structuring elements K_i $(i = 1, .., k)$;
> $\mathcal{A}_0 := \mathcal{A}_0 \setminus \mathrm{Inv}(\Phi_k)$;
> $\Theta_\psi := \mathcal{D}_\psi \cup \{K_k\}$;

A minimal generator basis is $\Theta_\psi = \{K_1, ..., K_k\}$.

Figure 1 is examples of the result obtained by this algorithm.

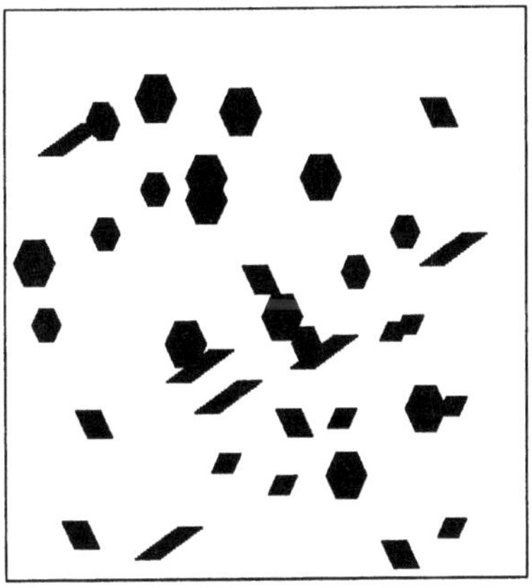

(1a) Test image 1

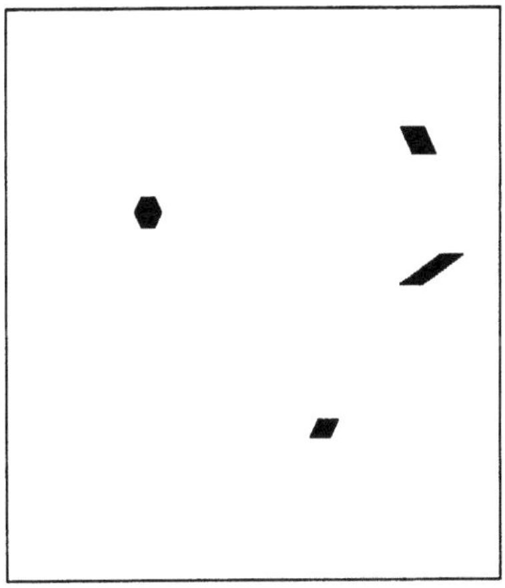

(1b) Minimal Generator Basis of image 1

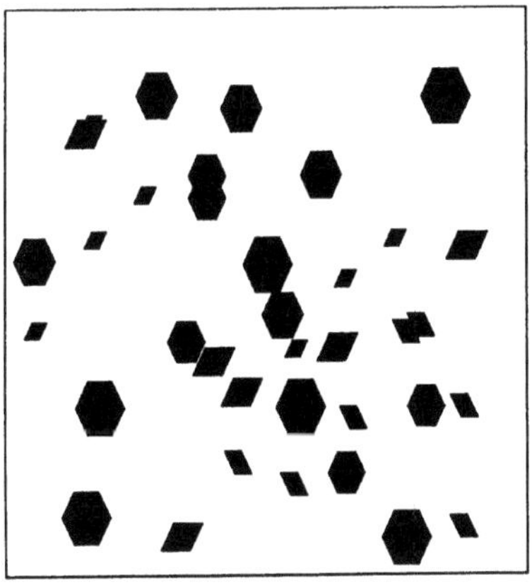

(2a) Test image 2

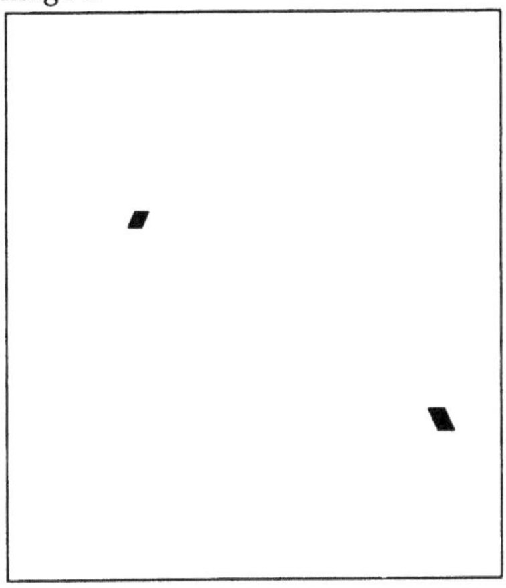

(2b) Minimal Generator Basis of image 2

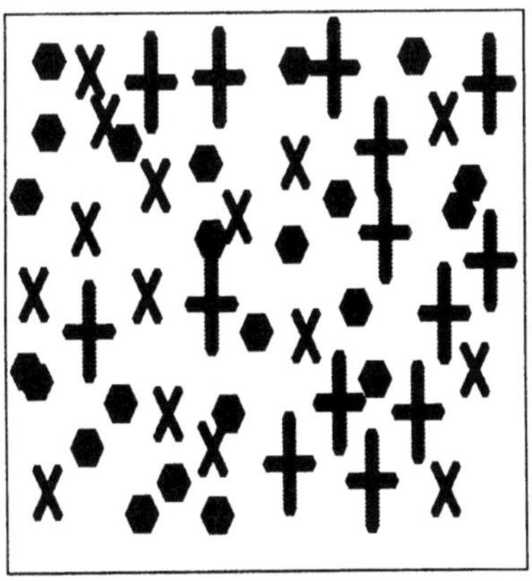

(3a) Test image 3

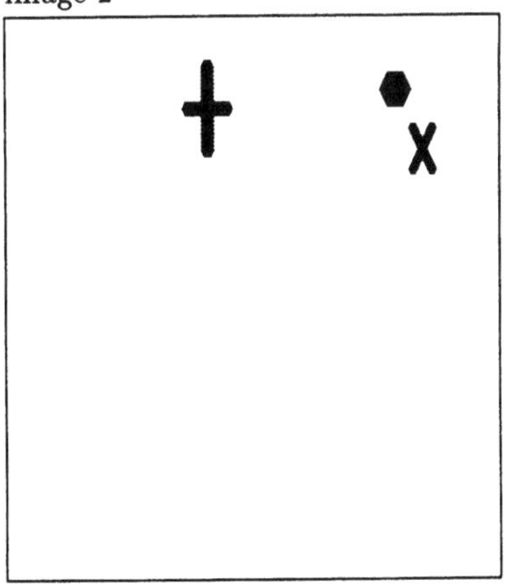

(3b) Minimal Generator Basis of image 3

Fig. 1. Example of the result obtained by the algorithm. Images (1a), (2a) and (3a) are generator basis of finite structural openings ψ_1 ψ_2, and ψ_3. Images (1b), (2b) and (3b) are respectively minimal generator basis of $\mathrm{Inv}(\psi_1)$, $\mathrm{Inv}(\psi_2)$ and $\mathrm{Inv}(\psi_3)$.

Acknowledgements

The author would like to thank Professors Jean-Pierre Aubin and Michel Schmitt for many encouraging, several useful suggestions and fruitful discussions. This work was supported by the DGA-DRET *Direction Générale de l'Armement, Direction des Recherches Études et Techniques.*

References

1. J.-P. Aubin. *Morphological and Mutational Analysis, Tools for Shape Regulation and Optimization.* Commett Matari Programme, CEREMADE, University of Paris-Dauphine, France, 1993.
2. F. Baccelli, G. Cohen, G. Olsder and J.-P. Quadrat. *Synchronization and linearity.* Wiley, 1992.
3. G.F. Banon and J. Barrera. Minimal representations for translation-invariant set mappings by mathematical morphology. *SIAM J. Appl. Math.*, 51(6):1782–1798, december 1991.
4. G.F. Banon and J. Barrera. Decomposition of mappings between complete lattices by mathematical morphology, Part I. General lattices. *Signal Processing*, 30:299–327, 1993.
5. N. Bourbaki. *Algèbre I. Chapitres 1 à 3. Éléments de mathématique.* Hermann, 1970.
6. S. Eilenberg. *Automata, Languages and Machines*, vol. A. Academic Press, 1974.
7. S. Gaubert. *Théorie des systèmes linéaires dans les dioïdes.* Thèse de docteur en mathématique et automatique, École Nationale Supérieure des Mines de Paris, 1992.
8. S. Gaubert. Introduction aux systèmes dynamiques à événements discrets. Notes de cours, ENSTA, 1994.
9. H.J.A.M. Heijmans. *Morphological Image Operators.* Academic Press, 1994.
10. H.J.A.M. Heijmans and C. Ronse. The Algebraic Basis of Mathematical Morphology : I. Dilatations and Erosions. *Computer Vison, Graphics, and Image Processing*, 50:245–295, 1990.
11. S. Lang *Algebra.* Addisson-Wesley, 1974.
12. S. Mac Lane and G. Birkhoff. *Algèbre : Structures fondamentales*, vol. I. Gauthier-Villars, 1970.
13. S. Mac Lane and G. Birkhoff. *Algèbre : Les grands théorèmes*, vol. II. Gauthier-Villars, 1971.
14. P. Maragos. A Representation Theory for Morphological Image and Signal Processing. *IEEE, Trans. on Pattern Analysis and Machine Intelligence*, 11(6):586–599, june 1989.
15. P. Maragos and R.W. Schafer. Morphological filters—part I: their set-theoretic analysis and relations to linear shift-invariant filters. *IEEE Transactions on Acoustics, Speech and Signal Processing*, 35(8):1153–1169, August 1987.
16. G. Matheron. *Random Sets and Integral Geometry.* John Wiley and Sons, New York, 1975.
17. G. Matheron. Filters and lattices. Technical Report 851, CGMM, École des Mines, September 1983.
18. G. Matheron. Filters and lattices. In J. Serra, editor, *Image Analysis and Mathematical Morphology, Volume 2: Theoretical Advances.* Academic Press, London, 1988.
19. G. Matheron. Les treillis compacts. Technical Report N-23/90/G, Centre de Géostatistique, École des Mines de Paris, Novembre 1990.
20. J. Mattioli. Domaine d'invariance d'une ouverture algébrique invariante par translation. Technical Report PER-94-2, L.C.R. Thomson-CSF, Orsay, France. 1994.
21. C. Ronse. Lattice-Theorical Fixpoint Theorems in Morphological Image Filtering. *Journal of Mathematical Imaging and Vision*, 4(1):19–42, january 1994.
22. C. Ronse and H.J.A.M. Heijmans. The Algebraic Basis of Mathematical Morphology : II. Openings and Closings. *Computer Vison, Graphics, and Image Processing*, 54(1):74–97, july 1991.
23. M. Schmitt and J. Mattioli *Morphologie Mathématique.* Masson, Paris, 1994.
24. J. Serra. *Image Analysis and Mathematical Morphology.* Academic Press, 1982.
25. J. Serra, editor. *Image Analysis and Mathematical Morphology, Volume 2: Theoretical Advances.* Academic Press, 1988.
26. J. Serra and L. Vincent. An overview of morphological filtering. *Circuits, Systems and Signal Processing*, 11(1):47–108, january 1992.

WATERSHED, HIERARCHICAL SEGMENTATION AND WATERFALL ALGORITHM

SERGE BEUCHER
Ecole des Mines de Paris, Centre de Morphologie Mathématique, 35, rue Saint-Honoré, F-77305 Fontainebleau Cedex, France

Abstract.
A major drawback when using the watershed transformation as a segmentation tool comes from the over-segmentation of the image. Over-segmentation is produced by the great number of minima embedded in the image or in its gradient. A powerful technique has been designed to suppress over-segmentation by a primary selection of markers pointing out the regions or objects to be segmented in the image. However, this approach can be used only if we are able to compute the marker set before applying the watershed transformation. But, in many cases and especially for complex scenes, this is not possible and an alternative technique must be used to reduce the over-segmentation. This technique is based on mosaic images and on the computation of a watershed transform on a valued graph derived from the mosaic images. This approach leads to a hierarchical segmentation of the image and considerably reduces over-segmentation.

Then, this hierarchical segmentation is redefined by means of a new algorithm called the waterfall algorithm. This algorithm allows the selection of minima and of catchment basins of higher significance compared to their neighborhood. A very powerful implementation of this algorithm using geodesic reconstruction of functions is also presented.

Finally, this approach is compared to another powerful tool introduced by M. Grimaud for selecting significant extrema in an image: the dynamics.

Key words: image analysis, mathematical morphology, watershed, hierarchical segmentation, waterfall algorithm, image reconstruction

1. Introduction

Image segmentation based on the use of the watershed transformation has proved to be an efficient method provided that the main drawback of this technique is suppressed. This drawback consists in the over-segmentation produced by the watershed transformation if applied directly on the images to be segmented. A solution for preventing this over-segmentation is well known and has been widely used in various examples [1, 2]. It consists in a prior selection of the objects or regions to be extracted in the image. This selection gives a collection of markers which are introduced in the watershed algorithm allowing the segmentation of the selected regions exclusively. Unfortunately, because of the complexity of the regions in a real scene, this marking is often difficult and sometimes even impossible. It is not always simple to associate obvious geometric or photometric characteristics with the objects to be segmented.

This paper deals with another approach for eliminating the over-segmentation problem. This approach is based on a hierarchical segmentation of the image aiming at merging the catchment basins of the watershed image belonging to almost homogeneous regions. This technique leads to various algorithms. The most efficient

J.Serra and P. Soille (eds.), Mathematical Morphology and Its Applications to Image Processing, 69-76

however, still uses the watershed transformation and the image reconstruction. Both tools are already used in the traditional process of segmentation in mathematical morphology.

The hierarchical segmentation will be described first (Sec. 2). It uses a simplified image called mosaic image. Then another algorithm, called the waterfall algorithm, will be presented (Sec. 3). The relationship between this algorithm and the hierarchical segmentation will also be emphasized. Finally, a comparison between these techniques and another transformation called dynamics will be made (Sec. 4).

2. The hierarchical segmentation

The best introduction of the hierarchical segmentation can be made by means of an image simplification process producing, from the original image f, a new image called the mosaic image or partition image [1].

2.1. Mosaic image: definition and building

Let f be a grey tone image and g be its morphological gradient. Let $W(g)$ be the watershed transformation of g. This watershed produces many catchment basins. Each catchment basin CB_i is associated with a minimum m_i of the gradient g. Let us calculate the average value f_i of the function f in the minimum m_i. In fact, in many cases, the minimum m_i corresponds to a zero-valued gradient and therefore f is constant and equal to f_i in m_i. A new function f' can then be defined by extending the value f_i to the entire catchment basin CB_i. This new function is called the mosaic image of f.

In practice, the watershed line C_{ij} separating two adjacent catchment basins CB_i and CB_j is given either the value f_i or the value f_j. This enables the definition of the mosaic image on the whole space and has no consequence on the following use of this simplified image. We notice that the watershed of this new image f is equal to the watershed of the initial image f.

2.2. Gradient of the mosaic image

Let us consider again two adjacent catchment basins CB_i and CB_j with respective values f_i and f_j. We define the gradient of the mosaic image h on every arc C_{ij} separating CB_i and CB_j by $h(C_{ij}) = |f_j - f_i|$.

2.3. Hierarchy and suppression of the over-segmentation

Starting from the mosaic image f' and from its gradient h, let us introduce a hierarchical process able to suppress the over-segmentation.

When we look at a picture, the distinction between more or less homogeneous regions is quite obvious despite the fact that these regions may be over-segmented by the watershed transformation. This over-segmentation is produced by low contrast variations inside these homogeneous regions. If we consider the arcs of the watershed inside the homogeneous regions, the value of the gradient of the mosaic image is lower than the values corresponding to the arcs separating different homogeneous regions. A solution for eliminating these arcs would consist in thresholding the watershed lines. However this solution is difficult to implement, because, on the one hand, a

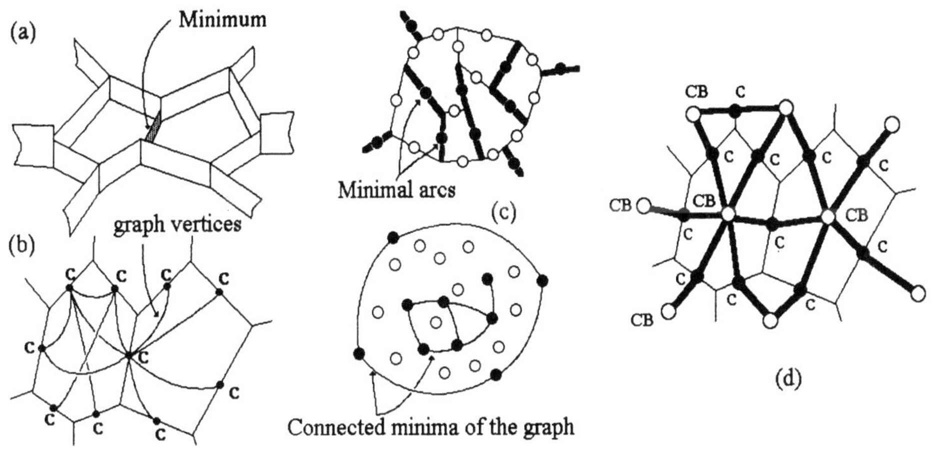

Fig. 1. a) 3D representation of the gradient of a simple mosaic b) associated graph c) minimal arcs and their correspondence on the graph d) planar 6 representation of the above graph.

suitable threshold value must be chosen and on the other hand, it is not sure that such a value exists. This is why the criterion used in the hierarchy is not a threshold but simply the fact that the gradient values are lower on the inside arcs than on the surrounding arcs. Consider Fig. 1a, representing the gradient of the mosaic image of a very simple homogeneous region split by a unique inside arc. The gradient value of this inside arc is lower than the gradient values of the arcs which contour the homogeneous region. If the over-segmentation of the homogeneous region was more severe, the resulting aspect of the gradient image would be the same: no inside arc greater than the surrounding ones or at least, no closed curve made of inside arcs all of them greater than the surrounding ones.

Let us define then a graph on the gradient of the mosaic image. Each arc C_{ij} of the watershed lines corresponds to a vertex of the graph. Then each vertex of this graph is the neighbor of another vertex if the arcs corresponding to these vertices surround the same catchment basin of the watershed (Fig. 1b). This graph is not a planar graph. However, each vertex can be valued with the gradient of the mosaic image (on each arc, it is a constant). The watershed transformation can be performed on this valued graph. The flooding starts from the arcs with a minimum valuation (the inside arcs, Fig. 1c) and propagates towards the other arcs. Finally, the watershed lines are made of those arcs which surround the homogeneous regions. This transformation produces exactly the desired result. The new catchment basins are made of all the inside arcs which are connected in the graph defined above. These arcs can be removed and the catchment basins of the primary watershed separated by these arcs can be merged. The result is a new segmented image where the over-segmentation of the homogeneous regions has been suppressed.

2.4. Hierarchical algorithms

The preceding graph is not easy to handle because it is not a planar graph. Although the watershed transformation can be extended in a straightforward way to 3D structures, in this particular case, it is possible to transform this non planar

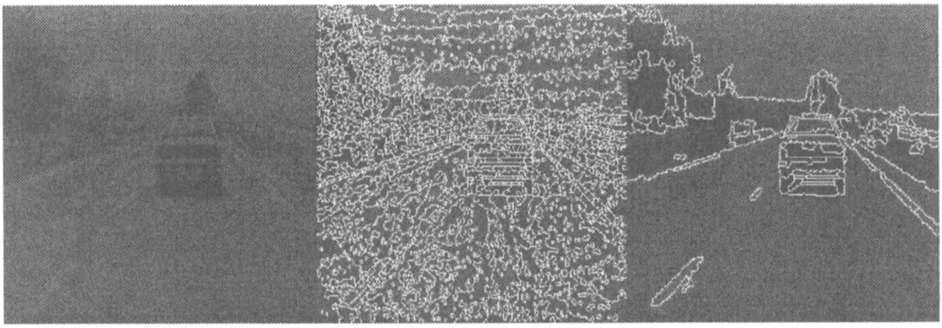

Fig. 2. a) initial road scene b) over-segmented watershed of the gradient image c) hierarchical segmentation, most of the over-segmentation has been removed.

graph into a planar one by adding vertices corresponding to the primary catchment basins (Fig. 1d). These new vertices provide an intermediary connection between the neighboring vertices of the non planar graph. These vertices, however must be valued. Their valuation $v(CB_i)$ is given by $v\,(CB_i) = \inf_j\,(h\,(C_{ij}))$. This valuation corresponds to the value of the lowest arc contouring the basin CB_i. Finally, this new representation leads to a third one which has the form of an image h', given by $h'\,(x) = h\,(C_{ij})$ iff $x \in C_{ij}$ and $h'\,(x) = v\,(CB_i)$ iff $x \in CB_i$.

This image h' is called the hierarchical image. The hierarchical process can then be performed on this image, in a very simple way, by performing the watershed transformation of h'. The only precaution consists here in replacing the watershed lines which do not belong to the initial watershed transform of g (they are inside an initial catchment basin) by the watershed lines which contour this catchment basin.

2.5. Example

Figs. 2a to 2c illustrate the efficiency of the hierarchical segmentation for reducing the over-segmentation. In this example, the road is a rather homogeneous object, but it appears nonetheless to be over-segmented (Fig. 2b). After the hierarchical processing depicted above, this over-segmentation has been removed and the road corresponds to a unique catchment basin which can be considered as the road marker in further processings.

3. Waterfall algorithm

Let us describe another hierarchical algorithm. This algorithm does not use the mosaic image but directly the initial function f.

3.1. The waterfall algorithm principle

Consider a function f as illustrated at Fig. 3.

Although the function used in this example is one dimensional, the notion introduced in the following is general and can be applied to any function. Among the various minima of the function f, three of them m_1 , m_2 and m_3 are interesting because they mark regions of higher importance in the image. If f is a gradient im-

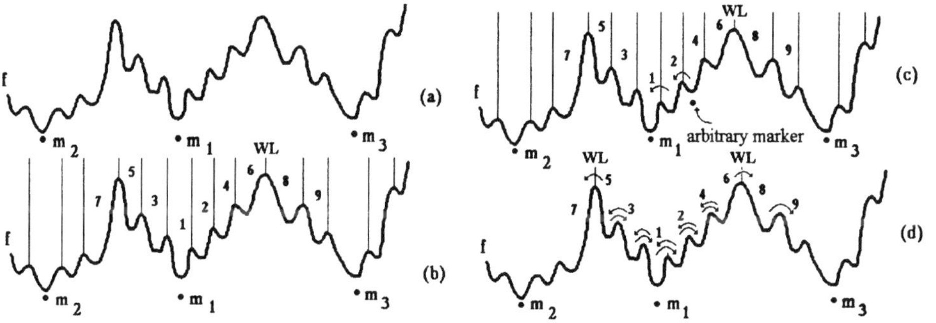

Fig. 3. a) primary watershed of the function f b) significant minima and the corresponding watersheds c) selection of a minimum and waterfalls towards the significant marker d) symmetrical waterfalls between adjacent catchment basins.

age for instance, m_1 could be the marker of an object to be segmented and m_2 and m_3 could be the outside markers. The other minima could be produced by noise. The watershed transformation of f produces as many catchment basins as there are minima (Fig. 3a). On the contrary, if only m_1, m_2 and m_3 are used by the watershed transform, only three catchment basins will appear (Fig. 3b). Two questions then arise. The first one is to characterize the minima m_1, m_2 and m_3. The second one is to find a way to determine automatically the catchment basin associated with the minimum m_1 for instance, without any a priori knowledge or construction of the primary watershed transformation. These two questions are answered through the notion of waterfall [1].

3.1.1. *Significant markers characterization*

One could think that the significant minima correspond to locally deepest minima of the function f. However, consider (Fig. 3c) a given minimum m. If we flood the catchment basin associated with this minimum, an overflow occurs when the lowest saddle point separating this catchment basin from an adjacent catchment basin is reached. This new catchment basin, then, is flooded and overflows either towards the preceding catchment basin or towards a new one. In the former case, the first minimum is a significant minimum. In the latter case, the first minimum is not significant. More generally, a minimum is said to be significant if the waterfall coming from its corresponding catchment basin pours in an adjacent catchment basin which, in turn, when flooded, overflows towards the first minimum. In fact, and for obvious reasons of symmetry, a significant minimum is not unique, and the minima linked by symmetrical waterfalls are equally significant. Moreover, it is equivalent to consider as a significant marker the arc of the primary watershed line separating the catchment basins linked by symmetrical overflows. This significant marker is an arc of minimum height of the primary watershed.

3.1.2. *Determining the catchment basin corresponding to a significant marker set*

A similar procedure based on waterfalls can be used to determine the entire catchment basin corresponding to a significant marker, made of primary catchment basins linked by symmetrical waterfalls. Consider the function f and a marker set made of at least two catchment basins CB_1 and CB_2 (see Fig. 3d). The arc C_{12} separating these catchment basins can be equivalently considered as the significant marker. Let us flood these two catchment basins. The water will pour into the basin CB_3. But if we flood CB_3, the water will pour into $CB_1 \cap CB_2$. So, because of the appearance of symmetric waterfalls over the arc C_{13}, this arc is removed and the three basins are merged. Let us continue our flooding process. The water coming from $CB_1 \cup CB_2 \cup CB_3$ will pour into CB_5. Finally all the catchment basins CB_1 to CB_6 will be merged because the waterfalls from a given basin to another one are symmetrical versus the arcs which separate them. On the contrary, the watershed line between CB_6 and CB_8 will not be removed because, if $CB_1 \cup \ldots \cup CB_6$ pours into CB_8, CB_8 pours into CB_9 first. At the end, the remaining watershed lines contour the catchment basin associated with the significant marker.

3.2. An efficient algorithm based on reconstruction

The main drawback of the previous algorithm comes from the fact that the waterfalls must be checked individually for every minimum or catchment basin of the primary watershed. This leads to a very slow and boring process. Fortunately, there exists a faster procedure based on image reconstruction.

3.2.1. *Image reconstruction*

Consider two functions f and g, with $f \geq g$. The reconstruction [1] by geodesic erosions $R^*(f,g)$ of f from g is defined by:

$$R^*(f,g) = E_f^{\infty}(g) = \lim_{n\to\infty} (E_f \circ \cdots \circ E_f)(g)$$

where $E_f(g) = \sup(g \ominus B, f)$.

3.2.2. *Reconstruction of a function by its watershed*

Let f be a positive and bounded function ($0 \leq f \leq m$) and let $W(f)$ be its watershed transform. $W(f)$ is the set of the watershed lines of f. Let us build a new function g with $W(f)$:

$$g(x) = f(x) \text{ iff } x \in W(f) \text{ and } g(x) = m \text{ iff } x \in W^c(f).$$

This function g is obviously greater than f. Let us now reconstruct f from g. It is easy to see that the minima of the resulting image correspond to the significant markers of the original image f (see Fig. 4).

In fact, the reconstruction fills in (partially) each catchment basin with a plateau at a height equal to the minimum height of the watershed line surrounding this catchment basin. Therefore, if there exists an adjacent catchment basin where the corresponding height is lower than the previous one, the waterfalls will not be symmetrical and the plateau generated in the basin will not be a minimum. Moreover, the watershed transform of $R^*(f,g)$ produces the catchment basins associated with these significant markers.

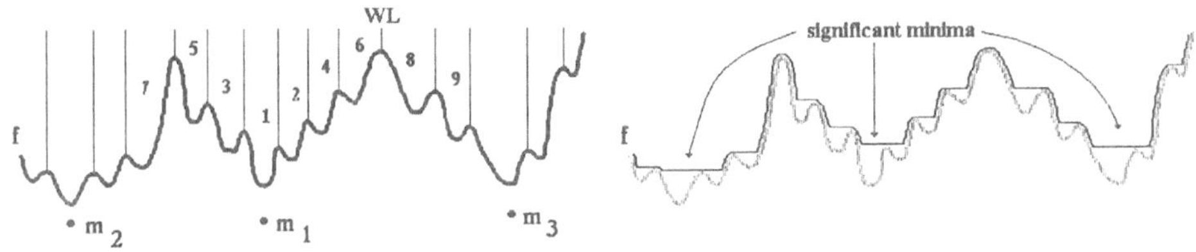

Fig. 4. Reconstruction from watershed lines and detection of the significant markers.

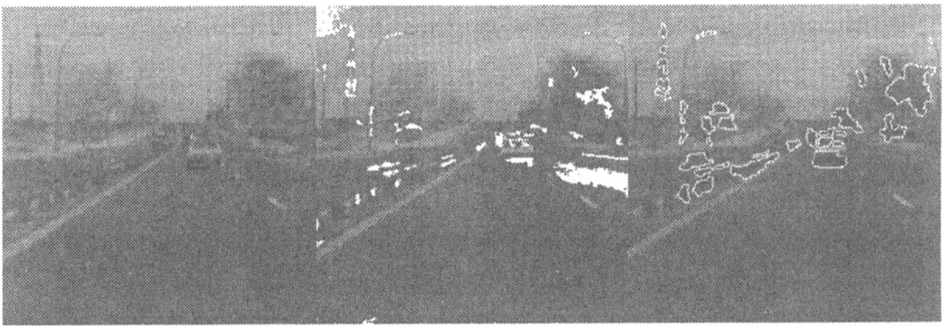

Fig. 5. The significant minima in an image are used as markers in the gradient watershed image.

4. Comparisons between these hierarchical segmentations

4.1. WATERFALLS AND MOSAIC IMAGES

When the initial image is the gradient of the mosaic image, the hierarchy settled by the waterfalls is identical to the hierarchy performed by the watershed applied to the graph defined by the gradient of the mosaic image. However, the waterfall is more general and can be applied to any image. This approach is particularly useful for detecting blobs in an image.

The following example (Fig. 5) illustrates this technique. The vehicles on the road are characterized by a front or rear dark region which can be detected by reconstructing the primary image with its watershed and by using the significant minima as markers in the segmentation. The watershed transform of the reconstructed image delineates the extension of the blobs. Then, by using both the significant minima and the watershed lines of this reconstructed image as markers in the watershed of the gradient image, we obtain the final result given at Fig. 5c. Further filtering of the blobs can be made based on their depth.

4.2. WATERFALLS AND DYNAMICS

The notion of dynamics of a minimum has been introduced by M. Grimaud [3]. The dynamics of a minimum is equal to the height we must climb before reaching any point in the function at a lower altitude than the minimum. If we compare the

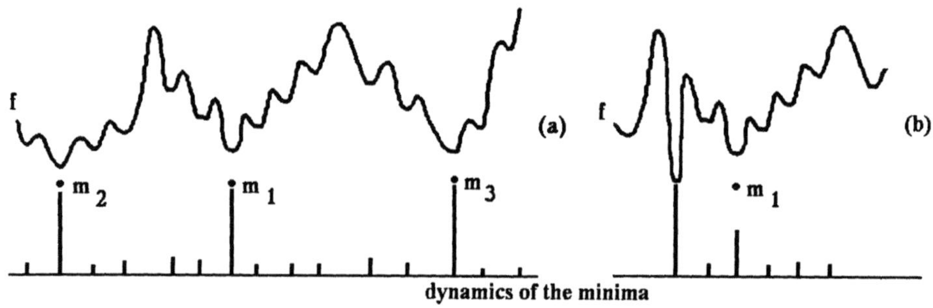

Fig. 6. Comparison betweeen the dynamics and the waterfall algorithm

dynamics and the significant minima of the function at Fig. 6a , we observe a strong similarity between the dynamics and the waterfalls, because the significant minima also correspond, in this example, to minima with high dynamics. This similarity, however, is misleading, as depicted in Fig. 6b. In fact, the two notions are based on two different characteristics: the dynamics is controlled by the relative altitudes of the minima. The waterfalls, on the contrary, are related to the relative heights of the watershed lines. Moreover, the dynamics is more difficult to handle because, in most cases, a threshold is needed to extract the minima with high dynamics. When applied to a gradient image, too, the dynamics give unsatisfactory results because most of the minima of the gradient are at level zero. Therefore, the definition of their dynamics is not simple.

5. Conclusion

In this paper, we have shown that the watershed transformation and the reconstruction of functions can be successfully used in hierarchical segmentation processes. The methodology described here for reducing the over-segmentation is rather simple, it is independent of scale and does not require the setting of any parameter. The final result provides almost homogeneous regions in the image. Further image processing applied on these regions allows us to filter them according to geometrical criteria and enables their possible selection as markers in more complex image segmentations.

References

1. S. Beucher: Segmentation d'Images et Morphologie Mathématique, Doctorate Thesis, Ecole des Mines de Paris, June 1990.
2. S. Beucher and F. Meyer: "The morphological approach to segmentation: the watershed transformation", in: E. Dougherty, ed. , Mathematical Morphology in Image Processing, Marcel Dekker Inc, 1992, pp. 433-481.
3. M. Grimaud: La géodésie Numérique en Morphologie Mathématique. Application à la Détection Automatique de Microcalcifications en Mammographie Numérique, Doctorate Thesis, Ecole des Mines de Paris, Dec. 1991.

MINIMUM SPANNING FORESTS FOR MORPHOLOGICAL SEGMENTATION

FERNAND MEYER
Ecole des Mines de Paris, Centre de Morphologie Mathématique, 35, rue Saint-Honoré, F–77305 Fontainebleau Cedex, France

Abstract. Image segmentation in mathematical morphology is essentially based on one method: the watershed of a gradient image from a set of markers. We show that this watershed can be obtained from the neighbourhood graph of the initial image. The result of the segmentation is then a minimum spanning forest of the neighbourhood graph. Powerful interactive and very fast segmentation methods are derived

Key words: segmentation, watersheds, markers, neighbourhood graph, minimum spanning forests

1. Introduction

The main tool used by Mathematical Morphology for image segmentation is the watershed. Watersheds were introduced in image analysis by Lantuéjoul & Beucher [1] and mathematically defined in [10,12]. However, except for a few simple cases, as in [1], the watershed cannot be applied directly. Generally used on gradient images, it produces a severe over-segmentation, which is difficult to overcome. In 1981, I suggested a solution to this problem which has proved very fruitful since. It consists in introducing markers and in flooding the relief formed by the gradient obtained from these markers. The principle of the watershed with markers and many examples of its use are given in [2,9]. The traditional way for introducing markers is a geodesic closing of the gradient function, leaving the markers as sole minima. A classical watershed algorithm is then applied to this image. The aim of the present paper is to give a definition and an insight into the properties of watersheds from a set of markers. To this purpose we use a weighted neighborhood graph, whose nodes are the regional minima of the image. Two minima are linked by an edge if the corresponding catchment basins are neighbours. The altitude of the pass between two catchment basins gives the valuation of the edge.

After giving a few reminders on minimum spanning trees and forests, we will show that the watershed associated with a set of markers is nothing but a forest of minimum weight on the neighbourhood graph. Each tree of the forest is of minimum weight, and a subset of the minimum spanning tree of the neighbourhood graph. We derive from this novel formulation new and remarkably efficient algorithms for interactive segmentation.

2. Graphs and trees, reminders [4]

Non oriented graph: A non oriented graph $G = [X, U]$ is a collection of a set X

J.Serra and P. Soille (eds.), Mathematical Morphology and Its Applications to Image Processing, 77-84

whose elements are called vertices or nodes and of a set U whose elements $u \in U$ are pairs of vertices called edges.

Adjacent edges: Two edges that share one or several extremities are said to be adjacent.

Degree: The degree of the vertex i, denoted $d(i)$ is the number of edges whose extremity is i .

Edges incident to $A \subset X$. *Cocycles:* Given a subset of vertices $A \subset X$, the cocycle associated with A is defined as the set of arcs whose initial extremity is in A and whose final extremity is in $\overline{A} = X - A$. It will be designated hereinafter as $\omega(A)$.

A chain of length n is a sequence of n edges $L = \{u_1, u_2, \ldots, u_n\}$, such that each edge u_i of the sequence $(2 \leq i \leq n-1)$ shares one extremity with the edge u_{i-1} $(u_{i-1} \neq u_i)$, and the other extremity with u_{i+1} $(u_{i+1} \neq u_i)$.

A cycle is a chain whose extremities coincide.

Trees: A tree is a connected graph without cycle.

Proposition: The graph $[X, T]$ is a tree if and only if there exists one and only one chain between any pair of vertices.

We can choose an arbitrary node r of a tree as a root. As the tree is without cycle, there exists for any other node x a unique path to the root.

Minimum spanning tree: Consider a graph $G = [X, U]$. Each edge $u \in U$ is associated a number $w(u)$ which is the weight of the edge u. Given a partial graph $G' = [X, U']$ of G, the weight of G' the number: $w(G') = \sum_{u \in U'} w(u)$. The minimum spanning tree is a tree of minimum weight. It is unique if all weights are different.

By removing the edge u from the tree $[X, T]$, we create two connected components of vertices $A \subset X$ and $\bar{A} = X - A$. The cocycle θ^u represents the set of edges that connect a vertex of A with a vertex of $\bar{A}$. Theorem 1 states that among all edges, the edge u is the one with minimum weight.

Theorem 1 : *A necessary and sufficient condition for* $[X, T]$ *to be a minimum spanning tree of* G *is that for all edges* $u \in T$ *the cocycle* θ^u *(such that* $\theta^u \cap T = \{u\}$*) satisfies:* $w(u) \leq w(v), \quad \forall v \in \theta^u \quad (v \neq u)$

Any edge u of $U - T$ connects two vertices x and y of G. There exists a path L in the tree T that connects the two vertices. According to theorem 2, the weight of the edge u is higher than the weight of all the other edges forming the path L. Thus, in the cycle $\mu^u = L \cup \{u\}$, the edge u is the edge of maximum weight.

Theorem 2 : *A necessary and sufficient condition for* $[X, T]$ *to be a tree of* G *of minimum weight is that for all edges* $u \in U - T$ *the cycle* μ^u *(such that* $\mu^u \subset T + \{u\}$*) satisfies:* $w(u) \geq w(v), \quad \forall v \in \mu^u \quad (v \neq u)$

Forests: A graph without cycle which is not connected is called a *forest.* Each connected component is a tree.

Spanning forest of minimum weight: Let $G = [X, U]$ be a connected valued and non oriented graph. Assume all valuations are positive or null. Given a sub-set of p distinct vertices $Y = [y_1, \ldots, y_p] \subset X$, we search for a forest $F = [X, V]$ with minimum total weight, in which each vertex $x \in X - Y$ is connected to one and only one vertex of Y.

A unique tree contains a forest: We can easily see that this problem can be transformed into a problem of a tree T of minimum weight on the following graph G'. An extra node z is added to the set of nodes X, which will be the root of the tree T: $X' = X \cup \{z\}$. In the graph G', z is connected to each vertex y_i by an edge of valuation -1. Let a_i be the edge (z, y_i). Then we can construct the minimum tree T of G'.

This tree necessarily contains all the edges of a_i of negative weight. By removing all edges incident to z from the tree T, we obtain a forest of minimum weight which has the required properties.

3. The neighbourhood graph of an image

The neighbourhood graph of a relief synthesizes the topography of a relief. Each vertex of the graph represents a catchment basin. Two vertices of the graph are linked by an edge if the catchment basins of the relief are neighbours. An edge represents the lowest pass found on the common boundary between two catchment basins; the valuation of the edge is equal to the altitude of this pass.

We have now to project the markers on this neighborhood graph. Markers are a collection of connected components with labels; each marker being assigned a distinct label. A marker may be split into several connected components with the same labels. Every time a catchment basin contains at most one marker or part of one marker, the corresponding node in the neighborhood graph will get the label of the marker and will be part of a graph marker. In the rare cases where a catchment basin contains more than one marker, one would change the homotopy of the corresponding catchment basin in order to produce two minima [2]. After this transformation, each catchment basin associated with a minimum contains at most one marker or part of a marker. Conversely, if a marker contains several connected nodes on the neighborhood graph, these may be replaced by a unique node with the same outside connections.

Structural changes are identical during the flooding of the initial relief or the neighborhood graph. Hence they yield the same watersheds.

3.1. The watershed from markers is a minimum spanning forest

We will establish the following proposition by an effective construction of a minimum spanning forest.

Proposition 1 *Constructing a watershed from a set of markers on a neighbourhood graph yields a partition. This partition is a minimum spanning forest, with each tree rooted at a marker.*

Proof: Our goal is to construct the watershed associated with a set of markers $Z = (z_k)_{k \in K}$ of a neighbourhood graph $[X, U]$, $X = (m_i)$, $U = (s_{ij})_{i,j \in I}$, where the $m_i$represent the regional minima of the initial image , and s_{ij} represent the height of the pass separating the neighbouring catchment basins i and j. The markers are labeled by a function $lab\,(z_k)$ (a marker may consist of several connected components, in this case they all have the same label). We add to the graph $[X, U]$ a fictitious root r linked to each marker by an edge of weight -1. Let us now construct the minimum spanning tree of this new graph; we choose for the construction the non optimal version of Prim's algorithms [4].

Input:

For each vertex $i \in X$, the list of incident edges $\omega(i)$ (this set is also called cocycle of i)

Method:

We construct a sub-set $A \subset X$ step by step.

(a) We start with the root r;

Initially: $A = \{r\}$, $\theta = \omega(r)$, $T = \emptyset$.

At any step of the algorithm A will contain the nodes of the already constructed part of the minimum spanning tree T; θ contains the boundary edges of A, i.e. the cocycle $\theta = \omega(A)$.

(b) Take in θ an edge u of minimum weight. Let j be the extremity of u which does not belong to A.

Do: $T \leftarrow T + \{u\}$, $A \leftarrow A + \{j\}$, $\theta \leftarrow \theta \Delta \omega(j)$ (symmetrical difference)

$lab(m_j) \leftarrow lab(m_i)$ and return to (b).

The tree constructed by this algorithm verifies the conditions of theorem 1. The first edges to be added to the tree T are all the edges of negative weight. After this first step all markers belong to A. In the following steps the algorithm exactly simulates the flooding from markers as does the classical algorithm for constructing watersheds. One chooses in θ an edge s_{ij} of minimum weight, among all edges linking an already flooded basin with an unflooded basin; the weight is chosen minimum, because the flood progresses through the lowest pass. As soon a catchment basin m_j is flooded, it gets the label of the minimum where the flood comes from; from now on m_j belongs to A and s_{ij}, being the pass taken by the flood, belongs to T. The purpose of the symmetrical difference $\theta \leftarrow \theta \ \Delta \ \omega(m_j)$ is more subtle: the boundary edges which existed between m_j and the set A before m_j were added to A and suppressed from θ; both extremities of these edges are already flooded. The same operation adds to θ the edges between m_j and zones which are not yet flooded.

After completion of the tree we cut the edges of negative weight and get a minimum spanning forest. Each tree of the forest having its root within a marker.

3.2. Corollaries

Since our problem has become one of minimum spanning trees, many classical algorithms may be used for their construction, in particular very efficient ones, such as Yao's algorithm. The following lemma is an example of the characterizations of watershed lines from markers which may be derived from theorems 1 and 2:

Lemma 1 : *Let A and B be the trees rooted in two different markers. Let s_{ab} be an edge of the neighbourhood graph, with one of the extremities a in A and the other, b in the set B; then s_{ab} has a valuation higher than any other edge inside the tree A or the tree B.*

3.3. MINIMUM SPANNING TREES AND FORESTS

Let $[X,U]$ be a graph and $(m_i)_{i\in I}$ be a set of markers. A minimum spanning forest $(A_i)_{i\in I}$ is associated with this set or markers, with each tree A_i rooted in m_i. We will establish that any such minimum spanning forest is a subset of the minimum spanning tree of the graph $[X,U]$.

We construct a new graph $[Y,V]$: the nodes represent the trees A_i of the forest and the edges represent the edges of U having their extremities in two different trees A_i and A_j of the forest. Let T' be a minimum spanning tree of the graph $[Y,V]$.

Theorem 3 : *The union of edges of the minimum spanning forest $(A_i)_{i\in I}$ and of the minimum spanning tree T' constitutes a minimum spanning tree T of the graph $[X,U]$.*

Robustness of the watershed from markers: For each set of markers, one gets a minimum spanning forest with a total weight between 0 and the weight of the minimum spanning tree of $[X,U]$. The weight will be zero if all nodes of the graph are markers ; this corresponds to the finest segmentation, where each catchment basin of the relief is taken. The weight will be maximum if only one marker is used, yielding the minimum spanning tree of $[X,U]$. The result of the segmentation is stable: modifying the position of the marker within a tree of a minimum spanning forest will neither change this tree nor the forest.

Drastic changes of the forest result from the adjunction, suppression or fusion of markers. We will see at the end of this paper how to deal with such events.

3.4. CONSTRUCTION OF A MINIMUM SPANNING FOREST FROM A MINIMUM SPANNING TREE

A minimum spanning tree of a neighbourhood graph has far less edges than the graph taken as a whole. Furthermore this minimum spanning tree is an overset of any minimum spanning forest associated with a set of markers. Taking this minimum spanning tree as a starting point will speed up the construction of a minimum spanning forest. As a first example, the Prim's algorithm presented above is greatly simplified and becomes linear with the number of edges. As a matter of fact, the operation $\theta \leftarrow \theta \;\Delta\; \omega(j)$ (symmetrical difference) had the effect of adding or suppressing numerous edges at each step.

- Suppressing an edge was necessary each time that two extremities of an edge were flooded before the flood passes through this edge. Now, this situation will only happen for the edges of the tree $[Y,V]$ introduced earlier.
- Adding an edge is necessary each time a new node is assigned to a tree of the forest: all incident edges linking this node with other nodes not yet in the forest have to be added to θ. In the present situation the number of such incident edges is most often 1 ; it may be higher than 1 if the pixel is a multiple point.

The simplification of the classical algorithm by Kruskal [4] is particularly striking.

3.4.1. *Algorithm of Kruskal by decreasing weight*

Let $[X,U]$ be a graph and $(z_i)_{i\in I}$ a set of markers. A minimum spanning forest $(A_i)_{i\in I}$ has to be constructed, with each tree A_i rooted in a different marker z_i. The starting point is the minimum spanning tree T of the graph $[X, U]$. The edges of T are first ordered in the order of their decreasing weights.

Method: The edge u_k of maximum weight is suppressed. If each connected component of the tree contains at least a marker z_i, the same operation is repeated recursively for each of the connected components. If not, the edge u_k is reintroduced and the next edge in decreasing order is processed.

Comments: This algorithm first suppresses the edges with the highest weights. For this reason it has the advantage to produce the great masses of the segmentation before the smaller details. In this way it constructs a pyramid of segmentations.

Best segmentation with n markers:

In particular, if one does not know how to get markers, one may wonder which segmentation is the best if one wishes to obtain a given number of regions. In absence of any other knowledge, we will take the the forest of minimum weight with n trees. In the absence of markers, Kruskal's algorithm becomes very simple: the (n-1) edges with the highest valuation are suppressed, yielding a forest with n trees. This forest has the minimum possible weight for any segmentation in n regions.

3.5. Interactive segmentation

Another situation frequently occurs: interactive segmentation. The user chooses interactively markers and asks for a segmentation associated with these markers. He can then, in a feedback loop add, delete or modify markers, until he reaches a satisfactory segmentation.

The question we ask now is the following: is it possible to edit markers interactively and obtain the associated segmentation without reconstructing it from scratch after each new modification? In other words are local reconstructions of the watershed possible? The answer is yes. The solution is based on two classical algorithms for constructing a minimum spanning tree. Both algorithms are called "disorder algorithms" because the edges are treated in any order, without being ranked according to their valuation.

3.5.1. *Algorithm by adjunction of edges*

The first algorithm for constructing a minimum spanning tree is based on the detection of cycles (theorem 2).We first present the algorithm and then we show how to use it to get a minimum spanning forest.

Let G be a valued graph, for which a minimum spanning tree is to be constructed.

Input: the list of edges of G in any order.

Method: The list of edges is read. Initially $T = \{u_1\}$. At step k do: $T \leftarrow T + \{u_k\}$. If T does not contain a cycle, continue. If T contains a cycle μ, and if v is an edge of maximum weight in μ, do $T \leftarrow T - \{v\}$ and continue.

The construction of a minimum spanning forest of G, with a family of roots $(z_i)_{i \in I}$ is performed as usual. A fictitious root z is added linked to all roots by an edge with negative weight. Adding a new edge from the list of edges may create a cycle in two different ways: a) either a cycle is created in the graph G itself without containing z. b) or the edge belongs to a chain linking two different markers. In this case, including the edges linking these markers and z creates a cycle. In both cases, one has to suppress the edge with the highest valuation in the cycle or in the chain.

Adding new markers in an interactive segmentation. The previous algorithm will show how to modify an already existing segmentation when a new marker is introduced. Introducing a new marker means creating a new edge between this marker and the fictitious root z.

First case: the marker consists in a unique node t. This node belongs to one of the trees A_i of the minimum spanning forest. There exists a chain in this tree linking the node t to the marker z_i of the tree. In application of the preceding algorithm, the edge of highest valuation has to be suppressed in this chain. This creates two trees: the one with the root z_i keeps its label, the other with the node t gets the label of t. Thus promoting a node t as a marker has the effect of cutting the tree containing t in two sub-trees. The other trees are not modified.

General case: a marker of label λ consists of several nodes. The same algorithm is applied to each node of the marker.

3.5.2. *Disorder algorithm suppressing edges*

Another disorder algorithm will show us how to modify a segmentation when a marker is suppressed. We first explain how this algorithm constructs a minimum spanning tree. The algorithm uses theorem 1. Let G be a valued graph, for which we want to construct the minimum spanning tree.

Input: the list of edges of G in any order.

Method:

Initially do: $T = U$. The list of edges is read. At step k, the edge $u_k = (i, j)$ is read. If the connectivity number of $G^k = [X, T - \{u_k\}]$ is equal to the number of G, then the edge u_k is removed from T. If the connectivity number of G^k is higher than the number of G, then G^k contains two connected components A and A' such that $i \in A$ and $j \in A'$. Let v be an edge of minimum weight linking A and A'. The edge v is added to T and the edge u_k removed: $T \leftarrow T + \{v\} - \{u_k\}$. The next edge is processed.

Application to the construction of a minimum spanning forest. The construction of a minimum spanning forest of G, with a family of roots $(z_i)_{i \in I}$ is performed as usual. A fictitious root z is added linked to all roots by an edge with negative weight. Considering that a node is not longer a marker is the same than suppressing an edge between this marker and the fictitious root.

Suppression of a marker. **Case 1:** the marker is reduced to one node. Suppressing a marker z_k means suppressing an edge between this marker and the fictitious root. Two connected components are thus created; one of them is precisely the tree A_k with the root z_k ; the other part is the union of all other trees. One has then to consider the cocycle of this tree inside the tree T, i.e. the set of edges linking this tree A_k to the other trees within T. Within this set of edges, the edge u with the smallest valuation is chosen. Adding this edge to the minimum spanning forest will link the tree A_k with another tree A_l; A_k will also take the label of A_l. All edges of the tree A_k have smaller valuations than the edge u. Thus the flooding coming from another marker passes through u and may flood entirely the tree.

General case: If the marker is not reduced to one node, two steps are necessary. The first step suppresses the links between the fictitious root and each node of the marker, as described above. The second step has to reintroduce the initial edges of the neighborhood graph between the nodes of the marker. For this the disorder algorithm introducing edges is used.

4. Conclusion

From all these results, it is not possible however to derive which set of markers is optimum for a given segmentation. This choice remains the intelligent part of the work, as pointed out in [2,9]. A minimum spanning forest with n trees is easy to obtain: it is sufficient to cut the edges with the highest weight until the desired number of subtrees is reached. This segmentation has the lowest weight among all segmentations in n regions but is not necessarily the best segmentation: it is not possible generally to spare oneself a thorough investigation in order to develop an algorithm giving a suitable and robust set of markers for the problem. But once the markers are obtained, the present paper shows how to obtain a very fast segmentation.

References

1. Beucher S., Lantuéjoul C., Use of watersheds in contour detection, Int. Workshop on Image Processing, CCETT/IRISA, Rennes, France, Sept. 79.
2. Beucher S., Segmentation d'images et Morphologie Mathématique, Thèse Ecole des Mines de Paris, 1990.
3. Grimaud M. La géodésie numérique en Morphologie Mathématique, Thèse de l'Ecole des Mines de Paris, décembre 1990.
4. Gondran M., Minoux M., Graphes et algorithmes, Eyrolles, Paris, 1979, chapitre 4: Arbres et arborescences.
5. Hanusse P., Guillataud P., Sémantique des images par analyse dendronique, Actes du 8ème Congres AFCET, Lyon-Villeurbanne, France, 1991, pp. 577-598.
6. Hu T.C., The maximum capacity route problem, Operations Research 9, 1961, pp. 898-900.
7. Kruskal J.B., On the shortest spanning subtree of a graph and the traveling salesman problem, Proc. Am. Math. Soc., 71, 1956, pp. 48-50.
8. Meyer F., Un algorithme optimal de ligne de partage des eaux, Actes du 8ème Congres AFCET, Lyon-Villeurbanne, France, 1991, pp. 847-859.
9. Meyer F., Beucher S., Morphological segmentation, JVCIR, Vol.11, N1, pp. 21-46, 1990.
10. Meyer F., Integrals, gradients and watershed lines, in "Mathematical Morphology and its applications to Signal Processing", Symposium held in Barcelona, May 1993, pp. 70-75.
11. Meyer F., Arbre des minima et dynamique, Note interne CMM, juillet 1993.
12. Najman L. and Schmitt M., Definition and some properties of the watershed of a continuous function, in "Mathematical Morphology and its applications to Signal Processing", Symposium held in Barcelona, May 1993, pp. 75-81.
13. Prim R.C., Shortest connection networks and some generalizations, Bell Syst. Techn. J., 36, 1957, p. 1389.
14. Vincent L., Graphs and Mathematical Morphology, Signal Processing, Vol. 16, No. 4, April 1989, pp. 365-389.
15. Yao A.C.C., An $O(|E| \log\log |V|)$algorithm for finding minimum spanning trees, Info. Processing Letters, 4., 1975, pp. 21-25.

THE FLAT ZONE APPROACH AND COLOR IMAGES

JOSÉ CRESPO*
Ecole des Mines de Paris, Centre de Morphologie Mathématique, 35, rue Saint-Honoré, F-77305 Fontainebleau Cedex, France

and

RONALD W. SCHAFER
School of Electrical Engineering, Georgia Institute of Technology, Atlanta, GA 30332, U.S.A.

Abstract. This paper treats the application of the flat zone approach for color images. For gray-level images, the flat zone approach was presented in (Crespo & Serra 1993) as a segmentation approach that imposes an inclusion relationship between the flat zones (or piecewise-constant regions) of the input image and the regions of the output partition. That is, a flat zone segmentation method behaves like a connected operator. Color images are formed by several (a priori) independent bands. In this paper we discuss how color images need a different treatment from that used for gray-level images. For gray-level images, the flat zone inclusion relationship preserves the shapes of the features that are observed in the input. On the other hand, for color images this desirable shape-preservation effect would not be obtained by forcing the inclusion relationship between the flat zones of *each* band and the regions of the output partition. A mask that contains the important regions of the color image, computed for each color band, is employed to restrict the flat zone inclusion relationship to those flat zones belonging to the mask. As in the gray-level case, the presented color segmentation method uses a hierarchical waiting queue algorithm that makes it computationally efficient.

Key words: Segmentation, flat zone approach, mathematical morphology and color images.

1. Introduction

The *flat zone aproach* is a segmentation approach that was presented in (Crespo & Serra 1993) as a proposed solution to some problems that appear in the *watershed approach* (Digabel & Lantuéjoul 1977). The watershed approach, or more specifically the watershed-plus-markers approach (Meyer 1986) (Beucher & Meyer 1993), is the traditional method to address the segmentation problem in mathematical morphology (Serra 1982) (Serra 1988). Whereas the flat zone approach as presented in (Crespo & Serra 1993) considered only gray-level images, this paper treats the case of color images, i.e., images composed of several (a priori) independent bands. As will be discussed later in the paper, the problem posed by color images is quite different to that by gray-level images.

The flat zone approach provides a solution to the *resolution problem* that occurs under the traditional watershed-plus-markers approach. In the watershed-plus-markers approach, some markers signal the location of the significant regions in the image. The need for locating each marker *inside* an image region poses an important limitation when features are very small or when their shape is quite elongated

* Formerly at the School of Electrical Engineering, Georgia Institute of Technology, Atlanta, GA 30332, U.S.A.

J.Serra and P. Soille (eds.), Mathematical Morphology and Its Applications to Image Processing, 85-92

and regions have thin parts on the order of one or two pixels wide. In these cases, there is virtually no inside part since all pixels are boundary pixels (this problem can be addressed within the watershed-plus-markers approach *when* the support of the image —the space of points— can be modified). Most often it is desired that small features be eliminated since large features are more visible and, likely, more significant. However, it is also true that segmentations in which some small but highly contrasted features have been eliminated are frequently not satisfactory. The prevention of an automatic and uncontrolled loss of small features is the motivation for this flat zone approach. The solution provided by this approach does not rely on providing better markers (which can reduce the problem but never eliminate it) but rather on abandoning the region marker concept.

In (Crespo & Serra 1993) this approach was presented for gray-level images. In this case, the flat zone approach establishes an inclusion relationship between the flat zones of the input image and the regions of the output partition. Color images are formed by several bands, and each one of them can be considered as a gray-level image. For color images the inclusion relationship between *all* flat zones of *each* band and the regions of the output partition is not appropriate and can lead to the loss of important regions. In this work we are going to employ an inclusion relationship that affects only the flat zones of all bands that are signaled as significant.

The outline of the paper is as follows. Section 2 further discusses the problems associated with the watershed approach. Section 3 discusses the flat zone approach and presents an extension for the color image case.

2. Watershed-Plus-Markers Approach: The Small Region Loss Problem

In the watershed-plus-markers approach, there are two well differentiated parts (Beucher & Meyer 1993):

(1) The computation of *regions markers.* A region marker is a connected set of pixels that are located inside a significant region.

(2) The *flooding* of a gradient function through region markers in order to compute its watershed. (The gradient function employed has as local minima only the region markers. This is achieved through a procedure called *homotopy modification.*)

From item (1) above, it is clear that a region marker does not contain all pixels of the flat zone they belong to, but rather a subset of it. After region markers have been computed, a watershed algorithm assigns neighboring pixels to the markers according to the relief defined by a gradient function (item (2)).

There are two problems inherent with the watershed-plus-marker approach. First, watershed algorithms do not guarantee that flat zones (regions) are not separated, not even the flat zone to which the marker belongs. The second and more severe problem arises when features have a very small size or when they have an elongated shape. It can happen that either a flat zone cannot be marked because it does not have *inside* pixels, or that it is marked with several markers.

These problems can be observed in Figure 1. The input image, in Fig. 1 (a), is an enlargement of the CAMERAMAN image. Fig. 1 (b) shows the output of the pre-filtering stage (a filter by reconstruction has been applied). Fig. 1 (c) displays two specified flat zones (white pixels) of Fig. 1 (b). In this example, the chosen markers

2	2	2	4
4	4	4	3
4	2	2	3
4	2	2	3

(a) Input gray-level function f

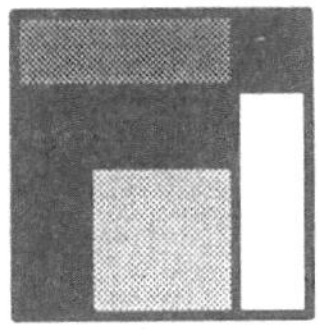

(b) Flat zones of f

EXAMPLE I
Flat zones. (a) Input gray-level function and (b) its four flat zones. All pixels in an image belong to a flat zone. Note: eight-connectivity has been used.

are the minima of the gradient of Fig. 1 (b), displayed in Fig. 1 (d). The watershed can be seen, in white, in Fig. 1 (e). Even using, as in this case, all the gradient minima as markers (which leads to a large number of markers and therefore of regions) the watershed-plus-markers approach fails to obtain a satisfactory segmentation because some significant features are only one- or two-pixels wide. In particular, the camera part signaled in Fig. 1 (c) has been practically lost.

3. The Flat Zone Approach

This section presents the flat zone approach as a simple solution to the small region problem. This solution abandons the region marker concept and requires neither the computation of a gradient function nor the modification of the support of the input image in order to increase the size of the features. A more detailed description, for the gray-level case, can be found in (Crespo & Serra 1993) (Crespo 1993).

3.1. General Principles and Definition: Gray-Level Image Case

The following definition states the proposed basic principle of a flat zone approach for gray-level functions. A gray-level function is a mapping $f : E \longrightarrow T$, where E is a space of points and T a completely ordered lattice (Birkhoff 1984) (Serra 1988). Because we use the concept of *connected component* for defining flat zone (Serra & Salembier 1993), it is assumed that the space E is provided with connectivity (or, in particular, that it is equipped with a point opening γ_x (Serra 1988)).

Definition 1 *The flat zones of a gray-level function are the connected components of pixels with the same funcion value.*

Example I illustrates the flat zone concept. The symbol F_x will be used to denote the flat zone to which the point (or a pixel, when E is a grid of points) x belongs to.

Definition 2 *Let f be a gray-level function, and let the symbol $\mathcal{F}$ denote the set of all f. A partition method $\Pi : \mathcal{F} \longrightarrow \mathcal{P}(\mathcal{P}(E))$ is said to be a flat zone approach when there is an inclusion between the flat zones of the input f and an element (a region) of the output partition $\Pi(f)$. That is,*

$$\forall x \in E, \exists \mathcal{R} \in \Pi(f) \text{ such that } F_x(f) \subseteq \mathcal{R}.$$

Thus, a flat zone segmentation algorithm behaves as a connected operator [1] (Serra & Salembier 1993) (Crespo, Serra & Schafer 1993). If a flat zone is to be preserved, then all its component pixels will be preserved. On the other hand, if a flat zone is not to be preserved then it is merged into another one in its entirety. The situation in which a region has lost some groups of pixels (the missing parts problem) cannot happen. From Definition 2, it is clear that *a flat zone approach is a flat zone growing method, i.e., a procedure that exclusively joins flat zones.*

Definition 3 *Flat zone mask M is the set of the flat zones of the input image to which all other flat zones are assigned.*

Note that this concept is different to that of the set of region markers in the watershed-plus-markers approach. Here (1) entire flat zones of the input image are marked, and (2) marked flat zones can be connected. Several criteria can be used for computing the flat zone mask, as explained in (Crespo & Serra 1993) (Crespo 1993).

A medical image example of the employment of the flat zone approach for gray-level images is shown in Figure 2.

3.2. Extension for Color Images

In this section, we discuss a possible extension of the flat zone approach for color images. Within mathematical morphology, other presented color segmentation techniques have been watershed-based techniques in (Meyer 1992) (Soille 1992) (Crespo 1993).

Color images are examples of mappings between a space and a product of totally ordered lattices (Serra 1992), i.e., mappings $f : E \longrightarrow T$, where $T = T_1 \times T_2 \times ... \times T_n$. An element t of T is expressed as $t = \{t_1, ..., t_n : t_1 \in T_1, ..., t_n \in T_n\}$.

Definition 4 *Let f be a multi-spectral function composed of bands f_i. The flat zone $F_x(f)$ of the point x is the largest connected component of pixels that contains x with the same function value in all bands.*

That is, $F_x(f) = \bigwedge_i F_x(f_i)$, where $\bigwedge$ denotes the infimum operator.

Let us first point out how a flat zone inclusion relationship between *each* band and the output partition is not appropriate for color segmentation. The inclusion relationship (Definition 2) was intended to avoid the loss of features. However, that principle, when applied literally to color images, is too restricted. Imagine a color image in which all the information (in this discussion, flat zones) is in one band (a strange case but possible). To simplify the problem, let us assume that we have two bands that are binary images: A_1 and A_2. Since all the information is in, for example, A_1, then A_2 is either the space E or the empty set, and the flat zone of any pixel in A_2 is the whole space. Thus, imposing the flat zone inclusion between *all* input bands and the output segmentation would force us to give as segmentation the whole space; all features in A_1 would be lost.

We are going to establish a flat zone inclusion relationship affecting only those flat zones that belong to an extracted feature. The feature extraction is performed

[1] An operator ψ is connected when, for all points x, $F_x \subseteq F_x\psi$.

in all bands. That is, flat zone masks are computed from all bands. Let us call the color bands I_R, I_G and I_B, and their corresponding flat zone masks, M_R, M_G and M_B. Consider in the following that the pixels in the masks M_R, M_G and M_B have a zero value if their corresponding flat zone is not in the mask and the maximum intensity value (for example, 255 for 8-bit images) otherwise. Let us build the following auxiliary image (assume that I_R, I_G and I_B are 8-bit images):

$$I_{aux} = (M_R \bigwedge I_R) \; + \; 2^8 \times (M_G \bigwedge I_G) \; + \; 2^{16} \times (M_B \bigwedge I_B)$$

The symbols + and × denote, respectively, the integer addition and integer multiplication operations. Note that the range of intensity values of the image I_{aux} is the sum of those in each of the bands (for implementation purposes I_{aux} must be, for example, an image of at least 24 bits if the images at each band are 8-bit images). A pixel of the image I_{aux} has a non-zero value if it appears in either M_R, M_G or M_B. In fact the flat zone of a pixel x in I_{aux}, $F_x(I_{aux})$, is the inf of the flat zones of x that are present in the inf of each band image with its mask:

$$F_x(I_{aux}) = F_x(M_R \bigwedge I_R) \; \bigwedge \; F_x(M_G \bigwedge I_G) \; \bigwedge \; F_x(M_B \bigwedge I_B).$$

Thus, the solution attempts to not lose the features marked by the masks. Very small regions (on the order of few pixels) should be eliminated from I_{aux} to diminish the number of regions in the output partition (the superposition of the three masks creates some regions belonging to the same feature that have only a few pixels).

What is needed now is to have *one* function on which to apply the flat zone assignment (or merging) procedure (Crespo 1993). Lacking a better solution, one band is chosen arbitrarily if no information is available about the characteristics of each band. It is at this point when all three bands are not treated equally that a decision must be made.

After selecting a color band, for example I_R, another image I'_R is computed *imposing* the non-zero flat zones of I_{aux} in I_R. For example, each non-zero flat zone in I_{aux} will be labeled in the image I'_R with the average of the intensity values (from I_R) of its components pixels. In the rest of the pixels of I'_R that are not in a non-zero flat zone of I_{aux}, the intensity values are just those of I_R. Since the average of a non-zero flat zone of I_{aux} can be the same of the label of a neighboring region in I_R (the feature is not in I_R), +1 or -1 can be added to that average to make less likely the loss of features. Then, the flat zone assignment procedure can assign all flat zones of I'_R to the non-zero flat zones of I_{aux} (which are now also flat zones of I'_R).

After the assignment, the output image is a mosaic whose number of regions is the number of non-zero flat zones of I_{aux}. This mosaic defines a partition (the flat zones of the mosaic) that can be used to compute mosaics for the remaining bands, in which the intensity values used to label a mosaic region are the average of the intensity values (taken from the corresponding band) of its component pixels. Figure 3 displays an example of flat zone color segmentation performed on AREAREA. In this example, a gradient-to-area criterion has been employed for computing the flat zone masks (the features) for the three bands.

A detailed description of the pseudocode of the flat zone assignment procedure, which uses a highly efficient hierarchical waiting queue algorithm (Meyer 1990), can be found in (Crespo 1993).

4. Conclusion

This paper began by discussing the inherent problems of the watershed-plus-markers approach: the possible separation of an input flat zone into several regions in the output, and the problem of obtaining markers for features that are one or two pixels wide. The flat zone approach appears as a simple solution to these problems. This approach resembles, for gray-level images, the connected operator concept in the sense that there is an inclusion of flat zones between the input and the output.

For color images the inclusion relationship between *all* flat zones of *each* band and the regions of the output partition is not appropriate and can lead to the loss of important regions. Instead, the color segmentation presented in this paper uses an inclusion relationship that affects only the flat zones of all bands that are signaled as significant.

5. Acknowledgements

We would like to thank the collaboration with Dr. Jean Serra as well as the comments and the help given by Dr. Christophe Gratin during the early stage of this work. This work has been supported by the Spanish government under the program *Formación de Postgrado y de Personal Investigador*, by the *École des Mines de Paris* and the *Centre de Morphologie Mathématique*, by the Digital Signal Processing Laboratory at the Georgia Institute of Technology, and by the Joint Services and Electronics Program under contract DAAH-04-93-G-0027.

References

Beucher, S. & Meyer, F. (1993), The morphological approach to segmentation: the watershed transformation, *in* E. Dougherty, ed., 'Mathematical morphology in image processing', Marcel Dekker, chapter 12, pp. 433–481.

Birkhoff, G. (1984), *Lattice Theory*, American Mathematical Society, Providence.

Crespo, J. (1993), Morphological Connected Filters and Intra-Region Smoothing for Image Segmentation, PhD thesis, School of Electrical Engineering, Georgia Institute of Technology.

Crespo, J. & Serra, J. (1993), Morphological pyramids for image coding, *in* 'Proceedings of SPIE, Cambridge'.

Crespo, J., Serra, J. & Schafer, R. (1993), Image segmentation using connected filters, *in* 'Workshop on Mathematical Morphology'.

Digabel, H. & Lantuéjoul, C. (1977), Iterative algorithms, *in* 'Proc. 2nd European Symp. Quantitative Analysis of Microstructures in Material Science, Biology and Medicine'.

Meyer, F. (1986), Sequential algorithms for cell segmentation, *in* 'Proc. International Symposium on Clinical Cytometry and Histometry'.

Meyer, F. (1990), Algorithmes à base de files d'attente hiérarchique, Technical Report NT-46/90/MM, Ecole des Mines de Paris, Centre de Morphologie Mathématique.

Meyer, F. (1992), Color image segmentation, *in* 'IEE Fourth International Conference on Image Processing and its Applications'.

Serra, J. (1982), *Mathematical Morphology. Volume I*, London: Academic Press.

Serra, J. (1992), *Mathematical Morphology in Image Processing*, Dekker, chapter Anamorphoses and Function Lattices.

Serra, J. & Salembier, P. (1993), Connected operators and pyramids, *in* 'Proceedings of SPIE, San Diego'.

Serra, J., ed. (1988), *Mathematical Morphology. Volume II: theoretical advances*, London: Academic Press.

Soille, P. (1992), Morphologie Mathématique: Du Relief à la Dimensionalité — Algorithmes et Méthodes—, PhD thesis, Université Catholique de Louvain.

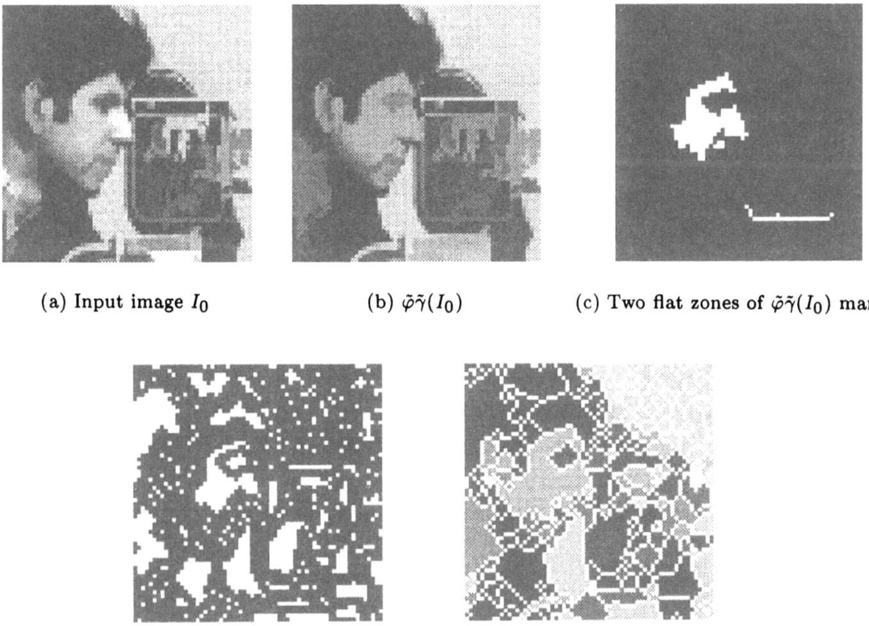

(a) Input image I_0 (b) $\tilde{\varphi}\tilde{\gamma}(I_0)$ (c) Two flat zones of $\tilde{\varphi}\tilde{\gamma}(I_0)$ marked

(d) Gradient minima of (b) (e) Watershed in white (markers: (d))

Fig. 1. Markers and the resolution problem. In the watershed-plus-markers approach, flat zones can be broken or separated, and features of small size (see, for example, the camera part marked in (c)) can be lost in the output partition (e).

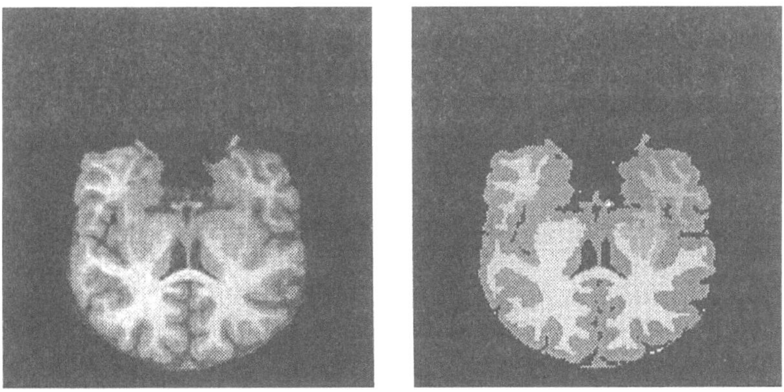

(a) Input image (b) Mosaic model

Fig. 2. Flat zone approach: gray-level example. This figure shows the mosaic model of a medical image that has been computed by using the flat zone approach. The labels of the output model (b) are the region averages. Image size: 170 × 170. (Image from the Department of Human Anatomy and Cell Biology, University of Liverpool.)

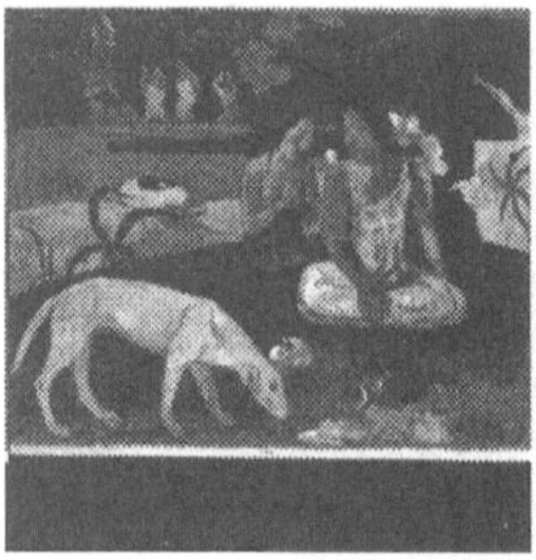

(a) Red band I_R

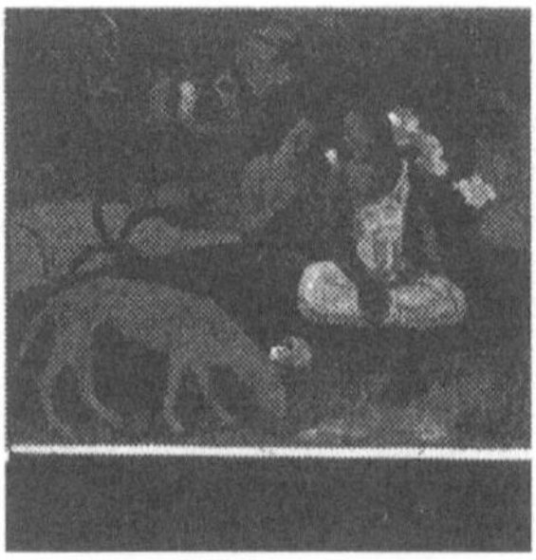

(b) Green band I_G

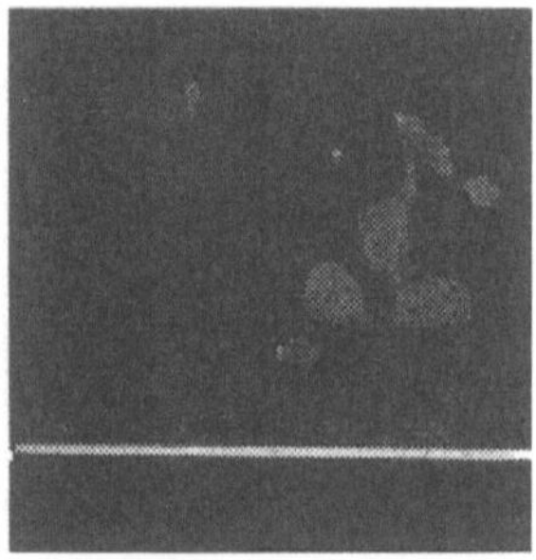

(c) Blue band I_B

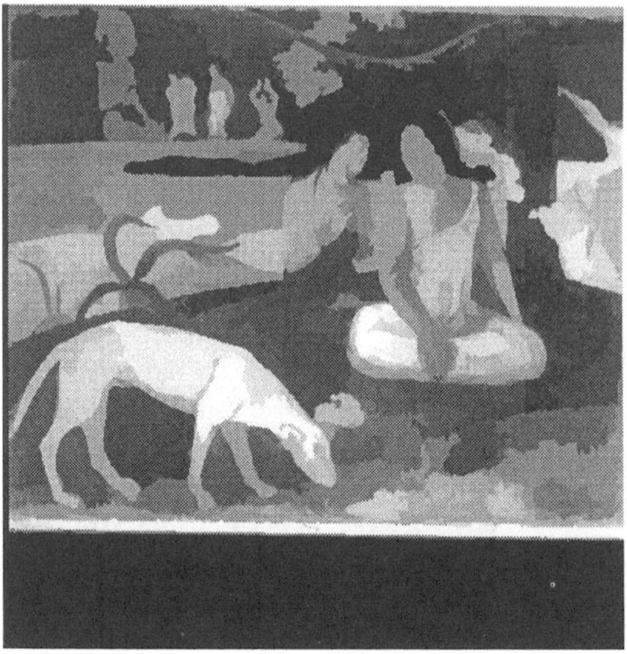

(d) Mosaic 690 regions

Fig. 3. Flat zone approach: color image example. Only a gradient-to-area criterion has been used in the computation of the flat zone mask. The output mosaic displays as labels, after histogram equalization, the region averages computed using the intensity values of the red band. Image size: 512 × 512. *(Note: because of publishing reasons, the true color result has not been reproduced.)* Image: AREAREA by P. Gauguin.

JOINT REGION AND MOTION ESTIMATION WITH MORPHOLOGICAL TOOLS

M. PARDAS and P. SALEMBIER
Dept. Teoria del Senyal i Comunicacions, ETSETB, UPC
Apdo. 30.002, 08080 Barcelona

Abstract. This paper presents a segmentation algorithm for image sequences oriented to very low bit rate video coding applications. The main issue of the process is to get a segmentation that is coherent in time and that solves the region correspondence problem. The morphological approach to this problem uses the temporal connectivity of the objects to establish the concept of "3D objects" and track the evolution of the regions in time. In this paper we propose a morphological time-recursive segmentation which introduces motion estimation within the segmentation process in order to better account for large motion and improve the tracking of objects.

Key words: Segmentation, Motion estimation

1. Introduction

Image sequence segmentation is an important issue in image processing for a large number of applications and, in particular, for second generation video coding techniques. For this purpose, a good segmentation should extract the visually important regions of the scene, be coherent in time, avoid as much as possible random fluctuations of the contour and solve the region correspondence problem. This last requirement indicates that one should be able to follow the time evolution of a given region (a given object).

In order to exploit appropriately the temporal relationship between frames, three dimensional (2D plus time) methods have been proposed in the past [1], [2]. However, the drawbacks of these methods (huge memory requirement, high computational load and introduction of a large processing delay) have lead to time-recursive methods [3]. A time-recursive method is based on the fact that most of the information contained in a frame is already present in the previous frame and that the changes are mainly due to object motion and the appearance of new objects.

In [3] we proposed a time-recursive method designed for coding purposes, which involves two modes of operation: intra-frame and inter-frame segmentation. During the intra-frame mode, the first frame is segmented. It is a purely 2D process. Then, during the inter-frame mode, each frame is recursively segmented using the segmentation of the previous frame. Two different steps can be distinguished in the inter-frame mode: first, define the time evolution of the regions that are present in the segmentation of the previous frame and second, detect the appearance of new regions.

J.Serra and P. Soille (eds.), Mathematical Morphology and Its Applications to Image Processing, 93-100

The definition of the time evolution of the regions is based on a connectivity criterion. That is, two objects in successive frames cannot belong to the same region if they are disconnected in time. Now, if the motion between successive frames is large, small objects can easily become disconnected. When the resulting segmentation is used for coding, the disconnection of objects introduces a large overhead of information to send in the coding process. To avoid this problem we propose a motion estimation step to be performed before the time evolution of the regions is defined. This motion estimation will modify the connectivity used for the extension of the previously segmented regions into the new image. On its turn, the segmentation obtained for the previous frame is used to find an accurate motion estimation.
The organization of this paper is as follows: Section 2 presents the intra-frame mode of the segmentation whereas section 3 is devoted to the time-recursive procedure. In this section the motion estimation process is described and also the inter-frame segmentation mode. Section 4 describes some results of segmentation. Finally, conclusions are reported in section 5.

2. Intra-frame Segmentation

The intra-frame segmentation relies on the hierarchical method proposed for still images in [4]. The algorithm first produces a simplified segmentation in the sense that it involves a reduced number of regions. Then, the segmentation is progressively improved by introducing more regions. Typically four segmentation steps are used. In the following, the principles of this method are summarized. More details can be found in [4].
Each segmentation step involves four basic transformations: simplification, marker extraction, decision and modeling.
- Simplification: In this step, images are simplified to make them easier to segment. The simplification controls the amount of information that is kept for segmentation at this level of the hierarchy. Different simplification tools can be used depending on the segmentation criterion. For coding applications, two visually important criteria are used: size and contrast. A "size" segmentation means that all regions larger than a given limit are segmented. Using a contrast criterion, regions of high contrast are extracted. Morphological filters by reconstruction or area filters are very efficient for size simplification. Rh-maxima or minima operators are suitable for contrast simplification [5]. These operators are very attractive for segmentation purpose because they simplify the signal by removing small or poorly contrasted regions without corrupting the contour information. Moreover, they belong to the class of "connected operators" [6] which are known to produce flat zones (zones of constant gray level value). The concept of flat zones is very useful for the marker extraction step.
- Marker extraction: This step is aimed to detect the presence of homogeneous regions. It produces markers identifying the interior of the regions that are going to be segmented. The marker extraction technique depends on the segmentation criterion. As explained in [5], for size-oriented segmentation, the marker extraction consists in labeling the interior of large regions after the simplification. This can be easily done thanks to the simplification process which has produced flat zones.

For contrast-oriented segmentation, the marker extraction relies on the labeling of specific flat zones produced by the Rh-maxima / minima operators [5].
- Decision: After marker extraction, the number and interior of regions to be segmented are known. However, a large number of pixels are not assigned to any regions. These pixels belong to the so-called uncertainty areas. Assigning these pixels to a given region can be viewed as a decision process that precisely locates the contours between regions. The classical morphological decision tool is the watershed [7]. Generally it works on the morphological gradient of the image to segment. However, as discussed in [1] the use of the morphological gradient results in a loss of information on the contour position of 1 pixel which is generally too high for coding application. To solve this problem, it was proposed in [1] to use a different version of the watershed algorithm working on the original image [8]. The resulting algorithm is a kind of region growing process: the set of markers is extended until they occupy all available space. During the extension, pixels of the uncertainty areas are successively assigned to a given marker. A point is assigned to a specific region because it is in the neighborhood of at least one marker and it is more similar (in the sense defined by a specific criterion) to this marker than to any other marker of its neighborhood.
- Modeling: The next hierarchical step in the segmentation process will have to deal with the regions that cannot be well represented by the coding process. In order to have information about these regions, each region is texture-coded, that is, filled with a gray level function which represents the coded version of the region the receiver will have. Then, the difference between the coded image and the original one, called the modeling residue, is computed. Since this residue concentrates all the information about the badly coded region, it is used as signal to segment by the next segmentation steps.
Typically four segmentation steps are used for the intra-frame processing. The three first ones deal with the size criterion and the last one with the contrast criterion. This hierarchical procedure has the following main advantages: it produces a good segmentation of the image taking into account the possibilities of the texture coding (it segments the coding residue). It allows the progressive estimation of the segmentation parameters, size and contrast, to get a segmentation result compatible with the coding objective (appropriate number of regions or of contour points, etc.).

3. Time-recursive Procedure

After the intra-frame segmentation, a time recursive procedure has to be performed in order to segment the successive images of the sequence in a coherent way. Two main steps can be distinguished in the segmentation: extension of the previously segmented regions into the current frame to segment and extraction of new regions that might have appeared in the scene. In order to have a suitable segmentation for very low bit rate coding, the extension of the previously segmented regions has to be performed in such a way that random fluctuations of the contour are minimized and every object correspondence is found. As it will be shown later, the extension of the previously segmented regions is based on a connectivity criterion. To avoid disconnection of objects in successive frames due to large motion, and also to produce more continuous contours, motion estimation is performed before segmentation.

3.1. Motion Estimation

The motion estimation is performed between the frame which has just been segmented and the next frame which is going to be segmented. Let us call these frames Ft-1 and Ft respectively. The procedure which has been used is a block-matching algorithm [9]. This algorithm involves the division of Ft into small square blocks. For each block of pixels, a search is conducted within a confined window in Ft-1, to locate a best matching block. Thus, it is assumed that all pixels within a block undergo a uniform motion. Even though this hypothesis is not strictly true, specially in blocks which include parts of different regions (corresponding to different objects which might have different motions) the approximation is good enough for our purposes. Actually, small blocks are used in order to have a more accurate estimation (8x8 pixels for QCIF format). Furthermore, there is the possibility of adapting the block sizes to the segmentation obtained previously. That is, the segmentation of frame Ft-1 is known. Let us call it St-1. When the location of the best matching block in Ft-1 for a given block in Ft is found to contain pixels belonging to more than one region, the block in the second frame can be split in smaller blocks, in order to better account for the motion of the different objects which it contains.
If motion is going to be used in other steps of the coding procedure (for contour or texture coding by compensation), it is possible to find, from the estimated motion vectors, a reduced number of parameters for every region. That is, when the segmentation of frame Ft (St) will be computed, a model including translation and zoom with four parameters can be defined for every region in St using the estimated displacement vectors for the blocks belonging to the region. The model parameters are easily computed minimizing the displacement error in the estimated vectors [10].

3.2. Motion Compensation

Once the motion vectors have been estimated for all the blocks of the image, the first image Ft-1 and its segmentation St-1 are motion compensated. That is, the motion vectors found for the original frame are also applied to the segmented image (a label image, with every label identifying a different region). Let us call the compensated images F't-1 and S't-1. However, as the motion estimation has been produced in a block basis, the compensation of the regions can produce disconnected regions in the compensated image S't-1. This effect can be particularly seen as small disconnected components close to the contours of the regions. As the compensated segmentation is going to be used for the extension of the labels into the new image, small disconnected parts could produce a wrong extension of these labels. Thus, small disconnected objects have to be eliminated. This is simply implemented by keeping from every region only its largest connected component. Of course, this produces non labeled pixels in the compensated segmentation S't-1, but, as this image is only used as initialization for the extension of the regions in the new image, it does not involve any problem.
This process is shown in Figure 1. The first column presents two original images (Ft-1 and Ft). The motion vectors obtained with a block-matching procedure between those originals frames are shown in the second column. The size of the blocks which

has been used is 8x8. The image obtained compensating the first original image with these vectors is in the second row of the second column (F't-1). Finally, the third row presents the segmentation of the first image (St-1) and its motion compensation (S't-1). The pixels in black correspond to the disconnected components of regions which have been eliminated.

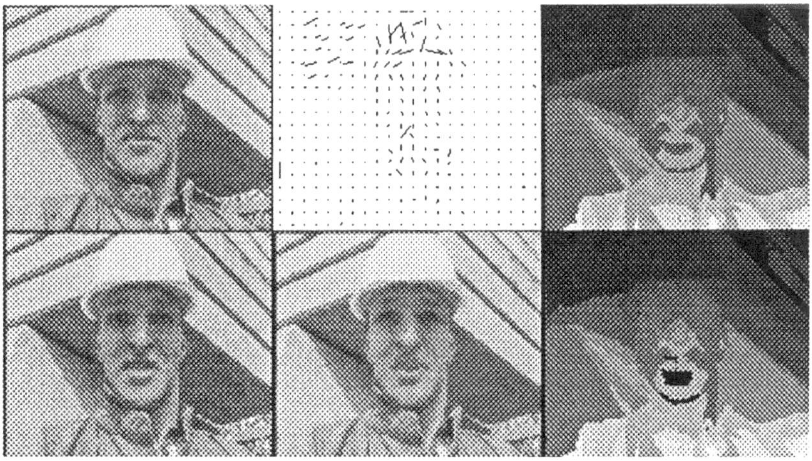

Fig. 1. Example of the motion compensation procedure

3.3. Inter-frame segmentation

As mentioned before, the first step in the inter-frame segmentation is the extension of the previously segmented regions into the current frame to segment. Second, new regions which might have appeared in the scene are extracted. These two points are discussed in the following:

3.3.1. *Extension of the previous segmented regions into the current frame*

This process is basically a projection problem. Assuming that St-1 has already been computed, our goal is to find the segmentation, St, at time t without introducing new regions. For this purpose, two 3D signals are going to be constructed using the compensated imaged generated before. Frames Ft-1' and Ft are grouped together to form a temporal block **F** of size 2 in the time direction. Similarly, the frame S't-1 is grouped with an empty frame So representing an entire frame of uncertainty. The resulting 3D signal denoted **S** is considered as the set of markers that should be used to segment the signal **F**. The extension itself is achieved by the decision algorithm used in the intra-frame segmentation. The only difference is the nature of the signals that are 3D signals. The watershed extends the markers defined by S't-1 into the empty frame So. Each pixel of the uncertainty area (that is of frame So) is assigned to a region of frame S't-1 based on a similarity criterion. It has to be mentioned that, the fact of compensating the original and segmented images Ft-1 and St-1 before computing the 3D watershed is equivalent to locally changing the connectivity in the computation of this watershed. That is, the connectivity in the

temporal dimension is modified in such a way that it takes into account the motion of the objects in the scene.
The similarity measure which has been used in the computation of the watershed consists mainly of the gray tone difference between the pixel of **F** under consideration and the mean of the pixels that have already been assigned to the region. However, this basic similarity measure has been modified to take into account the shape of the contours. As explained in [3] a measure of the straightness of the contours (in both spatial and time dimensions) is introduced in order to produce contours which are easier to code. Note that the straightness of the contours in the temporal dimension is equivalent to stability of the regions.

3.3.2. *Extraction of new regions*

Once the labels of the previously segmented regions have been propagated in the current image, new regions have to be extracted. From now on, the process is purely intra-frame. First of all, the residue image is computed. As for the intra-frame processing discussed previously, the residue image is obtained by texture-coding of the segmentation obtained from the extension of the past regions. Then, the difference with the original image gives the residue, where new appeared regions can be detected. The segmentation of new regions is performed with the method used for the intra-frame segmentation. That is, it consists on the basic segmentation steps: simplification, marker extraction and decision. The segmentation can be performed according to a size or a contrast criterion. Our experience has lead us to use a contrast segmentation only since, most of the time, large and non contrasted regions of the residue are not visually important.

4. Results

The tests performed show that this segmentation method performs better than a segmentation method without motion estimation for sequences with large motion. Furthermore, when the transmission rate is not 25 Hz, but of the order of 8 Hz, which is quite usual for very low bit rate video coding applications, the method allows to save a large amount of computation. That is, if motion compensation is not used, the sequence has to be segmented at 25 Hz in order to achieve enough continuity of the contours and avoid disconnection of objects. Afterwards, the sequences is coded at 8 Hz. Using motion compensation it is possible to segment the sequence directly at 8 Hz, without much loss of quality.
An example is shown in Figure 2. The first row presents three original images corresponding to the sequence "Foreman". Its segmentation without using motion estimation is shown in the second row. Every gray level corresponds to a different region. It can be observed that different new regions appear due to the large motion which this sequence presents. These new regions are represented by high gray level values (bright regions). Furthermore, some regions as the left eyebrow disappear without being recovered. On the contrary, in the segmentation performed using motion estimation, which is shown in the third row, these regions do not disappear and less new regions appear, due to the fact that they have been properly connected to their corresponding regions in the previous image. The forth and fifth row present

the same segmentation where every region has been filled with its mean value. The example presented in this figure corresponds to a sequence of 20 frames. The number of regions in the first frame is 84. For the whole sequence we obtain 105 regions without using motion compensation and 96 using motion compensation.

5. Conclusions

We have presented in this paper a time-recursive method based on morphological tools which uses motion information to improve the region tracking. It works in two different modes: intra and inter-frame. After an initial segmentation, a time recursive procedure is iterated. First, the motion between the already segmented image and the next frame is estimated. Following, the previously segmented regions are extended and new regions that might have appeared in the actual frame are extracted. The extension of old regions, which is the only 3D process in the segmentation, allows to exploit the temporal information present in the image sequences. It has been shown that this information is more efficiently exploited taking the motion into account before the extension of the regions. Furthermore, the motion information extracted can be easily used for further steps in the coding procedure.

Acknowledgements

This work has been performed within the framework of the RACE MORPHECO project and it has been partially supported by a grant of the Comissionat d'Universitats i Rcccrca, Generalitat de Catalunya.

References

1. M. Pardas, P. Salembier (1994), "3D Morphological Segmentation and Motion Estimation for Image Sequences", in EURASIP Signal Processing, Special Issue on Mathematical Morphology, Vol. 38, N. 2, September 1994.
2. P. Willemin, T. Reed and M. Kunt (1991), "Image sequences coding by split and merge", IEEE Trans. on Communications, Vol. 39, No12, pp 1845-1855.
3. M. Pardas, P. Salembier (1994), "Time-recursive Segmentation of Image Sequences", in Proc. of EUSIPCO-94, Edinburgh, September 1994.
4. P. Salembier (1994), "Morphological multiscale segmentation for image coding", in EURASIP Signal Processing (Special issue on Nonlinear Signal Processing), Vol 39, No 2, December 1994.
5. P. Salembier (1993), "Multi-criterion segmentation for image coding", Proc. of International Workshop on Mathematical Morphology and Its Applications to Signal Processing, Barcelona, pp.40-45.
6. J. Serra and P. Salembier (1993), "Connected operators and Pyramids", Proc. of SPIE Image Algebra and Mathematical Morphololgy, San Diego, Vol. 2030, pp. 65-76, 1993.
7. F. Meyer and S. Beucher (1990), "Morphological Segmentation", Journal of Visual Communication and Image Representation, Vol. 1, No.1 pp. 21-46.
8. F. Meyer (1992), "Color Image Segmentation", Proc. 4th International Conference on Image Processing and its Applications, Maastricht, 1992, pp. 303-307.
9. J.R. Jain and A.K. Jain (1981), "Displacement measurement and its application in interframe coding", IEEE Trans, COM-29, (12), 1981, pp. 1799-1808.
10. M. Pardas, P. Salembier (1994), "Motion and region overlapping estimation for segmentation-based video coding", submitted to First IEEE International Conference on Image Processing, Austin, Texas, November 94.

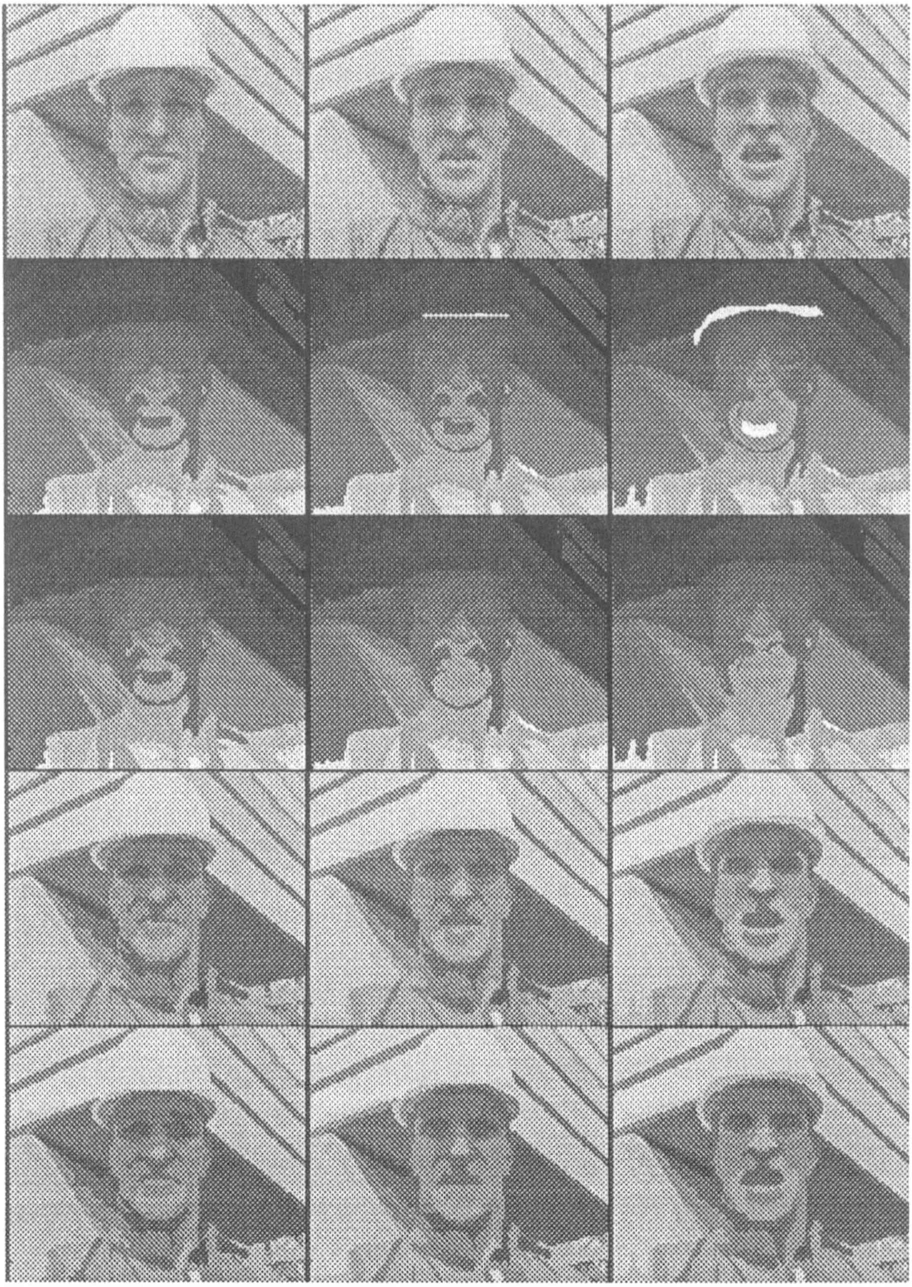

Fig. 2. Example of the segmentation results

MORPHOLOGICAL SEGMENTATION OF IMAGE SEQUENCES

B. MARCOTEGUI and F. MEYER
Ecole des Mines de Paris, Centre de Morphologie Mathématique, 35, rue Saint-Honoré, F-77305 Fontainebleau Cedex, France

Abstract. In image compression, object-based approaches are adapted to high compression rates, since they take into account the geometry of the objects and the human eye characteristics. Mathematical Morphology, dealing with geometrical features is a well suited technique for segmentation purposes. This paper presents a method to segment image sequences, first step of an object-oriented compression system, based on Mathematical Morphology.

Key words: Image Sequences, Segmentation, Mathematical Morphology, Image Compression.

1. Introduction

Classical methods of image compression use spectral decomposition inside spatial unities called blocks, which are not directly related with the image contents. These blocks produce artifacts in the coded image that prevent from reaching high compression rates with an acceptable quality. As an alternative, object-oriented methods have been developed [1]. In order to avoid block effects, these techniques split the image into semantic regions and then encode separately the shape and the contents of each region. Higher compression rates are expected, because the geometry of the objects and the human eye characteristics are taken into account.

The first step of an object-oriented approach is segmentation, on which is based the whole scheme. A good segmentation, with the visual contours and only them, maximizes the compression rate. In image sequences a good time continuity is the basis for a high compression rate.

Mathematical Morphology [2] [3], dealing with geometrical features is a well suited technique for segmentation purposes. This paper presents a method to segment image sequences, based on Mathematical Morphology. The first image of the sequence is segmented in an intra-frame mode, presented in section 2. In section 3 a method to reach maximum stability in image sequence segmentation is presented, as well as the possibility to include new regions, in the only cases when it is really necessary. Finally the problem of regulating the segmentation is discussed, in order to produce a bitstream compatible with the desired compression.

2. 2D segmentation

Dealing with image sequences, a 2D segmentation algorithm is also needed, in order to process intra frames (first frame of the sequence or initializing stage).

The segmentation algorithm may be split up into the following steps [4]:

– filtering step: the goal is to remove non perceptual features in order to simplify

J.Serra and P. Soille (eds.), Mathematical Morphology and Its Applications to Image Processing, 101-108

the detection of homogeneous regions. Morphological filters, (area opening and closing [5], and reconstruction filters) are used. They remove objects smaller than a given size preserving the contour of the remaining ones.

- feature extraction: the goal is to detect the existence of homogeneous regions.
- decision step: the goal is to place the contour of the objects that have been selected by the feature extraction. This decision is made by a watershed algorithm to a gradient image [6] [3] [7], which places the contour on the line of highest gradient between two objects.

A watershed algorithm applied directly on a gradient image produces a severe over-segmentation. Each gradient minimum becomes a region, and most of them do not match with visual regions. Gradient minima have to be classified according to their visual significance and the most significant ones have to be chosen in a number the system can afford. This is the aim of the feature extraction, the main difficulty of the segmentation.

The dynamic [8] applied to the gradient, classifies its minima according to their relative contrast. Figure 1 illustrates this ranking for a smooth function before and after adding noise. The two main structures have a high dynamics in both functions, while the noisy minima have a comparatively lower dynamics. This measure provides for feature extraction a selection criterion based on contrast. But pure contrast does not fit exactly with visual significance. Between two regions of same contrast, the larger one, would be more visible. For this reason, in order to get a more visual criterion, we have weighted the dynamics by a function of the region size.

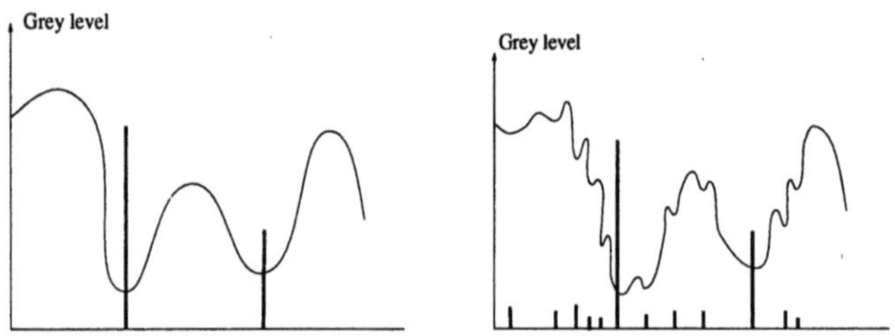

(a) Function's dynamics (b) Noisy function's dynamics

Fig. 1. Dynamics of function minima.

Some segmentations at different resolutions, based on a contrast-size criterion are shown in Fig. 2.

3. 3D segmentation

In order to reach a time stability, the successive frames of a sequence are segmented as a 3D volume [9]. In order to avoid unacceptable time delays, the time depth of the 3D volume has been reduced to 2 frames(previous and current frame); this means, a sliding window through the sequence [10].

A 3D segmentation algorithm transforms a sequence into a partition of the 3D space. Contours and texture of each region are subsequently coded. Coding cost of a region is minimum if it can be predicted (only a motion vector and prediction

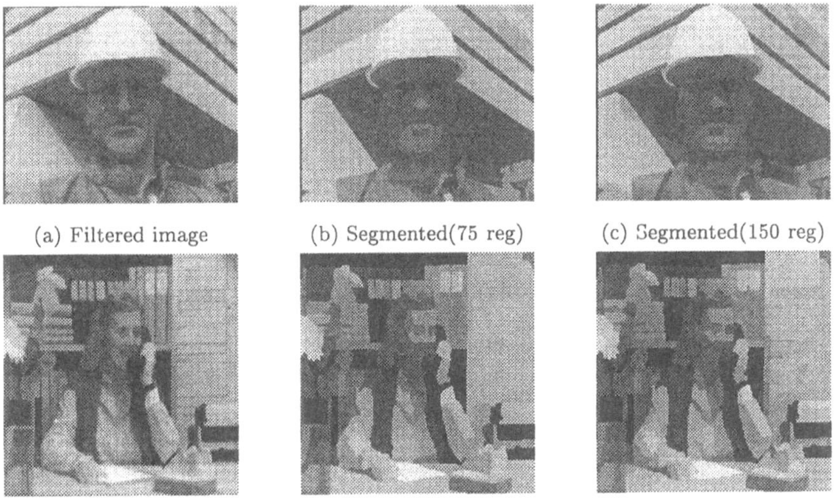

(a) Filtered image (b) Segmented(75 reg) (c) Segmented(150 reg)

(d) Filtered image (e) Segmented(150 reg) (f) Segmented(250 reg)

Fig. 2. 2D segmentations.

errors have to be coded). This is the case for any region keeping its label from the previous frame. On the other hand, contours and texture of new regions have to be completely coded, which is much more expensive. Therefore, to reach a high compression rate, segmentation algorithms have to favor time continuity accepting new regions only when they are really important.

3.1. Maximum stability

We first treat the ideal case, in which all regions are already present in the first frame and have been properly segmented in the intra frame mode. Thus, in inter frame mode, no further feature extraction is required. The previous segmentation works as a set of markers (put in the first frame of the sliding window) which invade the current frame.

The decision step, performed by the watershed algorithm, works on a gradient image in order to locate the contours of the selected markers. The gradient of thin objects does not contain contour information (see Fig. 3). In still images the filtering step removes the objects under the gradient resolution. In video sequences this problem worsens. The uncertainty of spatial contours is proportional to the object motion (Fig. 4). For this reason we perform the watershed on a time upsampled gradient (Fig. 5) which allows us to locate correctly the spatial contour.

Taking the previous segmentation as a set of markers, a watershed on a 3D time upsampled gradient, produces the contours we are looking for.

The image of foreman with a smooth motion (Fig. 6) is segmented in Fig. 7.

If motion is faster, some objects may not be connected with their markers. Those objects disappear in the segmentation. (The algorithm processes a disconnected object as two different objects). In Fig. 8 we have an example of this situation. The ping-pong ball disappears when the motion becomes faster. A high time dam in

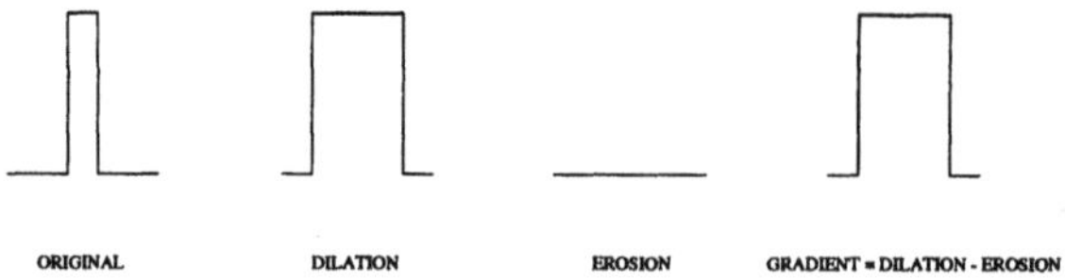

Fig. 3. Gradient of a thin object.

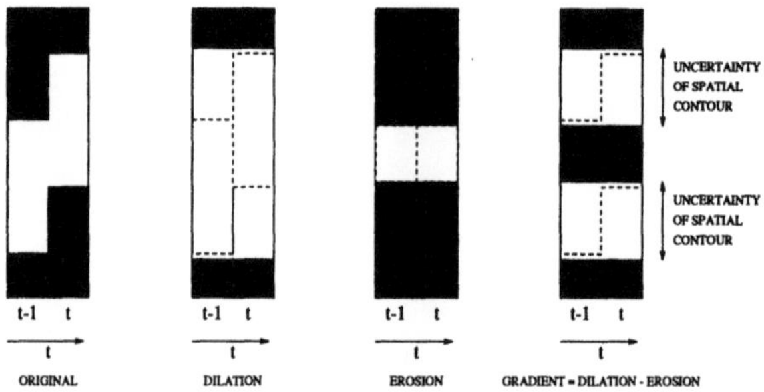

Fig. 4. 3D gradient of a moving object.

the gradient prevents the marker of the disappeared region from reaching the next frame.

This algorithm, intrinsically fails when a new object appears; the only markers we have are those of the previous frame. On the other hand, the algorithm is perfectly able to remove from the segmentation an object that has disappeared. Therefore the next problem to solve is the inclusion of new regions.

3.2. Inclusion of new regions

The algorithm presented in the previous section offers a maximum stability; it maintains permanent objects in the scene as long as possible, until they eventually vanish. Unable to let new regions appear, it has to be completed by a procedure for introducing new regions. Performing a feature extraction for each frame would introduce highly unstable segmentations, since the ranking of regions according to their visual significance would fluctuate one image to another. Stability will be introduced by a three step procedure:

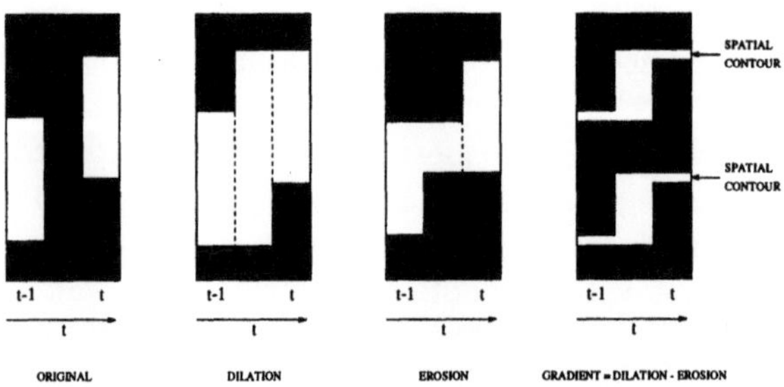

Fig. 5. 3D time upsampled gradient.

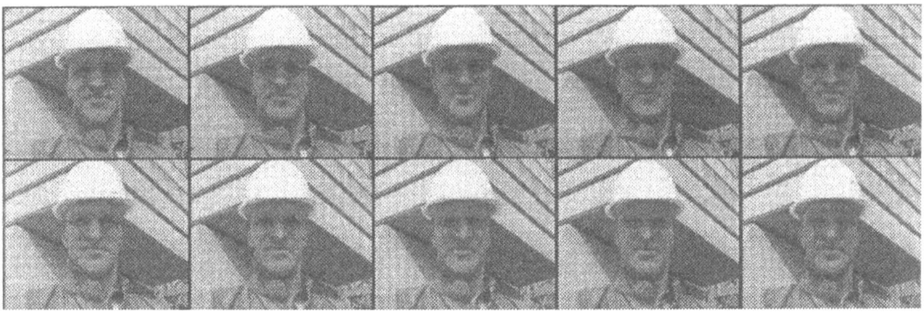

Fig. 6. Filtered image sequence

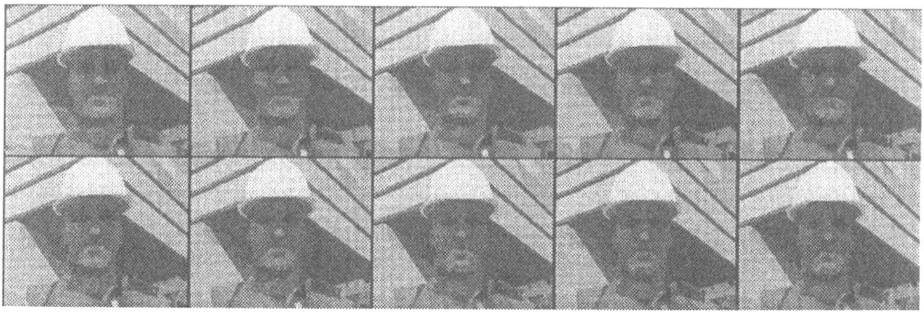

Fig. 7. Segmented image sequence

1. independent feature extraction.
2. validation of new markers.
3. merging new and old markers.

This procedure is hereafter explained in detail.

1. A feature extraction (with a contrast-size criterion, as presented in section 2) selects the objects visually important. This selection is performed without taking previous segmentations into account, and its result is taken as a provisional set of markers. Some of them already exist in the previous frame and they have not to be considered as new markers. Others are markers of new significant regions in the scene and have to be kept. The rest are ranking fluctuations and we want to reject them, in order to keep a good stability.
2. We want to introduce new regions only when they are justified by an important change in the scene. This criterion has been implemented by means of a moving mask, which removes those markers that are associated to regions that have not changed in time. The moving mask is generated as follows: the difference between two successive simplified frames is computed. Moving areas appear with a high grey level. The feature extraction step computes a contrast threshold, that corresponds to the required contrast of a region in order to be considered visually important. This threshold is applied to the difference image producing a mask of changing areas. Only markers under this moving mask will be kept as markers of new regions.

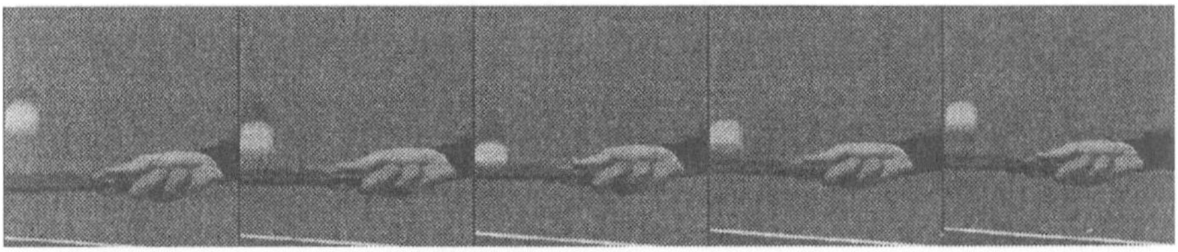

(a) Filtered image sequence

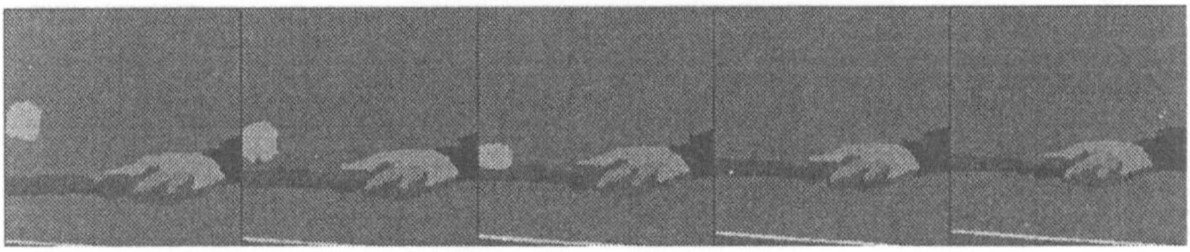

(b) Segmented image sequence

Fig. 8. No new regions.

3. Old and new markers are merged into a 3D image; in the first frame the previous segmentation (as markers of permanent objects) and in the frame corresponding to the current time, markers selected by the feature extraction that are under the moving mask (as markers of new regions).

After the feature extraction step, the decision step is performed in a 3D time upsampled image as explained in the previous section. Figure 9 contains a block diagram of this technique.

With this technique a new region appears only when an important change justifies it. In Fig. 10 a segmented image including new regions is presented.

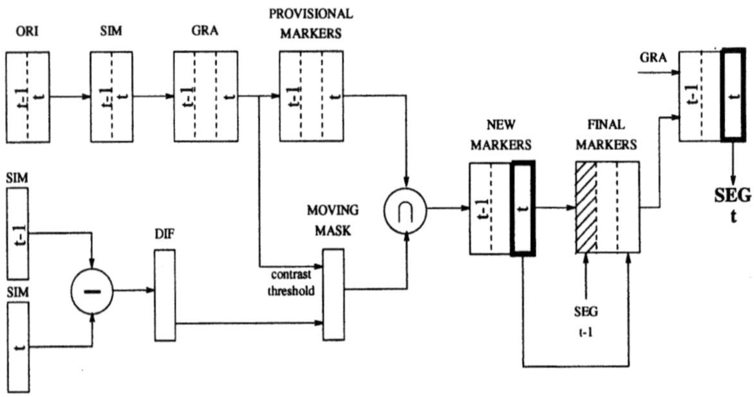

Fig. 9. Block diagram of inclusion of new regions.

3.3. Regulation of the segmentation

For a given compression rate the quality should be as high as possible. If motion in the sequence is predictable from the previous frames a fine segmentation is afforded.

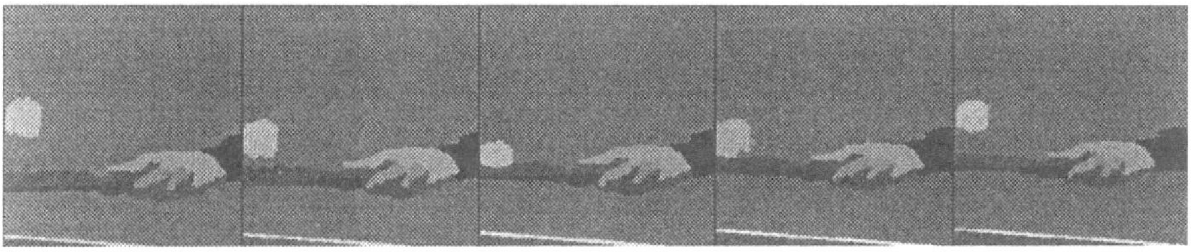

Fig. 10. Inclusion of new regions.

On the other hand if new significant regions appear all the time the accuracy of the segmentation have to be reduced. Therefore a mechanism should be provided enabling to introduce more regions upon request if predictable motion allows it or to merge them in order to assign bits for new significant regions. Several segmentations followed by coding step should be necessary before an optimum is reached. Complexity and processing time forbid this option. Another solution is to produce during the segmentation a more complete representation, such as a tree structure [11]. Each node of the tree represents a region linked by an edge to an ancestor region containing it and by two or several edges to daughter nodes representing all regions contained in it. Going down in the tree means merging regions, going up means splitting regions. Producing the best segmentation then simply results in cutting the tree at the level producing the required bitstream. For generating the initial tree in intra mode, the tree of increasing dynamics is a good candidate. We are currently developing algorithms for updating it in time: this means ranking the fusions according to their cost/benefit in inter mode and providing a mechanism for introducing new regions. In order to evaluate the stability of tree representations we have made the following experience. We consider the simple situation where no new regions appear. We construct from the first intra frame a tree of fusions and derive from it two segmentations: a fine segmentation (Fig. 11) included in a coarse one (Fig. 12). A 3D time recursive segmentation as presented in section 3.1 is applied, one using the fine segmentation and the other the coarse one; we obtain a fine and a coarse segmentations of the whole sequence. We then apply to all frames of the fine segmentation the same fusions of labels as defined in the initial intra frame; this gives us again a coarse segmentation. The coarse segmentation obtained by both methods are the same. This shows that our tree representation is indeed stable.

4. Conclusion

A morphological segmentation algorithm for image sequences has been presented in this paper. Good stability is reached, including new regions only when an important change in the scene justifies it. A way to regulate the segmentation accuracy is introduced. In future work we intend to generate a tree structure with a criterion taking into account not only visual significance but also coding cost. In that way we expect to maximize the quality/cost rate of the system.

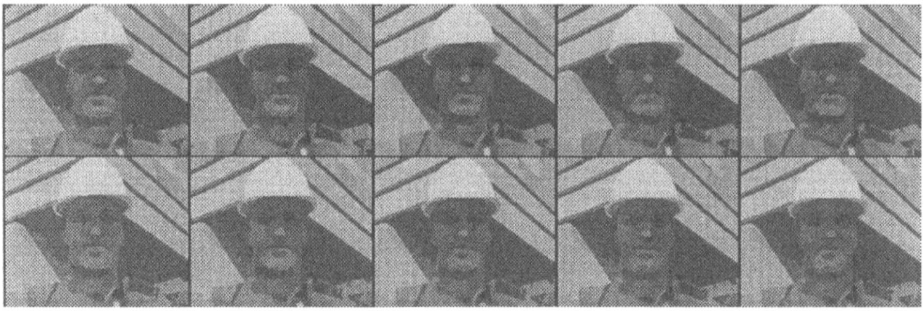

Fig. 11. Fine segmentation.

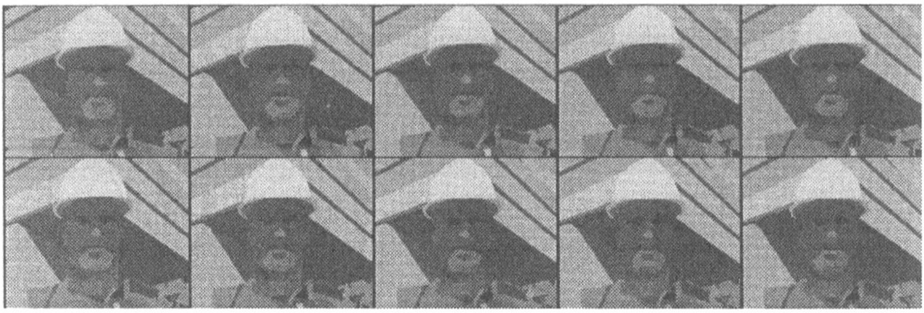

Fig. 12. Coarse segmentation.

References

1. M. Kunt, A. Ikonomopoulos, and M.Kocher, "Second-generation image coding techniques," *Proc. IEEE*, vol. 73, April 1985.
2. J. Serra, *Image analysis and mathematical morphology.* Academic Press, 1982.
3. S. Beucher, *Segmentation d'images et morphologie mathématique.* PhD thesis, Ecole des Mines de Paris, Juin 1990.
4. P. Salembier and J. Serra, "Morphological multiscale image segmentation," in *Visual Communications and Image Processing*, vol. 1818, SPIE, 1992.
5. L. Vincent, "Grayscale area openings and closings, their efficient implementation and applications," in *Mathematical Morphology and its Applications to Signal Processing*, (Barcelona), Mai 1993.
6. S. Beucher and C. Lantuéjoul, "Sur l'utilisation de la ligne de partage des eaux en détection de contours," Rapport Interne N-598, Ecole des Mines de Paris, Centre de Morphologie Mathématique, Mai 1979.
7. F. Meyer and S. Beucher, "Morphological segmentation," *Journal of Visual Communication and Image Representation*, vol. 1, pp. 21–46, Septembre 1990.
8. M. Grimaud, *La géodésie numérique en morphologie mathématique. Application à la détection automatique de microcalcifications en mammographies numériques.* PhD thesis, Ecole des Mines de Paris, Décembre 1991.
9. F. Friedlander, *Le traitement morphologique d'images de cardiologie nucléaire.* PhD thesis, Ecole des Mines de Paris, Décembre 1989.
10. M. Pardas, P. Salembier, and L. Torres, "3d morphological segmentation for image sequences," in *IEEE Winter Workshop on Nonlinear Signal Processing*, (Tampere), 1993.
11. F. Meyer, "Arbre des minima et dynamique," rapport interne, Ecole des Mines de Paris, Centre de Morphologie Mathématique, mars 1990.

CRITICAL MORPHOLOGICAL SAMPLING AND ITS APPLICATIONS TO IMAGE CODING

DINEI A. F. FLORÊNCIO and RONALD W. SCHAFER*

School of Electrical Engineering
Georgia Institute of Technology
Atlanta, GA - USA

Abstract. In this paper we introduce a new morphological sampling theory and show some of its applications to image coding. As in previous works on morphological sampling, we establish conditions that the signal should satisfy before (sub)sampling in order to meet a prescribed reconstruction error criteria. In contrast to previous theorems, however, the whole process is self dual. When compared to previous morphological schemes, Critical Morphological Sampling can save up to half the number of samples. We also establish a set of conditions under which the new theorem is Critical, i.e., a more sparse sampling grid could produce an unbounded reconstruction error (in a Hausdorff sense). We use the theorem to design a Morphological Pyramid Coder, similar to a Laplacian Pyramid Coder. The results not only are superior to the Laplacian Pyramid, but are found to be competitive with more complex linear coders, like the DCT-based JPEG.

Key words: Sampling, Critical Sampling, Morphology, Image Coding

1. Introduction

The traditional sampling theorem, also known as the Shannon Theorem, serves as the basis for most sampling (and subsampling) of signals when dealing with linear signal processing. However, in morphological signal processing, the traditional sampling theorem does not seem appropriate, because morphological systems are most commonly used where sharp contours are of primary importance and signals are inherently non-band-limited. Thus, a more appropriate sampling theory is required.

The subject of morphological sampling has been addressed by several authors. Heijmans and Toet [1], based on a specific definition for sampling ("probing element sampling"), presented a very general sampling strategy, but their unusual definition for sampling produces images that tend to wash out or darken when subsampled, therefore limiting the applications of their results. Using a more traditional sampling definition, Haralick et al. [2] provided many relations between the sampled signal and the original signal. From the results in that paper, one can establish relations between an appropriately filtered signal and its sampled version. Nevertheless, although giving sufficient conditions to preserve the information after the sampling, that work did not establish the necessity of those conditions. Earlier, Serra [3,

* This work was supported in part by CNPq (Brazil) under contract 200.246/90-9 and the Joint Services Electronics Program under contract DAAH-04-93-G-0027.

J.Serra and P. Soille (eds.), Mathematical Morphology and Its Applications to Image Processing, 109-116

pp216–] approached the problem for the particular case of binary signals from the point of view of preserving the homotopy of the sampled set (i.e. connected components map into connected components). His work yielded a sampling condition equivalent to Haralick's.

In this paper, we define a new sampling theory, which we call **Critical Morphological Sampling** [4], and show an application to image coding. This paper shows that the sampling conditions imposed in [2] were too strong, and that equivalent results can be obtained with half the number of samples. Therefore, in some sense, previous morphological sampling schemes **oversampled** the signal. The savings resulting from Critical Sampling have the potential of improving practically any multiresolution morphological algorithm.

In section 2 we define our sampling and reconstruction operators. In section 3 we state the Critical Morphological Sampling Theorem and some associated results. In section 4 we use these ideas to design anti-aliasing and associated reconstruction filters for a pyramidal image coder similar to the Laplacian Pyramid [5]. Simulation results in Section 5 show that the proposed coder not only outperforms the Laplacian pyramid, but it is competitive with more complex coding strategies, like the DCT-based JPEG.

2. Sampling and Reconstruction

The first step in obtaining a Sampling theorem is to define sampling. Although some authors have adopted slightly different definitions,[1] we use the traditional definition of sampling (the one in analog sampling). More formally, let $\mathcal{E}$ be our signal space, $F \subseteq \mathcal{E}$ our original signal, and consider the subspace $\mathcal{S} \subset \mathcal{E}$ as our sampling grid. With $\mathcal{P}$ denoting the power set, we define the sampling operator $\sigma : \mathcal{P}(\mathcal{E}) \to \mathcal{P}(\mathcal{S})$ such that:

$$x \in \sigma(F) \Leftrightarrow x \in F \cap \mathcal{S}. \tag{1}$$

Note that this defines a self-dual sampling, i.e., $\sigma(F) = (\sigma(F^c))^c$, where ^{c} denotes set complement.[2]

We place two additional constraints on the sampling grid:[3]

$$\mathcal{S} \oplus \mathcal{S} = \mathcal{S} \text{ , and} \tag{2}$$

$$\mathcal{S} = \check{\mathcal{S}}. \tag{3}$$

Finally, we define a reconstruction transformation $\rho : \mathcal{P}(\mathcal{S}) \to \mathcal{P}(\mathcal{E})$, as:

$$\rho(G) = G \oplus K \tag{4}$$

[1] Haralick et. al. [2] used a definition based on intersection, making set complementation in the sampled domain unclear. Heijmans and Toet [1] uses a *probing element* sampling, which is equivalent to a dilation followed by a sampling according to the usual definition.

[2] Note that this complement might be complement on $\mathcal{E}$ (if the set is defined on the original space $\mathcal{E}$) or on $\mathcal{S}$ (if the set is defined on the sampled space $\mathcal{S}$). The meaning will be clear from the context.

[3] We will be using the following definitions: Consider A and B sets in a space $\mathcal{E}$, and $x \in \mathcal{E}$. The *translation* of A by x is denoted by $A_x = \{y \mid \text{ for some } a \in A, y = a + x\}$. The *reflection* of A by $\check{A} = \{x \mid -x \in A\}$. The *dilation* of A by B is $A \oplus B = \bigcup_{x \in B} A_x$. The *erosion* of A by B is $A \ominus B = \bigcap_{x \in \check{B}} A_x$. The *closing* of A by B is $A \bullet B = (A \oplus B) \ominus B$, and the *opening* of A by B is $A \circ B = (A \ominus B) \oplus B$.

where $K \subseteq \mathcal{E}$ is the (reconstruction) structuring element (s.e.). The next proposition establishs the conditions under which this reconstruction operator will be self-dual.

Proposition 1 *The reconstruction by dilation defined in (4) will be self dual (i.e., $\rho(G) = (\rho(G^c))^c$) if and only if the associated s.e. K is such that:*

$$\mathcal{S} \oplus K = \mathcal{E} \qquad , \textit{ and} \tag{5}$$

$$\forall x, y \in \mathcal{S},\ x \neq y,\ K_x \cap K_y = \emptyset. \tag{6}$$

In other words, we require the translations of the s.e. K by all the points in $\mathcal{S}$ to form a partition of $\mathcal{E}$.

3. The Critical Morphological Sampling Theorem

We can now state some of the results associated with the defined sampling and reconstruction operators.

Proposition 2 *Let $\mathcal{E}$ be a signal space, $F \subseteq \mathcal{E}$ a signal in that space, $\mathcal{S}$ a sampling grid satisfying conditions (2) and (3), $\sigma(\cdot)$ the sampling operator defined in (1), and $\rho(\cdot)$ the reconstruction operator defined in (4), with the s.e. $K \subseteq \mathcal{E}$ satisfying (5) and (6). Then the following properties hold:*

$$F \ominus \check{K} \subseteq \rho(\sigma(F)) \subseteq F \oplus K \tag{7}$$

$$\sigma(F) = \sigma(\rho(\sigma(F))) \tag{8}$$

$$F = F \bullet K = F \circ \check{K} \Rightarrow \rho(\sigma(F)) \ominus K \subseteq F \subseteq \rho(\sigma(F)) \oplus \check{K} \tag{9}$$

Proposition 3 *If $F = F \bullet K = F \circ \check{K}$, the Hausdorff distance between F and $\rho(\sigma(F))$ is at most $r(K)$, where $r(K)$ is the radius of the smallest circle containing K.*

We are now ready to state the Critical Sampling Theorem:

Theorem 1 *Let $\mathcal{E}$ be a signal space, $F \subseteq \mathcal{E}$ a signal in that space, $\mathcal{S}$ a sampling grid satisfying conditions (2) and (3), $\sigma(\cdot)$ the sampling operator defined in (1), and $\rho(\cdot)$ the reconstruction operator defined in (4), with the s.e. $K \subseteq \mathcal{E}$ satisfying (5) and (6). Consider the classes of sets $\mathcal{P} = \{F \subseteq \mathcal{E} \mid F = A \oplus K \text{ for some } A \subseteq \mathcal{S}\}$, and $\mathcal{Q} = \{F \subseteq \mathcal{E} \mid F = F \bullet K = F \circ \check{K}\}$, then:*

1. *The samples of $F \in \mathcal{P}$ at the points in $\mathcal{S}$ are necessary and sufficient to perfectly reconstruct F.*
2. *The samples of $F \in \mathcal{Q}$ at the points in $\mathcal{S}$ are necessary to reconstruct F with bounded error (in a Hausdorff distance sense), and sufficient to reconstruct F with an error of at most $r(K)$.*

Note that some of these results may look similar to those reported in [2], but our results are less restrictive, allowing for using a smaller K. In the most common case of subsampling by two in a square grid, the results in [2] call for opening/closing the signal with a 3×3 s.e. For the same filtering, our results allow a subsampling by 3 (instead of 2) in each direction, therefore resulting in a 56% savings in the number of samples, while keeping the same (maximum) reconstruction error (in a Hausdorff sense). Looking at it another way, for subsampling by 2 in each direction, a 2×2 s.e. suffices according to our Theorem. We can therefore represent a larger class of signals with a smaller reconstruction error.

For simplicity, these results were established here for binary signals. The extension to gray level signals is possible if we define an operator similar to set complementation.[4] Details on the Critical Sampling Theorem, including proofs for the results and other interesting relations, can be found in [4]. An extension to Homotopy-preserving sampling can be found in [6].

4. Application to a Pyramidal Image Coder

The direct application of the morphological sampling theorem to subsampling followed by upsampling of an image, has been shown [4] to produce results that outperform previous morphological sampling schemes under several error criteria.[5] However, it performed worse than some linear techniques for the m.s.e. criterion.[6]

While edge preservation may be the most significant criterion in applications such as segmentation, this is not generally the case for image coding. In this section we adapt the ideas of Critical sampling to a non-linear coder which is competitive with other linear techniques, even under an m.s.e. criterion.

For this purpose, we developed a coder based on the Laplacian Pyramid Coder [5], depicted in Figure 1. In the Laplacian Pyramid, the analysis and synthesis filter are Gaussian filters. These filters are replaced by nonlinear operators in our scheme.

4.1. Pre-Sampling Filtering

The objective of the pre-sampling filter is to filter out the high frequency components of the signal in order to reduce aliasing in the subsampling process. In the Laplacian Pyramid Coder [5] this filtering is performed by a Gaussian filter. In morphological pyramids [7, 8, 9] openings, closing or dilations are generally used, with the structuring element chosen either empirically or based on some non-critical sampling strategy [1, 2]. The simple use of Critical Sampling reduced the entropy of the difference pyramids by about 14%, when compared with the pyramid proposed in [8].

Although better than previous morphological pyramids, these results were not yet competitive with other linear strategies. We then notice that there was an undefined region in the filtering process. Indeed, a picture formed by details that contain only two pixels has no detail that should be maintained. The problem can be associated with the fact that in Morphology we are dealing with shape, and removing a pixel from the signal does not necessarily mean reducing the energy, as in the linear case, since those pixels will, in fact become part of another shape in the picture. We

---

[4] For example, if the gray level is defined in a set $\mathcal{G} = 0, 1, 2, \cdots, N$ we define the *negative* f^* of a function $f : \mathcal{E} \rightarrow \mathcal{G}$ as $f^*(x) = N - f(x)$.

[5] (e.g., mean squared error (m.s.e.), mean absolute error (m.a.e.), and an edge-shift measure.)

[6] It outperformed linear techniques in the edge shift criterion and tied in m.a.e.

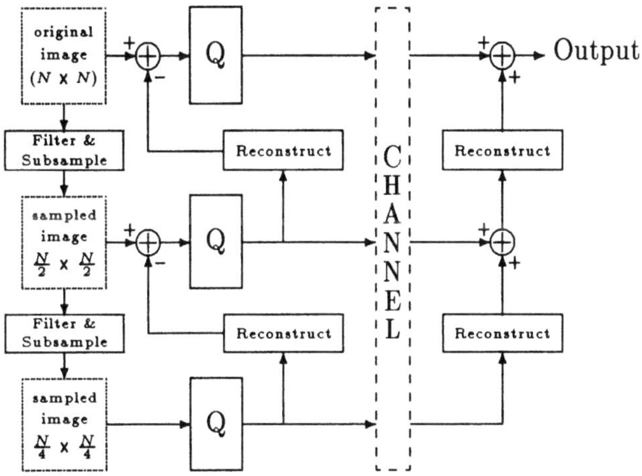

Fig. 1. Basic structure of a (3-level) pyramid coder

decided therefore to allow some amount of aliasing, in order to be able to keep some of the details that would be filtered out otherwise. After experimenting with several filters, we settled on a filter that preserves every feature that contains at least two pixels.[7]

4.2. The reconstruction Process

As mentioned earlier, we used a non-linear reconstruction process in order to produce the upsampled estimates at each level. To design the filter, we initially use Equation (9) to obtain upper and lower bounds for the image. We then use the hypothesis that the image is a low-detail image to make the final interpolation.

The reconstruction of the $2N \times 2N$ image Y from the $N \times N$ image X can be described in the following way:

1. For samples where both coordinates are even make $Y(2i, 2j) = X(i, j)$.
2. For samples with first coordinate even, and second coordinate odd, i.e., $Y(2i, 2j+1)$ compute a weighted median of $\{X(i-1, j), X(i-1, j+1), X(i, j), X(i, j+1), X(i+1, j), X(i+1, j+1)\}$ with weights $\{1, 1, 3, 3, 1, 1\}$.
3. For samples of the form $Y(2i+1, 2j)$, compute the symmetric of the previous item.
4. For samples in the form $Y(2i+1, 2j+1)$, compute the median of $\{X(i, j), X(i+1, j), X(i, j+1), X(i+1, j+1)\}$.

This reconstruction algorithm has shown capable of producing images with good subjective quality, and with smaller reconstruction error than the linear Gaussian filter.

[7] We used a filter $f(.)$ described by $f(x) = Median\{(x \bullet K) o K, \bigvee_{b \in \Lambda} x \bullet b, \bigwedge_{b \in \Lambda} x o b\}$, where "o" stands for opening, "•" stands for closing, "$Median\{w, y, z\}$" stands for the operation of pointwise median, i.e., chosing the median value among the 3 pixels corresponding to each of the three images w, y, and z, K is a 2x2 s.e., and "Λ" represents the four possible orientations for a 2 pixel element in thc square grid.

Level (# pels)	Quant. step	Entropy (bpp)	equiv. bpp	total bpp	SNR (dB)	Entropy (bpp)	equiv. bpp	total bpp	SNR (dB)
		Laplacian Pyramid				**Proposed Morph. Pyramid**			
$4(16^2)$	1	6.682	0.026	0.026	-	6.592	0.026	0.026	-
$3(32^2)$	2	5.164	0.081	0.107	-	4.941	0.077	0.103	-
$2(64^2)$	4	3.572	0.223	0.330	-	3.459	0.216	0.319	-
$1(128^2)$	8	2.044	0.511	0.841	-	1.976	0.494	0.813	-
$0(256^2)$	16	0.845	0.845	1.686	37.4	0.757	0.757	1.571	38.5

TABLE I
Entropy and SNR for the Laplacian and the proposed Morphological Pyramids

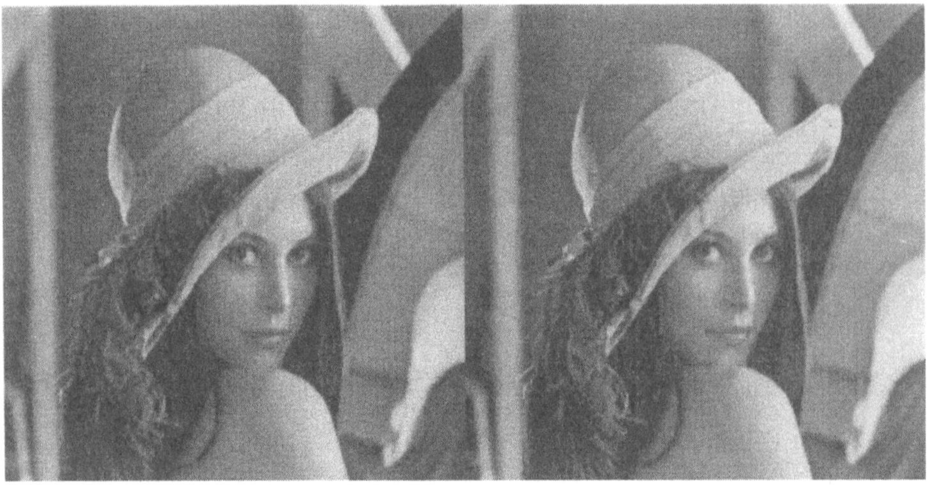

Fig. 2. Results with basic Quantization: (a) Laplacian Pyramid, (b) proposed coder.

4.3. Performance

To evaluate the performance of the coder, we implemented a 5-stage coder and compared it with the equivalent Laplacian pyramid coder and with a JPEG coder. We used the entropy of the quantized signal as an estimate of bit-rate. Of course, to attain that rate entropy coding has to be used. When comparing rates with JPEG, we allow for a 5% margin to account for the non-ideal coding.

To compare the proposed coder with the Laplacian Pyramid coder we set the quantization steps in both coders to 16, 8, 4, 2, and 1, at pyramid levels 0, 1, 2, 3, and 4 respectively. The results in Table I show the entropy at each level of the pyramid, beginning from the coarser image (16x16). Note that the proposed scheme produces a result 1.12 dB better than the Laplacian Pyramid, and yet, the entropy of the error pyramid is smaller (1.57 against 1.68 bpp). Figure 2 shows the corresponding images.

Probably more important than this small gain when compared to the Laplacian pyramid, is the ability of the proposed coder to produce sharp contours in any case, even when no information is transmitted for the finest pyramid level. We redesigned the quantizer for the proposed pyramid, and we obtained good results with reasonably smaller (estimated) bit rates. Table II shows the results of some simulations

Proposed Method		**JPEG**	
Entropy	SNR	Bit Rate	SNR
0.95	34.90	1.00	34.69
0.80	33.77	0.85	33.74
0.67	32.61	0.70	32.64
0.52	31.27	0.55	31.46

TABLE II
SNR comparison between JPEG and the proposed coder

on the image Lenna at a 256x256 resolution. The data corresponds to true bit rates for the JPEG coder, and entropy for the proposed coder. To compensate for the non-optimality of entropy coders, we allow a 5% margin when making the comparison. Observe that the performance of the two coders is practically identical in terms of SNR. The corresponding images (see Figure 3) show that JPEG introduces many artifacts in the image (blocking, ringing near the edges, false textures, etc), while the proposed coder introduces very few artifacts, the main distortion being the removal of some of the texture in some regions. This distortion seems to be less objectionable, producing images with higher subjective quality.

5. Conclusion

In this paper we introduced a new Morphological Pyramid coder, which combines elements of the recently developed theory of Critical Morphological Sampling with a non-linear reconstruction process which is capable of producing sharp images and reduce the raggedness of previous morphological reconstruction process. We have showed that the coder compares favorably to a Laplacian Pyramid coder in relation to both SNR and bit rate. When compared to a JPEG coder, we observed that the proposed coder (using a similar bit rate) produces an image with very few artifacts, with a higher subjective quality, even though it has a similar SNR.

Future work will be in the direction of further exploring the redundancy remaining in the difference pyramid, probably by using vector quantization. We are also working on improving some details of the reconstruction process, which could further reduce the energy in the difference pyramid, and therefore the bit rate.

References

1. H. J. A. M. Heijmans and A. Toet, "Morphological sampling," *CVGIP: Image Understanding*, vol. 54, pp. 384–400, Nov. 1991.
2. R. M. Haralick, X. Zhuang, C. Lim, and J. S. J. Lee, "The digital morphological sampling theorem," *IEEE Trans. Acoust., Speech, Signal Processing*, vol. 37, pp. 2067–2090, Dec. 1989.
3. J. Serra, *Image Analysis and Mathematical Morphology*, vol. 1. Academic Press, 1982.
4. D. A. F. Florêncio and R. W. Schafer, "Critical morphological sampling." under preparation.

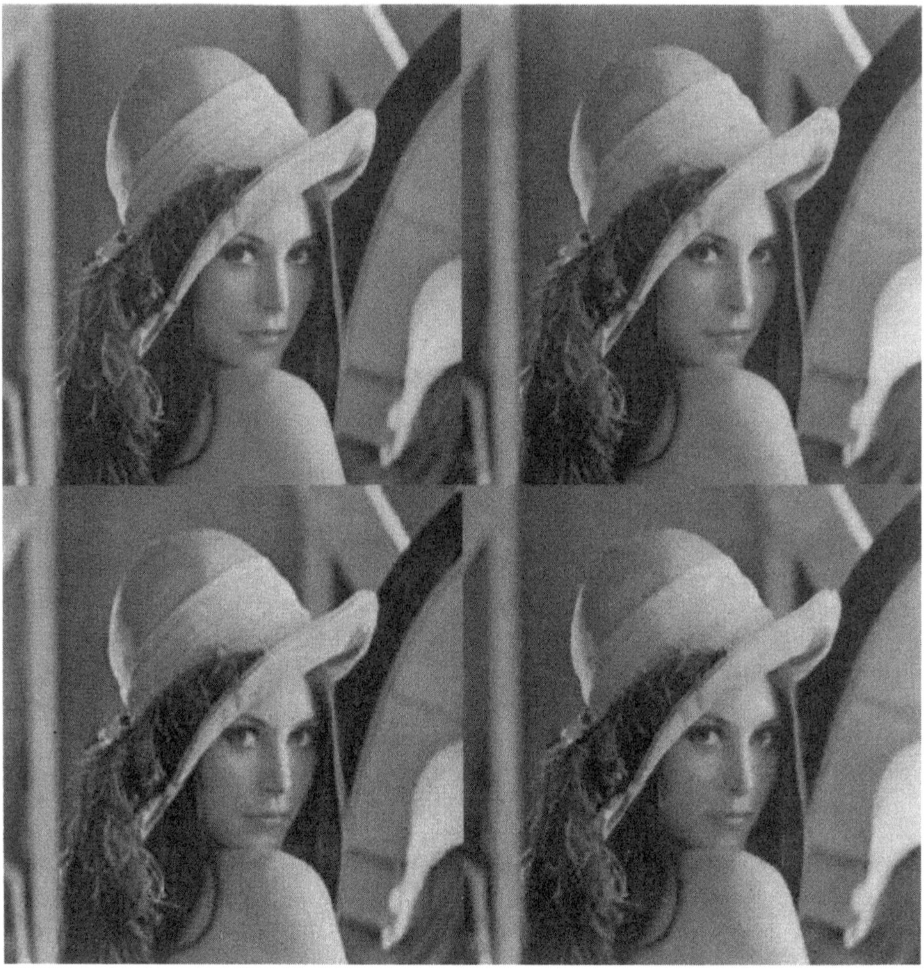

Fig. 3. (a) Original 256 x 256 image. (b) proposed M.P. Coder at entropy = 0.95 bpp (34.9 dB). (c) JPEG 0.7 bpp (32.6 dB). (d) Proposed M.P. coder at entropy=0.67 bpp (32.6 dB).

5. P. J. Burt, "The laplacian pyramid as a compact image code," *IEEE Trans. Commun.*, vol. 31, pp. 532–540, Apr. 1983.
6. D. A. F. Florêncio and R. W. Schafer, "Homotopy and critical morphological sampling." accepted to the 1994 Visual Communications and Image Processing Symposium, Sept. 1994.
7. L. A. Overturf, M. L. Comer, and E. J. Delp, "Color image coding using morphological pyramid decomposition," in *Human Vision, Visual Processing, and Digital Display III*, pp. 265–275, SPIE Vol. 1666, 1992.
8. F.-K. Sun and P. Maragos, "Experiments on image compression using morphological pyramids," in *Visual Communication and Image Processing IV*, pp. 1303–1312, SPIE Vol. 1199, 1989.
9. A. Toet, "A morphological pyramidal image decomposition," *Pattern Recog. Lett.*, vol. 9, pp. 255–261, May 1989.

A SAMPLING APPROACH BASED ON EQUICONTINUITY

JEAN SERRA
Ecole des Mines de Paris, Centre de Morphologie Mathématique,
35, rue Saint-Honoré, F-77305 Fontainebleau Cedex, France

Abstract. Our purpose is to design a sampling scheme that minimizes the number of sampling pixels in a grey tone image while ensuring a given accuracy. Moreover, this accuracy should be preserved under increasing and/or linear transformations. The convenient framework is that of the equicontinuous model, which is reminded in Secs. 2 and 3. It is then shown that the sampling problem requires a specific piece of information about the image under study. It is introduced and called inverse module. It is used to reduce by four the data points without visual degradation, and in a way that satisfies the imposed requirements.

Key words: equicontinuous function, mathematical morphology, image sampling, Hausdorff distances, morphological sampling.

1. Introduction

The sampling problems can be set in two ways, which are mutually converse:

– Given a sampling pattern, to which extent a given property is preserved?

– How to design the sampling pattern, when a given property is required?

In the present study, we shall consider successively both aspects of the problem, when the requirements are the following:

1. To provide an estimate f^* of a numerical function f such that, at any point x, the error between the two values is lower or equal to a given bound b:

$$\max_{x \in E} \{|f(x) - f^*(x)|\} \leq \psi_0.$$

2. To be able to predict the evolution of the maximum error when linear or morphological transformations are performed on both f and f^*.

There already exist several approaches for morphological sampling. The most classical one is geostatistics, but it does not ensure requirement 2. In [5] the two problems of accuracy after increasing mapping, and of 2-D homotopy preservation were treated in the binary framework only.

Other approaches were developed by Haralick *et al.* [2], on the one hand, and by Heijmans and Toet [3], on the other hand. The first study extends to grey tone images some sampling conditions already established in [5], the second approach involves a very useful multiresolution scheme. Both are based on an a priori (fixed or hierarchical) scheme for generating the sampling grid. The final operation of reconstruction is obtained by means of dilations or closings. Our approach differs from the previous ones in the sense that we will introduce, globally and locally, a piece of information stemming from the image under study, and that describes its degree of irregularity (namely the modulus of continuity and its inverse).

J.Serra and P. Soille (eds.), Mathematical Morphology and Its Applications to Image Processing, 117-124

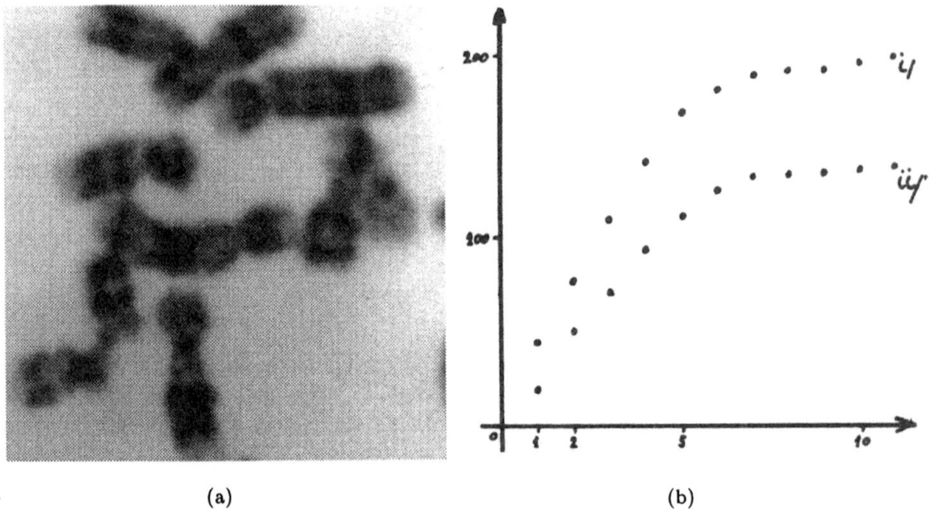

Fig. 1. (a) Chromosomes image. (b) Modulus of continuity of *(a)* i/ initial image, opening-closing size 1, opening size 10; ii/ opening-closing size 10.

2. Reminder on equicontinuous models

2.1. Modulus of continuity

With any numerical function f from a metric space E into $\overline{\mathbf{R}}$ one can always associate a second function, say φ, from $\mathbf{R}$ into $\overline{\mathbf{R}}$, as follows:

$$\varphi(h) = \sup\{|f(x) - f(y)|,\ x, y \in E, d(x,y) \leq h\}. \tag{1}$$

Equation 1 is absolutely general, and results in an increasing positive function. Now, if in addition f is supposed to be *uniformly continuous*, then, equivalently [1, pp. 1-17], we have

$$\lim_{h \to 0} \varphi(h) = 0,$$

i.e., φ is continuous near the origin. In this case, φ is called *modulus of continuity* and describes, in some sense, the degree of regularity of the function f under study. This approach can be compared with the use of the variogram, or the covariance, in the order two analysis. But, unlike the variogram, which provides the *quadratic mean* of the variation between two points, here we take into account the *maximum* absolute difference. For example, by adding to f a point impulse of maximum intensity, we do not change the variogram (in the Euclidean case) whereas the modulus is transformed into its horizontal asymptote, and becomes a Heaviside function.

In practice, the modulus φ is a meaningful descriptor. One can see from Figs. 1a and 1b how the range of φ reflects the sizes of the features in f, and its asymptote their dynamics.

Also, it is noticeable that Eq. 1 does *not* involve a possible translation invariance for the metric d of space E. Not only Eq. 1 is translation free, but it also applies to both continuous and discrete spaces. Actually, it will allow us to bridge the gap between the two cases. Therefore, we adopt the following notations: E denotes an arbitrary metric space of distance d ($\mathbf{R}^n$, $\mathbf{Z}^n$, their cond. versions, etc.) and T denotes a closed interval of $\overline{\mathbf{R}}$ or $\overline{\mathbf{Z}}$. For example [0,255] in the digital case, or [0,m] in the continuous one, or again $\overline{\mathbf{R}}$ or $\overline{\mathbf{Z}}$ themselves. By using E and T, we avoid the cumbersome distinction between discrete and Euclidean approaches.

2.2. Equicontinuous classes

The modulus of continuity turns out to be a tool for classifying the functions, and for grouping them into families that exhibit nice common properties. Here, the notion of equicontinuity w.r. to modulus φ, or more briefly, of φ-continuity, is used as a starting point.

Definition 1 *[1] A function $f : E \to T$ is φ-continuous when, given a modulus of continuity φ we have for all $x, y \in E$,*

$$|f(x) - f(y)| \leq \varphi[d(x,y)].$$

Similarly, the family of all functions $f : E \to T$ which satisfy the above inequality, for a given modulus φ is called φ-continuous, and denoted by $(T^E)_\varphi$.

Hence, the members of the φ-continuous classes are uniformly continuous functions, and

$$\varphi_1 \leq \varphi_2 \Rightarrow (T^E)_{\varphi_1} \subseteq (T^E)_{\varphi_2}. \tag{2}$$

As far as morphological treatments over $(T^E)_\varphi$, are concerned, the following results [8] provide an instructive guide line.

Theorem 2 *Given a modulus of continuity φ, the class $(T^E)_\varphi$ is a complete lattice for the usual* sup *and* inf *(i.e. the numerical* sup *and* inf *at each point $x \in E$).*

In other words, the type of variation, as described by φ-continuity is preserved under sup and inf operations.

We will now consider the transformations acting on an equicontinuous class $(T^E)_\varphi$. Every flat dilation or erosion is characterized by a structuring element mapping $K : E \to \mathcal{K}'$ that associates a non empty compact set with each point of E. Denote by ρ the Hausdorff distance, and assume that

$$\rho[K(x), K(y)] \leq d(x,y). \tag{3}$$

This hypothesis covers, among others, the conditional (or not) translation invariant cases. It allows us to state

Theorem 3 *Every* sup, inf, *and composition product of dilations or erosions by structuring elements that satisfies Eq. 3 applies $(T^E)_\varphi$ into itself and is continuous.*

For a more general statement, without the restriction of Eq. 3, refer to theorems 11—13 in [8]. As it is, theorem 3 says that all flat increasing mappings realized in practice preserve $(T^E)_\varphi$, and are continuous on it. Finally the modulus of continuity turns out to be *the* morphological invariant for numerical functions. Figure 1b illustrates this point. Neither an elementary close-open filter, nor an opening of

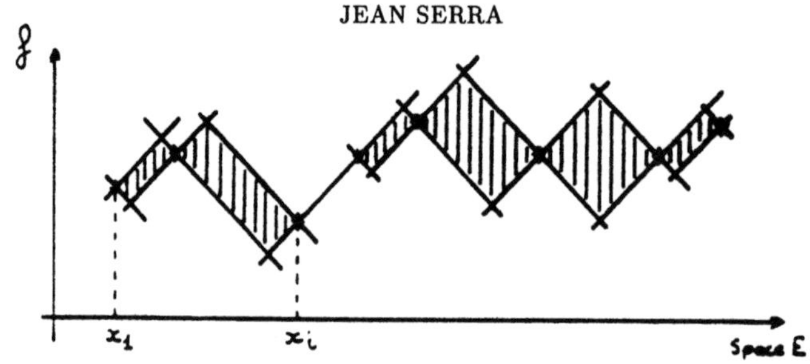

Fig. 2. Sampling of function f at points x_i. The modulus φ is the straight line of unit slope. The uncertainty zone is drawn in dash lines.

size 10 change the modulus of "chromosome" image; but if the opening is followed by a closing of the same size 10, then the modulus reduces appreciably. Then, according to rel. 2, this filtered image still belongs to the same class as the original "chromosome".

Concerning the linear transforms, some results are classical. If $f \in (T^E)_\varphi$ is convolved by a function g, with $v = \int |g(x)|\, dx$ then $f * g$ has a modulus $\varphi' = v\varphi$ (e.g. affinity, moving averages, etc.). In particular, in the digital case, Beucher's gradient

$$grad\,(f) = \frac{(f \oplus B) - (f \ominus B)}{2}$$

admits the same modulus as f itself.

3. Sampling

3.1. Global approach

φ-continuous functions perfectly lend themselves to sampling. Given a sampling pattern, if we know both the modulus φ of function f and the sampling $f^*$of f on the points of set S, then f is obviously comprised between the two envelopes of f^* by closing and by opening according to the cone of generator φ (see Fig. 2). This first Shannon type result, and also theorem 3, keenly suggest to look at the combination "sampling + image transformation". For increasing mappings, the approach is driven by the following result, due to Serra [9]:

Theorem 4 *Let K be a compact zone under study, S a sampling pattern for $f \in (T^E)_\varphi$ and let $\rho(K,S)$ be the Hausdorff distance between these sets. Then*

$$\left| \sup_{x \in K} \{f(x)\} - \sup_{x \in S} \{f(x)\} \right| \leq \varphi(\rho),$$

and dual result for inf. *Consequently, when S is a square grid of spacing a, for any compact infimum ψ of dilations on $(T^E)_\varphi$, whose restriction to S is $\psi^\star$, we have*

$$|(\psi f)(x) - (\psi^\star f)(x)| \leq \varphi(a\sqrt{2}/2) \qquad x \in E$$

The first part of the theorem is nothing but the algebraic version of conic openings and closings of Fig. 2. The underlying property is here that of the robustness of the grey tone lattice T for the distance $d(a,b) = |a-b|$, i.e.

$$\begin{cases} d(\bigvee_i a_i, \bigvee_i b_i) \leq \sup_i \{d(a_i,b_i)\} \\ d(\bigwedge_i a_i, \bigwedge_i b_i) \leq \sup_i \{d(a_i,b_i)\} \end{cases} \tag{4}$$

for all families (a_i, b_i) in $T \times T$. As a matter of fact, theorem 4 remains true for any ecart d that fulfills both inequalities in 4.

Another underlying background here, is the metric t associated with the uniform convergence, namely

$$t(f,g) = \sup_{x \in E} \{|f(x) - g(x)|\} \tag{5}$$

for every pair of functions f, g in $(T^E)_\varphi$. One can interpret geometrically distance t as a Hausdorff distance between functions, for balls reduced to the vertical segments.

Example: The initial image f_1 is the road scene presented in Fig. 3a. Its modulus of continuity values 60 at step 1 and ranges at 148 at step 20. Take the subgrid g_r that divides by four the number of pixels (one point out of two, one line out of two). Perform on the sampled image, first the square dilation of size 10, and second the square closing of size 10 followed by the square opening of the same size. Expand the sampled image by a small dilation of size one, to cover the empty zones between two samplings. This results in function f_r. The same expansion, applied to the 10-square dilation results in f_r and, to the 10-open closing, in f_4. The t-Hausdorff distances between f and the sampled expansions are

$$t(f, f_1) = t(f, f_2) = 60 \text{ and } t(f, f_3) = 40$$

a result that corroborates theorem 4. For functions f and f_2, whose grey tone variation ranges from 0 to 140, a t-distance of 60 is considerable, and noticeably alters the quality of f_2 (see Fig. 3b). We will try to correct this poor first result by a more local approach.

3.2. Local approach

In the previous approach, the local aspect of a point x operates through the respective geometrics of K and S. But there exist other features, useful for sampling, which are not purely geometric. The zone around x may be flat or fluctuating. Unfortunately the modulus φ gives only a *global* view of such variations, without informing us on the neighbourhood of a specific point x.

Now, an important sampling problem is that of local sub-sampling. It can be stated as follows: *Starting from the datum of the whole image f, what is the minimal number of values to be kept in order to ensure the knowledge of f within a given accuracy, and where must we implant the sampling points?*

This problem, which is the converse of that solved by theorem 4, requires some local piece of information. First, introduce a local version of the modulus φ by associating, with each point x, the maximum variation of f over the ball $B_x(h)$ of size h and centred at x:

$$\varphi_x(h) = \max\{(\delta_h f - f)(x) \; ; \; (f - \varepsilon_h f)(x)\} \tag{6}$$

where δ_h and ε_h are the dilation and the erosion by the $B_x(h)$'s.

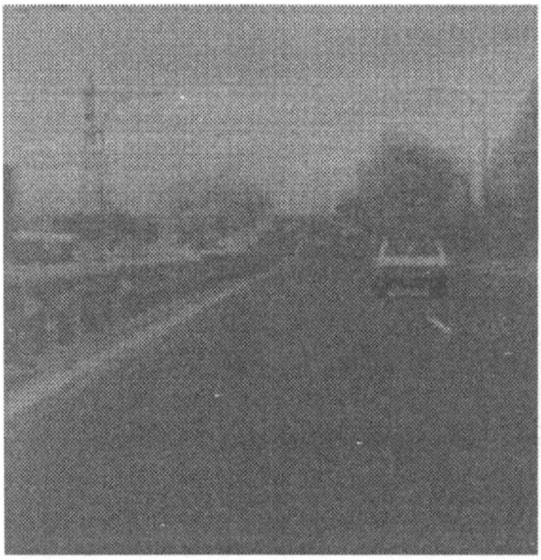

(a)

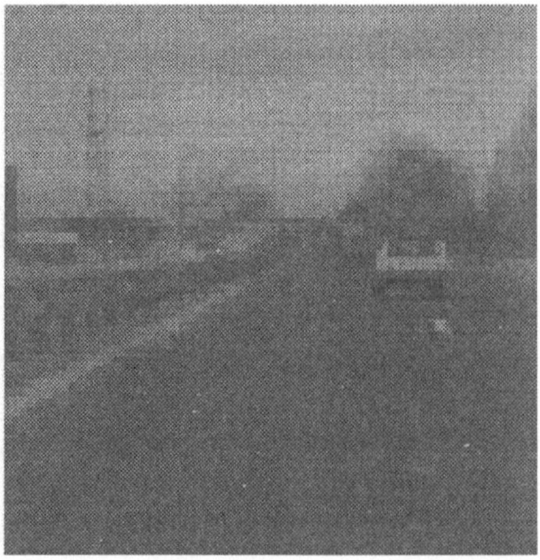

(b)

Fig. 3. (a) initial image f. (b) sampled version of f after a pixel reduction by four, following the square grid 2×2. The number of sampling pixels is $(128)^2 = 16,384$

Second, consider the so-called inverse $h_x(\varphi)$ of $\varphi_x(h)$. The value $h_x(\varphi)$ is the size of the minimum ball centred at x such that the fluctuation (in the sense of Eq. 6) be greater than or equal to the positive number φ. Function $h_x(\varphi)$ depends on two variables, but if we set the accuracy φ to be, say φ_0, then $h_x(\varphi_0) = h(x)$ becomes a numerical function of x only. The sampling protocol is then achieved by a downstream approach. Set $\varphi = \varphi_0$ and the value $a = 2^i$ for the largest sampling convenient spacing, and determine

$$X(a) = X(2^i) = \{x \,:\, h(x) \leq a\}\,.$$

Sample $X(2^i)$ with a grid $G(2^i)$ of spacing 2^i:

$$Y(2^i) = X(2^i) \cap G(2^i).$$

The points of $Y(2^i)$ have a certain zone of influence $k(i)$, hence the set $\delta_{k(i)}[Y(2^i)]$ indicates the zone of the space accessible from sample $Y(2^i)$. Iterate, by putting:

$$\begin{aligned} X(2^{i-1}) &= \{x \,:\, h(x) \leq a/2\} \setminus \delta_{k(i)}[Y(2^i)] \\ Y(2^{i-1}) &= X(2^{i-1}) \cap G(2^{i-1}) \end{aligned}$$

where $\setminus$ denotes the set difference. The dilation size $k(i)$ depends on the type of grid, and is calculated to make the influence zones contiguous, but not overlapping, at two successive steps. For square grids, for example, function $k(i)$ is given by the recurrence formula:

$$k(i) + k(i-1) = 2^i - 1 \tag{7}$$

with $k(0) = 0$ as initial condition, since grid $G(1)$, associated with value $i = 0$, must correspond to the full sampling. Figure 4a shows the result of this iterative sampling

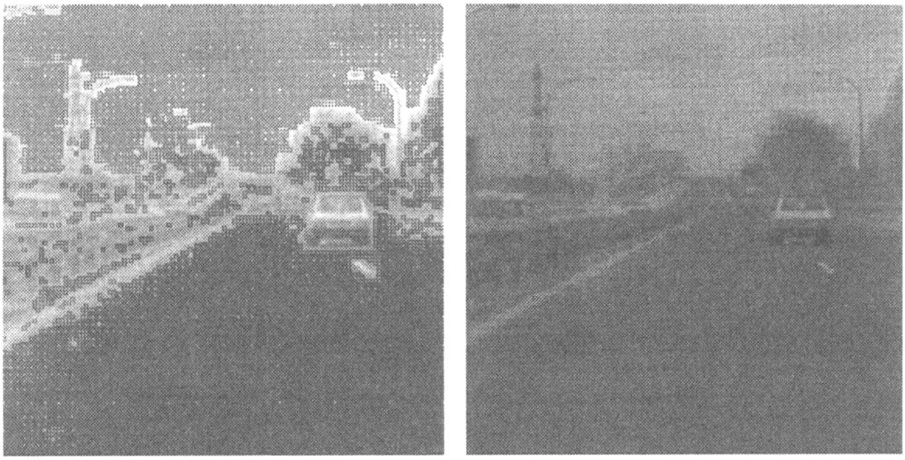

(a) (b)

Fig. 4. (a) Sampling grid G derived from the inverse modulus h. The number of sampling pixels is 15, 992. (b) Sampled image obtained from grid 5. Compare the quality with that of Fig. 3 (whereas the latter is obtained by more sampling pixels).

scheme, when applied to the road image, and where the white points are those of grid G:

$$G = \cup \{Y(2^j), 1 \leq j \leq \log a\}$$

The estimation $f^\star$ of f is obtained by dilating f at the sampling points $Y(2^j)$ by the square $k(j)$, and by taking the max for $j \in [1, \log a]$. This leads to Fig. 4b.

At each point x, the quantity $|f(x) - f^\star(x)|$ is by construction $\leq \varphi_0$. Hence the t-Hausdorff distance between f and its estimate is in turn $\leq \varphi_0$: $t(f, f^\star) \leq \varphi_0$.

When the final grid G is determined, there are several ways to affect grey tone values to the pixels. In the overlapping zones, one can give any value between the min and the max associated with the squares which overlap. The distance criterion 5 always remains satisfied. Visually speaking, the arithmetic mean is softer than the max, and allows us to enlarge φ_0 for a same visual quality. Also, we are not obliged to keep φ_0 constant. By reducing it for large spacings we can improve the look of the flat zones.

4. Optimal sampling and downstream operations

Let $f^\star$ be obtained from $f \in (T^E)_\varphi$, for a given accuracy φ_0, by the sampling scheme 3-2. We remark, first, that $f^\star$ belongs to $(T^E)_\varphi$, i.e. admits φ as modulus of continuity. Indeed, the squares of sizes $k(i)$ are always smaller than the spacings 2^i; therefore, the accuracy φ_0 is extended beyond the size of each square $k(i)$, for $i \geq 1$. Hence, if the module of continuity $\varphi(i)$ is larger than $2\varphi_0$, for $i \geq 1$, the sampling process cannot increase it.

Consider now an increasing and vertically invariant mapping ψ. It is known [6] that one can always represent ψ as an inf of dilations δ_j, $j \in J$. With each point x, and for each $j \in J$, the transform (ψf) is given by the relation

$$(\psi f)(x) = \bigwedge_{j \in J} \bigvee \{f(y) + g_j(y,x), y \in E\},$$

where the structuring function $g_j(*,x)$, depending on point x, characterizes the dilation δ_j. Since lattice T is robust, we may apply both inequalities of rel. (4), and write

$$|(\psi f)(x) - (\psi f^\star)(x)| \leq \bigvee_{y \in E} |f(y) - f^\star(y)| \leq \varphi_0.$$

Hence, the accuracy φ_0 is preserved under increasing mapping. The case of linear operations is treated in a similar way. At each point x, we have

$$(\psi f)(x) = \int f(x) g(y,x) dx,$$

for a function $g(*,x)$, that depends on the location x. Introducing the scalar range

$$r = \bigvee \left\{ \int |g(y,x)| \, dx, y \in E \right\}$$

we see that, for all $x \in E$

$$|(\psi f)(x) - (\psi f^\star)(x)| < r \bigvee \{|f(y) - f^\star(y)|, y \in E\} < r.\varphi_0$$

$$i.e.\ t(\psi f, \psi f^\star) \leq r.\varphi_0.$$

For example, if ψ is an affinity of ratio 3, the accuracy will be multiplied by 3.

Theorem 5 *Let $f^\star$ be the result of the sampling scheme 3-2, when applied to function $f \in (T^E)_\varphi$. Then $f^\star$ belongs to $(T^E)_\varphi$ and we have, for every increasing mapping ψ,*

$$t(\psi f, \psi f^\star) \leq \varphi_0,$$

and for every linear mapping ω of scalar range r:

$$t(\omega f, \omega f^\star) \leq r.\varphi_0 .$$

References

1. G. Choquet. *Topology.* Academic Press, 1966.
2. R.M. Haralick, X. Zhuang, C. Lin, J.S.J. Lee. The digital morphological sampling theorem. *IEEE Trans. Acous. Speech, Signal Proc.*, Vol. 37, pp. 2067-2090, December 1989.
3. H. Heijmans, A. Toet. Morphological sampling. *CVGIP: Image Understanding*, Vol. 54, pp. 384-400, November 1991.
4. G. Matheron. *Les treillis compacts,* Technical report, Ecole des Mines de Paris, 1990.
5. J. Serra. *Image Analysis and Mathematical Morphology,* Vol. 1, Academic Press, 1982.
6. J. Serra. Mathematical Morphology for complete Lattices. In J. Serra, editor, *Image Analysis and Mathematical Morphology. Volume 2: Theoretical Advances*, chapter 1, pp. 13–35. Academic Press, 1988.
7. J. Serra. Lipschitz lattices and numerical morphology. *SPIE Conf. Image Algebra and Morphological Image Processing,* San Diego, July 1991.
8. J. Serra. Equicontinuous functions: A model for mathematical morphology. *SPIE San Diego Conf.* Vol. 1769, pp. 252-263, July 1992.
9. J. Serra. Les treillis de fonctions équicontinues. *Colloque Géométrie Discrète et Imagerie,* Chassery et al. Eds, ULP, IMAG; CNRS publ., Strasbourg, September 1993.

APPLICATION OF MORPHOLOGICAL FILTERS FOR CONTOUR IMAGE SEQUENCE CODING

CHUANG GU and MURAT KUNT
Signal Processing Laboratory
Swiss Federal Institute of technology
CH-1015, Lausanne, Switzerland
Tel: +41 21 693 4682, Fax: +41 21 693 7600, Email: cgu@ltssun4.epfl.ch

Abstract. In this paper, an improved method for contour image sequence coding is described [1]. It is based on motion estimation, compensation and morphological filters. In order to exploit the high temporal redundancy of the contour image sequence, motion estimation and compensation are used for the correspondent label image sequence. The first frame is directly coded by using lossless Chain-Code method. All the following frames are coded in motion compensation mode. Within each frame, labels are divided into foreground and background labels. Only the prediction error for the foreground labels are coded. Morphological filters are applied to clean the prediction error for the foreground labels. Afterwards, an efficient prediction error coding algorithm is shown. For contour simplification purpose, a new Morphology-like filter is introduced. Experimental results have demonstrated outstanding performance in the coding of contour image sequence for very low bitrate coding.

Key words: contour coding, D-filter, motion compensation, region adjacent graph, chain-code, occurrence coding.

1. Introduction

Recently, there is an increasing interest in the field of very low bitrate image sequence coding in order to develop new applications such as multimedia database, videophone, etc. Unfortunately, existing standards such as H.261 does not produce satisfactory results on that low band width. New techniques based on the second generation methods [1] taking into account the characteristics of the human visual system is a focus of the current researches. This kind of methods attempt to describe an image in terms of contour and texture. These entities seem to be more natural in that they coincide with psychological concepts of vision. Each object in a natural scene is characterized by its borders (contours) surrounding its surfaces (texture).

During the past few years, many researches have been carried out towards that direction. Traditional segmentation [2] by split and merge of variable block size does not provide precise partition along the object boundary, which leads to visual block artifacts. Meanwhile, Mathematical Morphology has demonstrated outstanding performance as a non-linear image processing tool [3] [4]. It is particularly powerful for the image(s) segmentation [5] [6] [7]. In [6], an unsupervised image segmentation algorithm based on a multiscale approach is proposed which allows a hierarchical processing of the data ranging from the most global scale to the most detailed one. Later [8], this concept is extended to 3D images (2D plus time) as a three dimen-

[1] This work was done within European RACE/Morpheco project.

J.Serra and P. Soille (eds.), Mathematical Morphology and Its Applications to Image Processing, 125-132

sional segmentation of the video sequence. This approach successfully avoided the random fluctuations of the contours and solved the region correspondence problem.

The contour coding represents really a bottleneck for low bit-rate coding. In the 2D case, the well known chain code [9] method needs roughly 1.2 bits per contour pixel, under some constraints [10]. In [11], a modified Chain-code method was developed which takes into account the location of "triple-point" thus improves the coding efficiency. In the 3D case, the spatial-temporal contours make situation even worse. There is few work existing in literature to code the contour image sequence. Although the binary-tree algorithm described in [2] can code the still boundary parts of 3D contours the same way as quadtree coding in 2D situation, it does not work well for moving boundary parts. Actually, it is too costly and not necessary to code contour image sequence losslessly. The high temporal redundancy should be exploited.

On the other hand, motion estimation and motion compensation successively exploit the temporal redundancy for graylevel image sequence. Motion estimation analyses the movement of objects in an image sequence, and this interframe displacement information allows for the improvement of predictive and interpolative coding. To estimate the displacement vector of a moving object from two successive frames, several techniques have been developed, which essentially belong to two main groups: block-based or region-based algorithms. Based on the segmentation algorithm chosed here, a region-based method is naturally used in order to obtain more realistic motion.

The main idea of our method is to code the first contour frame losslessly by Chain-code and make the prediction for the following frames by motion compensation and only code the prediction errors. Several methods [12] [13] were presented to reduce these prediction errors and to code them efficiently. In this paper, an improved version of the codec with extensive use of Morphological filters will be introduced. Finally, the number of bits needed to code the contour for successive frames reduce drastically.

In Section 2, motion estimation and compensation algorithm is described. The application of Morphological filters is presented in Section 3. In Section 4, an efficient coding method for the prediction error is shown. The problem of how to reconstruct the background labels after the reconstruction of foreground labels is solved in Section 5. A new Morphology-like filter for contour simplification is introduced in Section 6. Finally, the experimental results are demonstrated with a conclusion remark.

2. Motion estimation and compensation

2.1. Region-based motion estimation algorithm

In order to achieve high compression ratio, the temporal redundancy of the contour image sequence should be exploited. After the time-recursive three dimensional morphological segmentation [8] is applied to the original image sequence, a labeled image sequence is obtained. A region with the same label indicates a homogeneous region. From this labeled image sequence, we can immediately get the contour image sequence and vice versa. It is obvious to find the high redundancy existing in two successive frames. Motion estimation and compensation are introduced here to predict the current label frame from the previous received label frame.

A simple translational motion model is used here to reduce the supplementary cost due to the coding of the motion parameters. It is easy to find that an accurate estimation of the label movement will considerablely reduce the prediction error. For each region, the prediction error is calculated as the total number of label pixels which are not correctly motion compensated in the current frame. A fast full-search motion estimation algorithm for label images [14] was developed in order to minimize the prediction error. It avoids to estimate the motion of each region separately, but deals with all them together. Comparing to traditional full-search motion estimation algorithm, there is a significant improvement of the speed with a fact of:

$$k = \frac{O(old)}{O(new)} = \frac{2 \cdot S_x \cdot S_y \cdot L_x \cdot L_y \cdot R}{S_x \cdot S_y \cdot (L_x \cdot L_y + R)} = \frac{2 \cdot L_x \cdot L_y \cdot R}{(L_x \cdot L_y + R)} \approx 2 \cdot R \tag{1}$$

where R is the total number of regions, S_x, S_y are the lengths of the searching window, L_x, L_y are the sizes of the current image. At last, a translational motion vector is assigned to each labeled region.

2.2. Separation of foreground and background

Since the forward motion estimation is used, adjacent regions in the previous frame will cause overlapped prediction regions in the current frame, which need even more bits to represent them. In order to solve this problem, a region adjacency graph (RAG) which represents the adjacency relation between different regions is constructed in the current frame, see Figure 1. Depending on thc quantity of prediction error, an order list is built to indicate the order to translate each region, for example, $R_1R_4R_3R_2R_5$ where R_1 has the minimal prediction error and R_5 has the maximal prediction error. Based on the RAG and this order, the regions in the current frame can be easily separated into foreground and background regions. By using a stack structure, each time a region is popped out to be checked. If all of it's surrounding regions are foreground regions, it is defined as a background region. If not, it is defined as a foreground region. In the case of Figure 1, $R_1R_4R_5$ will be defined as foreground regions and R_2R_5 as background regions. Only the prediction errors for the foreground regions need to be transmitted. The boundary of background regions are naturally defined by the reconstructed foreground regions. By eliminating the background regions, the prediction error components are greatly reduced, which leads to a very efficient representation.

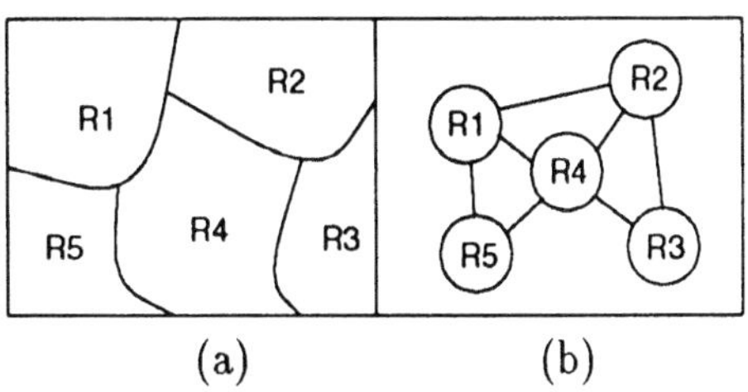

Fig. 1. (a) Labeled image in current frame; (b) Region Adjacent Graph (RAG)

3. Morphological filters with size of 2 by 2

After motion estimation and compensation applied to the foreground regions, the resulting prediction errors are still rather noisy. Morphological filters are introduced to purge these binary regions. As we know, a simple opening can delete objects with a certain size. But it will also cause the boundary degradation for the large regions. Fortunately, the opening by reconstruction [15] does not have this drawback. Afterwards, the size of the structural element should be determined. The opening by reconstruction of 3 by 3 will erase those objects of size two, in other words all objects which can not contain the 3 by 3 structural element will be removed. In the case of our contour coding scheme, this will cause a maximal two-pixel error for the contour location which is too large for very low bitrate application. So, a 2 by 2 structural element is used. Then the deviation problem will occur, see Figure 2. A simple method is developed by upsampling first and using 3 by 3 structural element followed with a downsampling.

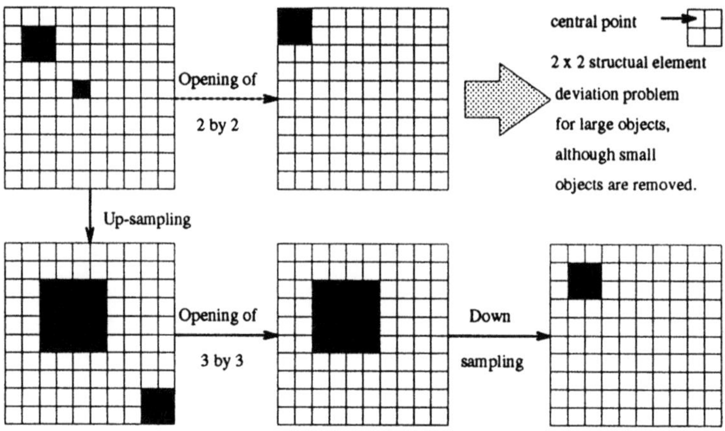

Fig. 2. Comparison of using 2 by 2 structural element directly and an up-down method

So, the morphological opening by reconstruction of size 2x2 is used to clean the prediction error of each foreground region. This step ensures the preservation of the boundary for large prediction error while erasing those small noisy errors. Here, the loss of information is introduced with a tolerable maximal one-pixel error for the contour location.

To further reduce the prediction fragments for the foreground regions, a mask is incrementally constructed in the current frame to indicate the region where boundaries have already been settled. Therefore, any prediction fragment which falls into this mask should not be considered.

4. Prediction Error Coding

An efficient coding method has to be found to code the prediction error. From Figure 3(a), it is easy to find that the boundaries of the prediction error area are composed of motion compensated boundaries and the new boundaries in current frame. Only the new boundaries need to be coded. These new boundaries are divided into two groups: boundaries which define the area to be added (R2) and boundaries which define the area to be deleted (R1). From Figure 3(b), we can find that actually only the thick curves need to be coded. For the coding of a single and continues digital curve, the derivative Chain-code [10] is the most efficient method. Instead of using differential position coding method to code the starting points, occurrence coding method [14] is used. The idea is to code the correct occurrence number of new boundaries. In the case of Figure 3, only a number 1 needs to be coded which means the first possible position to put the thick curve is the correct one. The new occurrence coding method significantly improves the coding efficiency of the starting points.

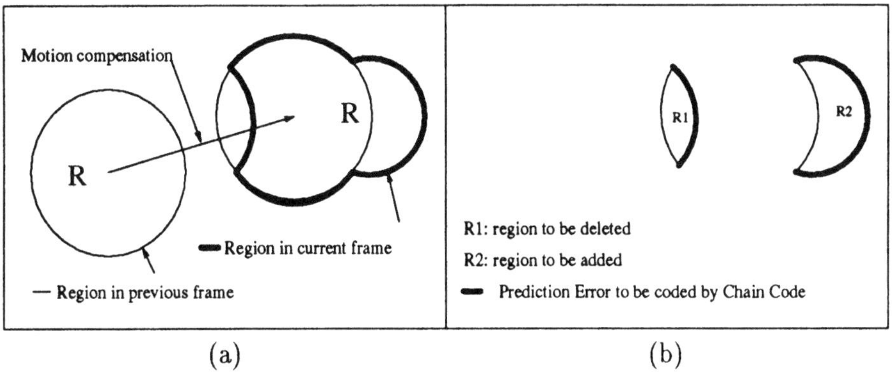

Fig. 3. (a) Region-based motion compensation; (b) Prediction error coding

It should be mentioned that the new appeared regions in the current frame are directly coded by the modified Chain-Code [11] since there are no correspondent regions in the previous frame which can be used to predict them. At last, only the motion vectors, the prediction error and the order for the foreground regions need to be coded and transmitted.

5. Reconstruction of foreground and background regions

At the decoder side, the foreground regions are constructed based on previous label frame, motion vectors, prediction error and order for foreground regions. As in the encoder part, a mask is constructed incrementally to indicate the area where boundaries have already been settled. Any compensated part which falls into this area should be neglected.

After the reconstruction of the foreground labels, a reference mask in the current frame can be obtained indicating the background area which needs to be reconstructed. In order to erase those cracks which are caused by opening by reconstruction of size 2 by 2 for foreground prediction errors, an opening of size 2 by 2 is applied to the background area to get this reference mask. Then, a mark image for the background labels in the current frame is obtained by motion compensation for the background labels from the previous frame within the reference image. It can be considered as a partially reconstructed background labels. Afterwards, a geodesic dilation of this label marks within the reference mask leads to the complete reconstruction of the whole background labels, see Figure 4. Thus, for still part of the image, zero

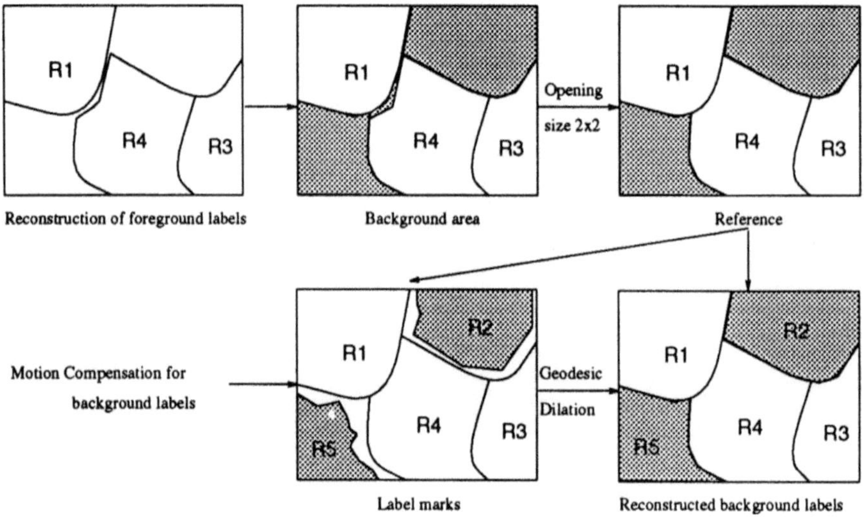

Fig. 4. Reconstruction of foreground and background

valued motion vector needs to be transmitted. For moving part of the image, only those contours of foreground regions which can not be motion compensated need to be transmitted. The effects are two-fold: the contour points which need to be transmitted for each frame reduce drastically and small or noisy impulsive contours will be suppressed.

6. Pre/post-processing of contour

In many cases, contours are needed to be simplified both before (pre-processing) and after (post-processing) the coding in order to delete those small sparks which are insensitive to human visual system but cost much for contour coding. A multi-scale Morphology-like filter (D-filter) [16] is designed as follows to filter the label image in order to simplify the contours:

Assume point P is the label pixel under consideration, structural element R indicates an area surrounding P, and there are n different labels $(L_1, L_2, ..., L_n)$ existing in R with the total number of $N_1, N_2, ..., N_n$ for each label.

IF $N_i > N_j, 1 \leq j \leq n, j \neq i$
THEN label(P) = L_i
ELSE keep original label.

This operator is continuely applied on the label image until nothing changes in the label image (in practice, ten iterations is enough).

Actually, the D-filter chooses the dominant label (with the maximum number) around the point as the label for this point. It is obvious to find that the result is independent of the assignment of the labels in a segmentation. It only relys on the shape of the contours. The size and shape of the structural element R is variable, which can provide a multi-scale simplification. Meanwhile, the geometric structure of the segmentation is strictly preserved after applying the D-filter. In practice, the structural element of 3 by 3 square or cross shape are used to obtain the acceptable simplification effect. In this case, an imperceptible contour position error of one pixel will occur, while the bits for contour reduces at an average rate of 20%. Spark contour will disappear which results in a much more pleasant smoothed contour image. This simplification procedure is applied to the current label image both before and after the coding. Furthermore, the D-filter can be used in the upsampling part when the QCIF label image is converted into CIF format for display purpose. In this case, a 3 by 3 square structural element is used in order to smooth the zig-zaged label image after the upsampling procedure.

7. Results

Experiments have been carried out on two typical videophone sequences: Miss America and Carphone, with the segmentation algorithm proposed in [8]. The image format is QCIF at 5 Hz. A first order adaptive arithmetic coder is used for derivative chain code, occurrences and motion vectors. It is meaningless to only give a number of bitrate to compare the efficiency of the new contour coding algorithm with the traditional one, because the result also relies on the amount of contours appeared in the original segmentation. In Figure 5, 6, the comparison between lossless Chain-code (dashed line) and our method (solid line) with a maximal contour location error of one pixel is shown. The average number of bits for contour coding in interframe reduce 4 times less respectively. As for the texture coding part, a second order cosine orthonormal basis function is used. The final bitrate for Miss America and Carphone are 12 Kbits/s and 22 Kbits/s respectively. A video demo will be shown during the conference.

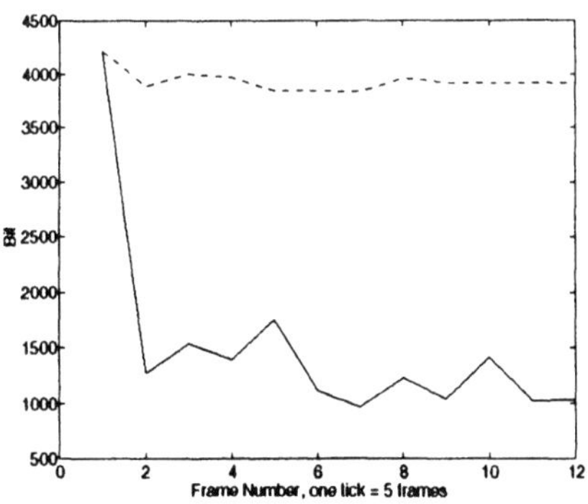

Fig. 5. Simulation result on Miss America

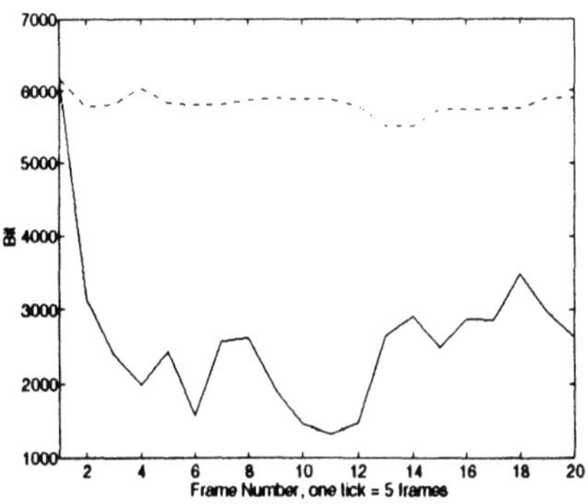

Fig. 6. Simulation result on Carphone

8. Conclusion

An efficient method for the coding of contour image sequence is presented in this paper. It aims at solving the bottleneck problem for the very low bit-rate applications based on contour-texture approach. Experimental results have shown a high compression ratio for contour image sequence while keeping good visual quality.

Acknowledgements

The authors wish to thank Dr. P. Salembier for his helpful comments and are grateful to Dr. H. Nicolas for the proofreading of this paper.

References

1. M. Kunt, A. Ikonomopoulos, and M. Kocher. Second generation image coding techniques. *Proceedings of the IEEE*, Vol. 73, No. 4, pp. 549–575, April 1985.
2. P. Willemin, T. Reed, and M. Kunt. Image sequence coding by split and merge. *IEEE Trans. Communications*, Vol. 39, No. 12, pp. 1845–1855, December 1991.
3. J. Serra (Ed). *Image analysis and Mathematical Morphology, Volume II*. Academic Press, Inc., London, 1988.
4. J. Serra and L. Vincent. An overview of morphological filtering. *Circuit Systems and Signal Processing*, Vol. 11, No. 1, pp. 47–108, 1992.
5. F. Meyer and S. Beucher. Morphological segmentation. *Journal of Visual Communication and Image Processing*, Vol. 1, No. 1, pp. 21–46, Sept. 1990.
6. P. Salembier and J. Serra. Morphological multiscale image segmentation. In *VCIP'92*, pages 1818–65, 1992.
7. C. Gu and M. Kunt. Multi-criterion segmentation for image sequence coding. In *EUSIPCO'94*, Edinburgh, U.K., September 1994.
8. M. Pardas, P. Salembier, and L. Torres. 3D morphological segmentation for image sequence processing. In *IEEE Winter Workshop on Nonlinear Signal Processing*, Tampere, Finland, January 1993.
9. H. Freeman. On the encoding of arbitrary geometric configurations. *IRE Trans. Electron. Comput.*, Vol. EC-10, pp. 260–268, June 1961.
10. M. Eden and M. Kocher. On the performance of contour coding algorithm in the context of image coding. part I: Contour segment coding. *Signal Processing*, Vol. 8, pp. 381–386, 1985.
11. F. Marqués, J. Sauleda, and T. Gasull. Shape and location coding for contour images. In *Picture Coding Symposium, PCS'93*, Lausanne, Switzerland, March 1993.
12. C. Gu and M. Kunt. Contour image sequence coding by motion compensation and morphological filters. In *International Workshop on Coding Techniques for Very Low Bit-rate Video, VLBV'94*, page 7.1, Cochestor, United Kingdom, April 1994.
13. C. Gu. 3D contour image coding by morphological filters and motion estimation. In *ICASSP'94*, Australia, April 1994.
14. C. Gu and M. Kunt. Efficient contour prediciton error coding. In *Picture Coding Symposium, PCS'94*, California, U.S.A., September 1994.
15. P. Salembier and M. Kunt. Size-sensitive multiresolution decomposition of images with rank order based filters. *Signal Processing*, Vol. 27, No. 2, pp. 205–241, May 1992.
16. C. Gu and M. Kunt. Contour simplification by a new nonlinear filter for region-based coding. In *VCIP'94*, Chicago, U.S.A., September 1994.

THE GEODESIC MORPHOLOGICAL SKELETON AND FAST TRANSFORMATION ALGORITHMS*

P. BRIGGER and M. KUNT
Signal Processing Laboratory
Swiss Federal Institute of Technology
CH-1015 Lausanne, Switzerland
Email: brigger@lts.de.epfl.ch

and

F. MEYER
Ecole des Mines de Paris, Centre de Morphologie Mathématique,
35, rue Saint-Honoré, F-77305 Fontainebleau Cedex, France

Abstract. A new method to encode and reconstruct the contours of a segmented image is described in this paper. Encoding is based on the morphological skeleton which is extended using geodesic distance functions. This allows us to fully take into account already coded labels and hence known contours and to avoid coding a contour twice. Moreover, fast algorithms for skeleton reconstruction based on hierarchical queues will be presented.

The algorithm is used for image sequence coding at very low bit-rates. The experimental results validate the chosen approach.

Key words: Morphological skeleton, geodesy, image sequence coding, very low bit-rates

1. Introduction

Contour coding is a bottle-neck in second generation based image coding approaches. Such methods consist in segmenting an image or image sequence into its pertinent objects of which contours and textures are coded and transmitted [5]. The Human Visual System is very sensitive to image contours and therefore they have to be well represented. The direct consequence is that the information assigned to contours represents a large part of the coded information.

The skeleton is a shape representation that has been known for a rather long time and it has been successfully used in many analysis applications. Lantuéjoul [6] has developed the formal definition in terms of morphological operations, given in the equation:

$$S(X) = \bigcup_{\rho>0} s_\rho(X) = \bigcup_{\rho>0} [\epsilon^\rho(X) \setminus \gamma^1(\epsilon^\rho(X))], \tag{1}$$

where $\epsilon^\rho(X)$ is an erosion of size ρ, and $\gamma^1(X)$ stands for the elementary opening. This formula applies in the case of the discrete space. The skeleton is found by

* This work was supported by the European RACE/Morpheco project 2053

J.Serra and P. Soille (eds.), Mathematical Morphology and Its Applications to Image Processing, 133-140

taking the centers of all maximal inscribed disks. A disk is maximal if there is no larger disk which can be inscribed into X and which contains the first disk.

The skeleton allows a lossless way of coding contours. It is composed of the skeleton points, which are the center points of the maximal inscribed disks. For each point, the size of the disk has to be known, which is called the quench function.

This definition has been employed for compact representation of one region [7]. The authors showed that the so defined skeleton contains redundant points, due to entirely overlapping structuring elements. Indeed, roughly 50% of the skeleton points can be eliminated while still guaranteeing a perfect reconstruction. In [4], morphological techniques are given for a partial elimination of these points.

In this paper, the skeleton will be extended to the geodesic skeleton in Section 2. This will allow its efficient use for the representation of boundaries of segmented images containing many regions. An algorithm for fast skeleton reconstruction and elimination of redundant points will be presented in Section 3 and Section 4. Results for applications at very low bit-rates are shown in Section 5 and conclusions drawn in Section 6.

2. The geodesic morphological skeleton

In [9], Meyer presents and develops some results established by Matheron [8], leading to a new definition for the skeleton on the digital grid. It characterizes the skeleton points as a special, well defined set on the distance function and leads to an extremely fast algorithm. In the following, we will give a short summary and show how it can be used in the context of image coding.

The skeleton is based on the distance function. Given a set X, then the distance function ρ at a point x of X is defined as:

$$\rho_X(x) = d(x, X^c) = \inf_{y \in X^c} d(x, y). \tag{2}$$

It can be easily seen, that there exists always at least one point y_0 on the boundary of X such that $d(x, y_0) = \rho_X(x)$. Starting from a point x, we call *upstream* of x, the set of points y satisfying the relationship

$$\rho(y) = \rho(x) + d(x, y). \tag{3}$$

If the upstream of x consists of just x itself, then x is a skeleton point. It leads to the following definition:

The skeleton is the set of points without other upstream than themselves.

or

The skeleton is the set of points without any higher neighbors.

The neighborhood relationship in the second definition is defined by the distance measure which is used. From this definition, we can derive the geodesic skeleton. It is obtained by restricting the point y_0 to some specific boundary points of X.

This proves very efficient in the case of segmented images. Here, the image space is partitioned into n different regions and every region is given a different number, going from 1 to n. In what follows, such a numbered region will be called a label and denoted X_i. As soon as one or several labels are coded, some boundaries are known at the receiver side and they do not have to be considered again. Thus, for the computation of the distance function in (2), the point y_0 may only occupy boundary points which are still unknown to the receiver.

If Z is the label to be skeletonized and if $m < n$ labels are already coded, the following distance function has to be computed:

$$\rho_S(z) = \inf_{y \in S^c} d(z,y), \tag{4}$$

where $S = (Z \cup (\cup_{i=1}^{m} X_i))$ and $z \in Z$. All points of $\rho_S(z)$ without higher neighbors are skeleton points. Therefore, as the coding proceeds, more and more labels and borders are known and it is taken into account for the remaining labels. The set S grows as the coding proceeds and thus S^c gets smaller with each coded label. In the distance function, less points without other upstream than themselves are present and therefore less skeleton points are needed for the coding of the remaining labels. An illustrative example is given in Fig. 1, where the dashed area represents labels that have already been coded. Therefore, all boundaries to a dashed area are known. The skeleton points are marked by a circle and they represent the minimal skeleton after removal of the redundant skeleton points.

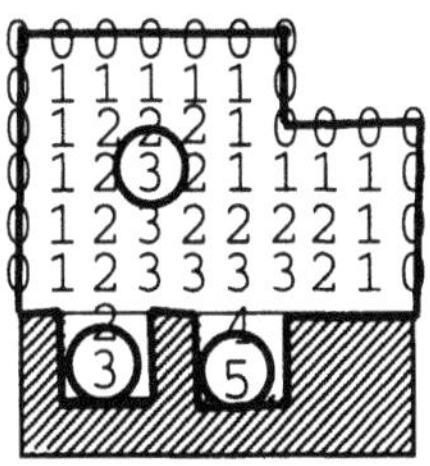

Fig. 1. Example of the geodesic skeleton

Experiments show that reductions of more than 50% of the skeleton points are obtained. Results on real segmented images are reported in Fig. 2 where a label image, its ordinary skeleton and its geodesic skeleton are shown.

The distance function can be implemented using a sequential algorithm requiring one image scan and then propagation of values using queues. Determining pixel without higher neighbors in the distance function requires only one more image scan resulting in an extremely fast skeleton computation. In order to obtain a minimal skeleton, redundant points have to be eliminated. This can be done individually for each skeleton disk using the reconstruction algorithm that will be presented in the next section.

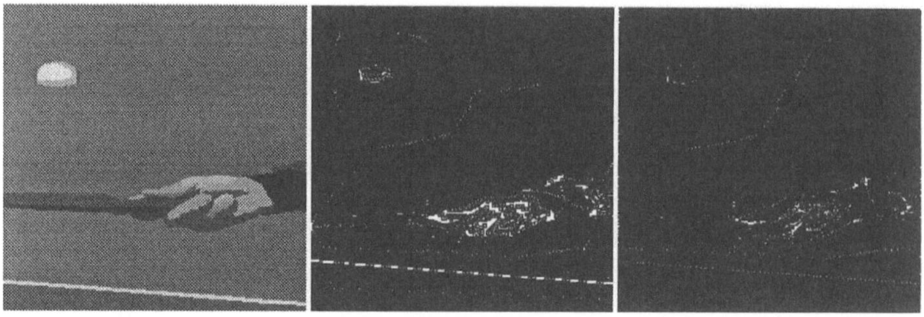

Fig. 2. Label image of the table tennis player (left) ordinary skeleton (middle) and geodesic skeleton (right)

3. Fast algorithm for decoding of the skeleton subset

In almost all image coding applications, the decoder ought to be working in real time. This requirement implies a structure which is (i) simple and (ii) efficient.

The geodesic skeleton allows an exact reconstruction of the original label image containing n labels by the following procedure:

$$X = \bigcup_{i=1}^{n} X_i, \qquad (5)$$

$$X_i = \bigcup_{\rho>0} \delta_R^{\rho}[s_{\rho}^{i}(x)],$$

where X_i represents label i in the segmented image, R is the reference set composed of the unknown area, $R = (\cup_{i=1}^{m} X_i)^c$ assuming that m labels are already coded. δ_R^{ρ} denotes geodesic dilation of size ρ with respect to reference R, s_{ρ}^{i} represents the skeleton points with corresponding quench function ρ for every label i. The order in which the reconstruction takes place has to be identical to the one used for the skeleton decomposition.

Thus, a simple reconstruction based on unions of dilations is guaranteed. However, the reconstruction process as defined in (5) is not efficient. The skeleton guarantees that every inscribed disk covers at least one point which is not covered by any other disk, but many points will be covered by several disks. It implies that during the reconstruction by dilation procedure, many points will be processed several times. In order to avoid this and to provide a most efficient dilation algorithm, we propose the use of hierarchical queues. The image will be scanned only once to put all skeleton points into the queue and only points involved in the dilation are processed.

Hierarchical queues are an excellent tool for such a task [2]. These are simply several FIFO (FirstInFirstOut) queues which are ordered according to a certain criterion. In our case, this is the size of the dilation.

Fig. 3a shows the original label. Its skeleton decomposition is shown in Fig. 3b. It consists of one point with quench function three, one point with quench function

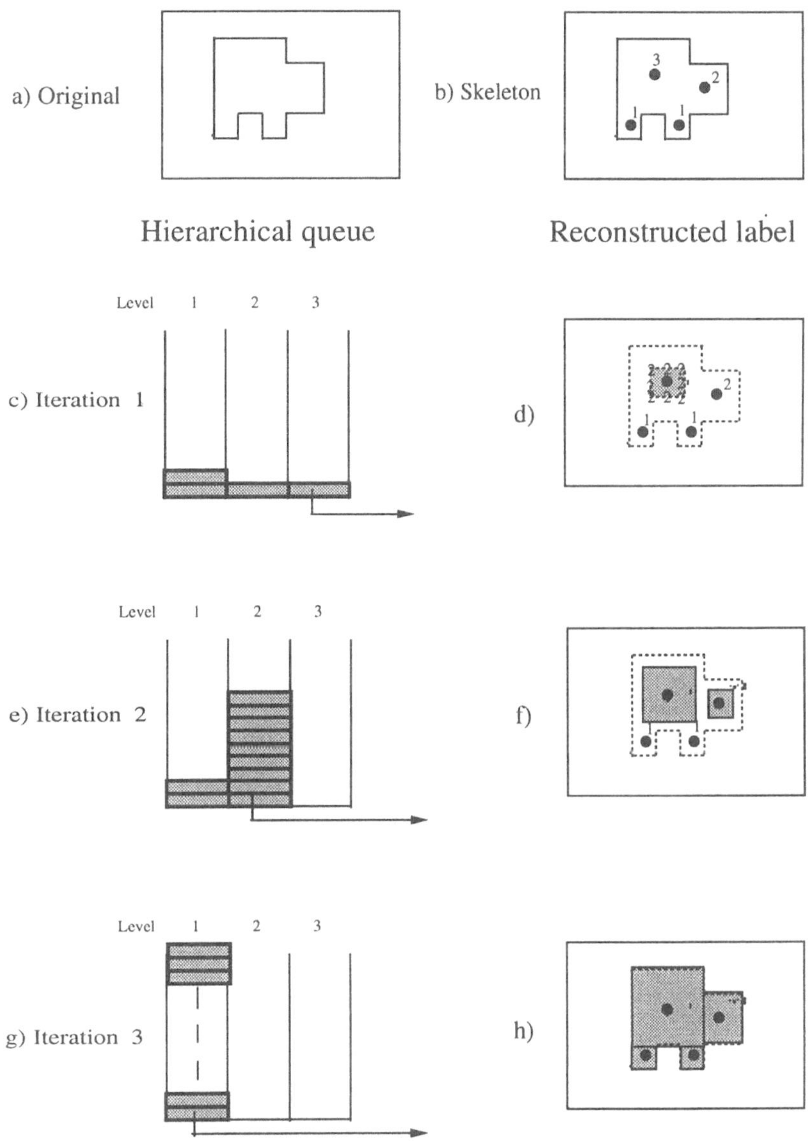

Fig. 3. Reconstruction using hierarchical queues

two and two points with quench function one. The image is initially scanned and the points put into the hierarchical queue. Thus, on the highest hierarchy level, there is one point. On level two there is one point and on level one there are two points, Fig. 3c.

The process starts by extracting the first element out of the queue, i.e. the skeleton subset point with quench function three, and to dilate it by one unit, Fig. 3c and Fig. 3d. If all neighbors are within the reference set, then eight new points are created, each of which will have to be dilated by size two and they are put into the queue at level two. Therefore, the queue at level two now contains nine elements, Fig. 3e. If queue number three is empty, dilation is continued at level two. Each element of queue two is taken out and dilated by one unit, Fig. 3f. The neighbors which have not yet been processed are put into queue at level one. When queue two is empty, queue one will contain 26 elements, Fig. 3g. They are extracted and dilated by one, Fig. 3h. The iteration stops when queue one is empty and the label reconstructed.

4. Elimination of redundant points

The skeleton computed using (4) contains redundant points, as pointed out in [7]. Using the results of the previous section, they can be detected efficiently. The redundancy elimination process takes place individually for each label right after the skeletonization process and consists of two steps.

1. A redundancy matrix is computed. For every pixel, the number of structuring elements that cover it are counted.
2. All skeleton points that cover an area that is already completely covered by other maximal structuring elements are removed.

Let us assume that m labels have already been coded, the reference set is $R = (\cup_{i=1}^{m} X)^c$. By $s_\rho^i(x)$ we denote the skeleton points of quench function ρ of label i. The redundancy matrix is then computed as:

$$D^i = \sum_\rho \sum_x \delta_R^\rho [s_\rho^i(x)], \tag{6}$$

where D^i is the redundancy matrix for label i and R is given as in (5). The dilation is a binary dilation with values 0 and 1. The redundancy matrix indicates for each pixel how many times it is covered by a structuring element.

In the second run, for each skeleton point it needs to be checked whether the redundancy matrix is ≥ 2 on the support defined by $\delta_R^\rho[s_\rho^i(x)]$. If this is the case, $s_\rho^i(x)$ can be removed as well as its contribution to the sum of D^i in (6). For the dilation, the fast algorithm with hierarchical queues is used. Furthermore, it is important to define the scan used for the second run. For coding purposes, a large area should be covered by as few skeleton points as possible. Thus, skeleton points with small quench function have to be removed first and therefore the scan has to start with $\rho = 0$.

5. Results

In the following, the skeleton decomposition was used as the contour coding element in a morphological image coding system [3]. The segmentation algorithm works on a sliding temporal window and produces a correspondence between labels in different frames [10].

Contours are motion compensated using an affine transformation [1] and the prediction residues are coded with the geodesic skeleton. In Fig. 4 the first four coded frames of the Miss America sequence are shown. The coding rate is 5 Hz, thus they correspond to frames 6, 11, 16 and 21 in the original frame . In Fig. 5 the skeleton points which have to be transmitted are shown. The corresponding bit-rates are given in Table I for QCIF image sequences (176 × 144) and 50 frames.

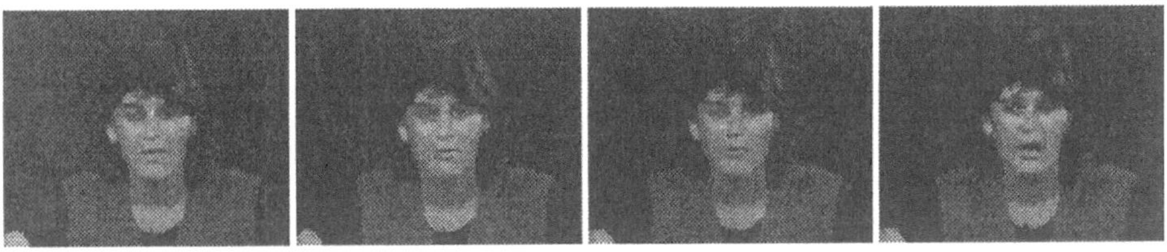

Fig. 4. First four coded frames (Coding rate: 5 Hz)

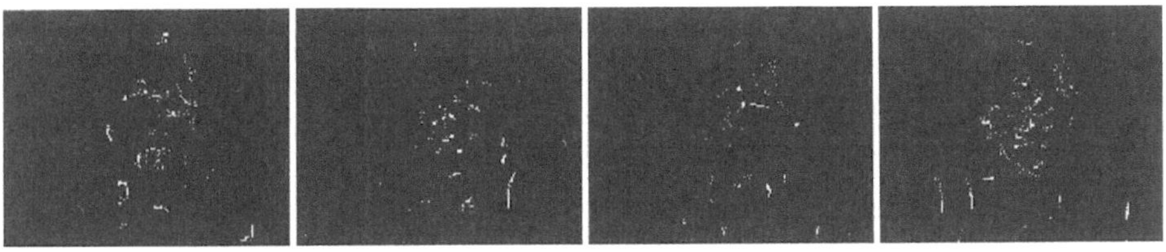

Fig. 5. Skeleton points to be transmitted for the sequence shown in Fig. 4

TABLE I
Bit rates for QCIF image sequences

	INTRA (kbits)	INTER (kbits/s)
MissAmerica	10	15
CarPhone	14	24
Foreman	13.5	30

6. Conclusions

In this paper, the extension from the ordinary to the geodesic skeleton is established. A new shape representation is found that can be used to code the contours of a segmented image. It guarantees that all contours are coded only once. The skeleton decomposition and the decoding procedure are described and fast algorithms proposed.

Implementation of the method in a morphological image coder produces good quality of the decoded sequences at very low bit-rates.

References

1. S. Ayer and P. Schroeter. Hierarchical robust motion estimation for segmentation of moving objects. In *Eigth IEEE Workshop on Image and Multidimensional Signal Processing*, Cannes, France, September 1993.
2. S. Beucher and F. Meyer. The morphological approach to segmentation: the watershed transformation. In E. Dougherty, editor, *Mathematical morphology in image processing*, chapter 12, pp. 433–481. Marcel Dekker, 1993.
3. P. Brigger and M. Kunt. Contour image sequence coding using the geodesic morphological skeleton. In *International Workshop on Coding Techniques for Very Low Bit-rate Video*, pp. 3.1–3.2, Essex, Colchester, April 1994.
4. R. Kresch and D. Malah. Morphological reduction of skeleton redundancy. In J. Serra and P. Salembier, editors, *Mathematical Morphology and its Applications to Signal Processing*, pages 145—150, Barcelona, Spain, May 1993. Universitat Politècnica de Catalunya.
5. M. Kunt, A. Ikonomopoulos, and M. Kocher. Second-generation image coding techniques. *Proc. IEEE*, 73, No.4, April 1985.
6. C. Lantuéjoul. Sur le modèle de Johnson-Mehl généralisé. Technical report, Centre de Morphologie Mathématique, Fontainebelau, France, 1977.
7. P. A. Maragos and R. W. Schafer. Morphological skeleton representation and coding of binary images. *IEEE Transactions on acoustics, speech and signal processing*, 34(5):1228–1244, October 1986.
8. G. Matheron. Examples of topological properties of skeletons. In J. Serra, editor, *Image analysis and mathematical morphology. Volume 2: theoretical advances*, chapter 11, pp. 217–238. Academic Press, 1988.
9. F. Meyer. Skeletons and watershed lines in digital spaces. *SPIE*, 1350:85–102, 1990.
10. M. Pardas, P. Salembier, and L. Torres. 3d morphological segmentation for image sequence processing. In *Proc. of IEEE Winter Workshop on Nonlinear Signal Processing*, Tampere, Finland, 1993.

MULTI-PARAMETER SKELETON DECOMPOSITION

R. KRESCH and D. MALAH
Department of Electrical Engineering
Technion - Israel Institute of Technology
32000, Haifa, Israel

Abstract. In this work we propose a further generalization of the *Morphological Skeleton Decomposition* on Boolean Lattices. In this generalization, the family of structuring-functions which determines the decomposition has its scalar index λ replaced by a *generic* index i from a totally *or partially* ordered set I. This enables, for example, skeleton decompositions by richer and more complex families of shapes, characterized by several scalar indices (i.e., a multi-dimensional index), instead of just a single scalar index.

Particular cases and applications are discussed.

Key words: Skeleton, Mathematical Morphology, Boolean Lattices, Set Decomposition, Image Representation

1. Introduction

The study of the Morphological Skeleton was divided historically into two main branches: topological and algebraic [2]. While characteristics like skeleton connectivity and shape concern the topological branch, the main interest of the algebraic branch in the Skeleton is in it being a compact error-free representation of the original set. In this work, we relate basically to the latter.

According to Serra [2], in order to obtain an appropriate representation, from the above algebraic point of view, the following requirements concerning a Skeleton Decomposition are expected to be satisfied:

1. *Existence and uniqueness* of the Skeleton of a set, for a given family of structuring-functions.
2. *Perfect reconstruction* of the original set from the Skeleton subsets.
3. An *explicit formula* for computing the Skeleton.

These requirements were shown by Lantuéjoul (see [5, Chapter 11]) to be fulfilled when the family of elements are open balls in the Euclidean space, and the sets to be decomposed are open sets in the same space. With the generalization of Mathematical Morphology to Complete Lattices, sufficient conditions for the fulfillment of the requirements were stated in [1, Chapter 2]. Yet, with the advent of new developments in the Skeleton theory [6, 8], Serra recently updated those conditions in [2], providing a quite general framework for the Skeleton Decomposition on Boolean Lattices.

During the above historical development, the family of decomposition elements was always indexed by a non-negative *scalar* parameter λ. The fact that no attempt was made previously to replace this scalar parameter by a vector one can be explained, perhaps, by the interest in obtaining a meaningful Skeleton from the

J.Serra and P. Soille (eds.), Mathematical Morphology and Its Applications to Image Processing, 141-148

topological and *geometrical* points of view (having, for instance, a related *quench function*, which maps every skeleton point to the radius of the respective maximal element). However, the Multi-Structuring-Element Skeleton (MSES) proposed by the authors in [3] (see also [7]) *cannot* be considered as a particular case in Serra's framework (it demands a partial ordering of the indices of the decomposition subsets), and, nevertheless, it satisfies the three *algebraic* requirements stated above.

Our purpose in this paper is to propose a generalized definition of the Skeleton, having as particular cases both Serra's general Skeleton, and the MSES. Therefore, we generalize the above parameter λ (and, therefore, extend the Skeleton scope), while adapting the conditions stated in [2], to assure that the above three requirements are still satisfied. This provides a more flexible analysis tool, and new decompositions besides the above mentioned ones - Multi-Parameter Skeletons and Hybrid Skeletons, as described in the sequel.

The proposed generalization of the Skeleton Decomposition is presented in section 2.1. In section 2.2, theorems assuring that the algebraic requirements are met are presented. In section 3, particular cases of the general decomposition are presented, and in section 4, some applications are discussed.

2. Proposed Generalization

2.1. Generalized Skeleton Definition

Let us consider a set E and the Boolean Lattice defined by $\mathcal{P}(E)$ (the set of subsets of E), *inclusion* order, and *union* and *intersection* as the supremum and the infimum, respectively.

Let I be a set of indices i, totally *or partially* ordered by an order $\geq$. The set I can be, for instance, a d-dimensional space, so that the indices i are vectors.

We choose an arbitrary family of structuring-functions (i.e. functions from E into $\mathcal{P}(E)$), indexed by I, $\{\delta_i(x)\}_{i \in I}$. This choice uniquely determines the families of dilations $\{\delta_i(X)\}$, adjoint erosions $\{\varepsilon_i(X)\}$ and morphological openings $\{\gamma_i(X)\}$, where $X \in \mathcal{P}(E)$.

We define an *element* with "radius" $i \in I$ and "center" $x_0 \in E$, $\delta_i(x_0)$, as the image of x_0 by the structuring-function $\delta_i(x)$, and a *maximal element* in a set $X \in \mathcal{P}(E)$ as an element contained in X but not contained in any other element which is contained in X.

As usual, we define the Skeleton of a set $X \in \mathcal{P}(E)$ as the collection of the centers of all the maximal elements contained in it. It always exists and it is unique for the chosen family of structuring-functions and the given set X. The sets $\{S_i(X)\}_{i \in I}$, each containing the centers of the maximal elements of "radius" i, are called *Skeleton Subsets*.

The above definitions (and also the theorems in next section, and their proofs) are a direct generalization of those given in [2]. The main difference is that, in [2], the set of indices I are restricted to $\mathcal{R}_+$ or $\mathcal{Z}_+$ and its order $\geq$ to the usual total order, whereas here I and $\geq$ are not restricted. Because of lack of space, we do not present first the main results of [2], but proceed with our generalization. However, since the work here follows to a great extent the work in [2], one can easily recover the earlier results by setting $I = \mathcal{R}_+$ or $I = \mathcal{Z}_+$ throughout this paper.

2.2. Calculation and Reconstruction Formulæ

The following theorem provides an explicit formula for calculating the skeleton subsets $\{S_i\}_{i \in I}$:

Theorem 1 *If the family of structuring functions $\{\delta_i(x)\}_{i \in I}$ satisfies the following two conditions:*

1. $i \leq j \Rightarrow \gamma_i \delta_j(x) = \delta_j(x), \forall x \in E$ *(i.e., the family is* granulometry-generating *in a generalized sense),*
2. *For all $i, j \in I$ and $x, y \in E$:*

$$\delta_i(x) \supseteq \delta_j(y) \Rightarrow \begin{cases} i > j, & \text{if } x \neq y \\ i \geq j, & x = y \end{cases}$$

then, for any $X \subset \mathcal{P}(E)$, and for all $i \in I$:

$$S_i(X) = \varepsilon_i(X) - \bigcup_{j > i \in I} \gamma_{[i,j]} \varepsilon_i(X) \tag{1}$$

where $\gamma_{[i,j]}$ is the morphological opening associated with the structuring function $\delta_{[i,j]}(x) \triangleq \varepsilon_i \delta_j(x)$.

Equation (1) is a direct adaptation of the generalized Lantuéjoul's formula in [2]. The proof is given in the appendix.

A similar direct adaptation of the conditions for lossless reconstruction proposed in [2] guarantees perfect reconstruction from the proposed generalized Skeleton Subsets. In order to state this, by means of a theorem, we consider the following definitions:

- Let L_X be the set of all the elements contained in X, i.e., $L_X \triangleq \{\delta_i(x) \mid i \in I, x \in \varepsilon_i(X)\}$.
- A subset $\{\delta_{i_k}(x_k)\}_{k \in K}$ of L_X is called an *increasing chain* in L_X, if K is a totally ordered set of indices, and if $k < k'$ implies $\delta_{i_k}(x_k) \subseteq \delta_{i_{k'}}(x_{k'})$.
- We say that an increasing chain $\{\delta_{i_k}(x_k)\}$ *converges* to an element $\delta_{i_0}(x_0)$, if $\bigcup_{k \in K} \delta_{i_k}(x_k) = \delta_{i_0}(x_0)$.
- L_X is said to be *inductive for inclusion* [2], if *every* increasing chain in L_X converges to a unique element in L_X.
- Let J be any subset of the set of indices I. We say that J is an *anti-umbra* in I if the conditions $j \in J$ and $i \geq j$ imply $i \in J$.
- For an anti-umbra J in I, we define the following opening: $\forall X \in \mathcal{P}(E), \gamma_J(X) \triangleq \bigcup_{j \in J} \gamma_j(X)$

Theorem 2 *Let $\{S_i(X)\}_{i \in I}$ be the skeleton decomposition of X, according to the family of structuring functions $\{\delta_i(x)\}_{i \in I}$. If L_X is inductive for inclusion, and J is an anti-umbra in I, then*

$$\bigcup_{i \in J} \delta_i(S_i(X)) = \gamma_J(X) \tag{2}$$

The perfect reconstruction is assured whenever $X = \gamma_J(X)$. Equation (2) also provides a *partial reconstruction* formula for the skeleton, in case that $\gamma_J(X) \neq X$. The proof of theorem 2 is also given in the appendix.

3. Multi-Parameter Skeleton

As stressed before, choosing I to be a totally ordered set of indices, such as $\mathcal{R}_+$ or $\mathcal{Z}_+$, brings us to the standard skeleton decomposition, as defined in [2]. The purpose of this paper is to propose decompositions which are *not* based on totally ordered sets.

We consider in this section the following particular case:

- I is a set of d-dimensional vectors, i.e., every index i is in the form $i \triangleq (i_1, i_2, \ldots, i_d)$. More specifically, $I = \mathcal{R}_+^d$ in the continuous case, and $I = \mathcal{Z}_+^d$ in the discrete case.
- The order of I is chosen to be its *strong order*, i.e., for any two indices $i^{(1)}$ and $i^{(2)}$ in I, $i^{(1)} \geq i^{(2)}$ iff $i_n^{(1)} \geq i_n^{(2)}$ for all $n = 1, 2, \ldots, d$.
- The conditions of theorems 1 and 2 hold.

We denote a skeleton associated with such case a *Multi-Parameter Skeleton.* If we denote as k_n the d-dimensional vector having its n-th component equal to 1 and all the others equal to 0, then the *continuous-case* Multi-Parameter Skeleton subsets are given by:

$$S_i(X) = \varepsilon_i(X) - \bigcup_{n=1}^{d} \left[\bigcup_{\lambda_n > 0} \gamma_{[i, i+\lambda_n k_n]} \varepsilon_i(X) \right], \qquad i \in \mathcal{R}_+^d \tag{3}$$

where λ_n, $n = 1, \ldots, d$, are *scalar* variables. Notice that the union in (1), which is performed over the *vector* variable j, is replaced in (3) by unions performed over *scalar* variables, n and λ_n, $n = 1, \ldots, d$.

The unions performed over λ_n in (3) express, actually, convergence towards a supremum, when $\lambda_n \to 0$. In the *discrete case*, these unions converge to maxima, which are reached when $\lambda_n = 1$, $n = 1, \ldots, d$. Therefore, in the discrete case, (3) becomes:

$$S_i(X) = \varepsilon_i(X) - \bigcup_{n=1}^{d} \gamma_{[i, i+k_n]} \varepsilon_i(X), \qquad i \in \mathcal{Z}_+^d \tag{4}$$

We consider now a more specific particular case. Let us select d convex structuring-elements B_n, $n = 1, \ldots, d$, and define for each i in I:

$$A_i \triangleq i_1 B_1 \oplus \ldots \oplus i_d B_d, \tag{5}$$

where $\oplus$ denotes Minkowski addition, and $i_n B_n$, $n = 1, \ldots, d$, denote $(i_n - 1)$ times the dilation of the structuring-element B_n by itself. If the structuring-functions used for the skeletonization are in the form:

$$\delta_i(x) = A(i) \oplus \{x\}, \; i \in I \tag{6}$$

then the associated Multi-Parameter Skeleton is called *Multi-Structuring-Element Skeleton* (MSES) [3, 7]. In the *discrete case* ($I = \mathcal{Z}_+^d$), the morphological openings $\gamma_{[i,i+k_n]}(X)$ associated with a MSES are independent of i, and equal to $X \circ B_n$ (where $(\cdot) \circ B$ denotes translation invariant morphological opening by the structuring-element B). Therefore, if we denote by $(\cdot) \ominus B$ the translation invariant erosion by

B, the associated MSES subsets $S_i(X)$ are given by:

$$S_i(X) = X \ominus A_i - \bigcup_{n=1}^{d} [X \ominus A_i] \circ B_n, \qquad i \in \mathcal{Z}_+^d. \tag{7}$$

3.1. Example

As an example, let us consider a MSES with $d = 2$, B_1 equal to the unit *vertical* open segment, and B_2 equal to the unit *horizontal* open segment.

The related Skeleton decomposition of an open set X yields the centers of the maximal open *rectangles* inscribable in X (note that $(i_1 B_1 \oplus i_2 B_2)$ in this case is a rectangle with vertical side i_1 and horizontal side i_2).

In the discrete case ($I = \mathcal{Z}^2$), the decomposition is with respect to rectangles with sides of discrete lengths only, and it can be calculated using (7).

A question which can be asked at this point is: Would we get the same decomposition as above if, instead of using (7), we calculated the Skeleton w.r.t. the family $\{\lambda B_1\}_{\lambda \in \mathcal{R}_+}$ of vertical open segments, and then, *on the resultant subsets*, the Skeleton w.r.t. the family $\{\lambda B_2\}_{\lambda \in \mathcal{R}_+}$ of horizontal open segments? The answer is no; composition of skeletons do not give centers of *maximal elements*. For a decomposition into maximal elements, the composite skeleton must be calculated.

4. Applications

The applications of the conventional skeleton (I being a totally ordered 1-dimensional space), are well known. In this section, we present some applications of skeletons based on partially ordered sets, such as Multi-Parameter Skeletons.

From the *topological* and *geometrical* points of view, a Multi-Parameter Skeleton may have little interest. First, it is far less connectivity-preserving than the conventional skeleton. Also, it fails to exactly provide a *Medial Axis* of the shapes under study. And, finally, a Multi-Parameter Skeleton usually can *not* be characterized by a *quench function*, because a point $x \in E$ may be the "center" of two (or more) different maximal elements. The latter is consequence of I being *partially* ordered.

On the other hand, from the *algebraic* point of view, a Multi-Parameter Skeleton can be very useful. First, it can decompose an image into an assortment of shapes richer than the one a conventional skeleton is able to provide. Moreover, if we consider the element indices i to be a degree of "importance", or as a "category classifier", as is often done regarding the conventional skeleton, then a Multi-Parameter Skeleton can provide finer distributions and classifications. In addition, there is greater diversity of possible partial reconstructions, where their proximity to the original image are controlled by the choice of the anti-umbra J in (2). Finally, each of the scalar parameters of the multi-dimensional index i may have a different physical interpretation, such as size, time duration, gray-level, etc., in contrast to the conventional skeleton decomposition, where different physical characteristics of the image can not be treated independently.

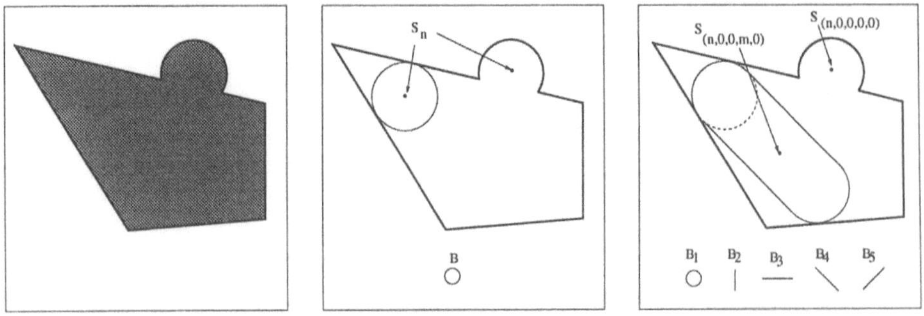

(a) (b) (c)

Fig. 1. (a) A binary image containing a partially occluded disc, (b) elements detected by a conventional skeleton, (c) elements detected by a 5-parameter skeleton.

4.1. Pattern Recognition

Suppose we are interested in finding a pattern in a binary image, and that this pattern is not corrupted with holes but may be partially occluded. E.g., the disc in Figure 1(a).

In order to detect the shape, let us consider a family of translation invariant structuring-functions, with the structure shown in (6). If the pattern we are interested in is one of the shapes of the family $\{A_i\}$, then it should be easy to locate such a pattern using the associated skeleton decomposition, since it provides the centers of maximal elements from that family in the given image. In other words, we consider patterns to be located as maximal elements, and define a proper family of shapes $\{A_i\}$ for decomposition. Thus, in order to detect the disc in Fig. 1, we may calculate the skeleton w.r.t. a family of increasing discs.

However, for a conventional skeleton, the above idea does not work well. In Fig. 1(b) we see that we may find, in the subsets S_n of the skeleton, maximal elements other than the pattern we are looking for.

On the other hand, a MSES could give better results. For the example in Fig. 1, we choose a 5-parameter skeleton, based on 5 structuring-elements: a unit disc (which we want to detect), and 4 unit lines in four different directions. In this case, we are interested in the subsets of the form $S_{(n,0,0,0,0)}$ only. As seen in Fig. 1(c), most of the "false alarms" obtained by the conventional skeleton are now in different subsets than $S_{(n,0,0,0,0)}$.

4.2. Coding

Let us compare a Multi-Parameter Skeleton, w.r.t. a partially ordered family of structuring-functions $\mathcal{F}$, to a conventional one-parameter skeleton w.r.t. a totally ordered sub-family $\tilde{\mathcal{F}}$ *contained* in $\mathcal{F}$. For example, if we consider the family of open rectangles defined in section 3.1 to be $\mathcal{F}$, then $\tilde{\mathcal{F}}$ could be the family of open squares. Because of the partial ordering, the number of skeleton points in the multi-parameter skeleton is expected to be larger than the number of skeleton points in the one-parameter skeleton. But after removing redundant points in both skeletons (see [4, 7] for redundancy reduction approaches), the situation is inverted; the multi-parameter skeleton is expected to contain considerably fewer points than the one-parameter skeleton, which appears to be of great advantage for Coding purposes.

However, since the number of subsets in the multi-parameter skeleton is usually much bigger than the number of subsets in the one-parameter skeleton (about N^d in comparison to N), this turns out to be too costly in terms of coding efficiency. Moreover, its computational burden, usually of order $\mathcal{O}(d)$, is very high if compared to $\mathcal{O}(1)$ of the one-parameter skeleton.

However, the General Skeleton Decomposition presented in section 2.1 does not restrict us to either a one-parameter or a multi-parameter skeleton; combinations of them are also possible. For example, instead of considering a decomposition w.r.t. the family of *all* the rectangles, as presented in section 3.1, or w.r.t. the family of squares only, We can *arbitrarily* select *any* sub-family of rectangles for the skeletonization. This combines, at some extent, the advantages of both the multi-parameter and the one-parameter skeletons. We call such decomposition a Hybrid Skeleton.

As opposed to a full multi-parameter decomposition, which in the general case is not substantially advantageous when compared to the one-parameter skeleton, Hybrid Skeletons showed promising results in preliminary simulations. Methods for optimal (or sub-optimal) determination of the sub-family of structuring-functions (given a full multi-parameter family) are presently being examined.

5. Conclusion

The scope of the Morphological Skeleton definition is further extended, so that the family of structuring-functions which determines the decomposition can be indexed by a *generic* index, instead of a *scalar* one only. Conditions for the morphological calculation of the Generalized Skeleton subsets and for the reconstruction of the original image are determined, and the respective formulæ derived.

Particular cases of the general definition (which are called Multi-Parameter Skeletons, Multi-Structuring-Element Skeletons (MSES's), and Hybrid Skeletons) are considered, and potential applications of such skeletons, with comparisons to the application of conventional skeleton, are also presented.

References

1. J. Serra, *Image Analysis and Mathematical Morphology, Volume 2: Theoretical Advances.* London: Academic Press, 1988.
2. J. Serra, "Skeleton Decompositions", *SPIE Vol. 1769, Image Algebra and Morphological Image Processing III*, pp. 376-386, 1992.
3. R. Kresch and D. Malah, "Morphological Multi-Structuring-Element Skeleton and its Applications", *Proc. of ISSSE'92*, Paris, pp. 166-169, September 1992.
4. P. Maragos and R.W. Schafer, "Morphological Skeleton Representation and Coding of Binary Images", *IEEE Trans. ASSP*, Vol. 34, No. 5, pp. 1228-1244, October 1986.
5. J. Serra, *Image Analysis and Mathematical Morphology.* London: Academic Press, 1982.
6. G. Sapiro and D. Malah, "Morphological Image Coding Based on a Geometric Sampling Theorem and a Modified Skeleton Representation", *Journal of Visual Communication and Image Representation*, Vol. 5, No. 1, pp. 29-40, March 1994.
7. R. Kresch and D. Malah, "Morphological Redundancy of Skeleton Redundancy", *Proc. of the International Workshop on Mathematical Morphology and Its Applications to Image Process-*

ing, Barcelona, pp. 145-150, May 1993, to appear in Signal Processing, 1994.
8. D. Schonfeld and J. Goutsias, "Morphological Representation of Discrete and Binary Images", *Trans. Signal Processing*, Vol. 39, No. 6, pp. 1369-1379, June 1991.

Appendix

Proof of Theorem 1:

A maximal element from a family $\{\delta_i(x), i \in I, x \in E\}$ inside a set X is an element $\delta_i(x)$ contained in X, such that, for any $j \neq i$ and $y \in E$, if $\delta_j(y) \subseteq X$, then $\delta_i(x) \nsubseteq \delta_j(y)$. But since condition 2 of the theorem makes it impossible for $\delta_j(y)$ to contain $\delta_i(x)$ if $j \not> i$ (unless $i = j$ and $x = y$), we need to check only for $j > i$. The skeleton subset $S_i(X)$ is the set of points x, such that $\delta_i(x)$ is maximal in X.

The following is always true:

$$\delta_i(x) \subseteq X \Leftrightarrow x \in \varepsilon_i(X) \tag{A.1}$$

$$\delta_i(x) \nsubseteq \delta_j(y) \Leftrightarrow x \notin \varepsilon_i\delta_j(y) = \delta_{[i,j]}(y) \tag{A.2}$$

It is always true also that $\delta_j(y) \subseteq X$ implies $\varepsilon_i\delta_j(y) \subseteq \varepsilon_i(X)$, but the equivalence is usually not assured. However, since the family of structuring-functions is granulometry-generating (condition 1 of the theorem), for $j > i$ the equivalence is obtained, which can be written in the following way:

$$\delta_j(y) \subseteq X \Leftrightarrow \delta_{[i,j]}(y) \subseteq \varepsilon_i(X) \Leftrightarrow y \in \varepsilon_{[i,j]}\varepsilon_i(X) \tag{A.3}$$

Therefore, according to (A.1), (A.2) and (A.3), $x \in S_i(X)$ iff $x \in \varepsilon_i(X)$ and $x \notin \gamma_{[i,j]}\varepsilon_i(X)$, $\forall j > i$. This leads to (1).

Proof of Theorem 2:

The left side of (2) can be written in the following way:

$$\bigcup_{i \in J} \delta_i(S_i(X)) = \bigcup_{i \in J} \bigcup_{x \in S_i(X)} \delta_i(x) \tag{A.4}$$

which means that it is equal to the union of all the maximal elements contained in X, with "radius" in J. Therefore, we need to proof that $x \in \gamma_J(X)$ iff x belongs to some maximal element with "radius" in J.

If $x \in X$ belongs to a maximal element $\delta_j(y)$, $j \in J$, then $x \in \gamma_j(X) \subseteq \gamma_J(X)$, which proves one way.

If $x \in \gamma_J(X)$ then there is $j \in J$ such that $x \in \delta_j(y) \in L_X$ (for some $j \in E$), which is not necessarily a maximal element. But, since L_X is inductive for inclusion (condition of the theorem), every increasing chain in L_X converges to a unique element, and therefore, by Zorn's Lemma, $\delta_j(y)$ (and hence x too) is contained in a maximal element. The radius of this maximal element is obviously greater or equal to j and belongs to I. Thus, since J is an anti-umbra in I (condition of the theorem), the radius of the maximal element containing x belongs to J, which proves the way back.

The above proofs are an extension of those in [2].

MORPHOLOGICAL SYSTEMS THEORY: SLOPE TRANSFORMS, MAX–MIN DIFFERENTIAL EQUATIONS, ENVELOPE FILTERS, AND SAMPLING

PETROS MARAGOS *
School of Electrical and Computer Engineering
Georgia Institute of Technology, Atlanta, GA 30332–0250, USA

Abstract. In this paper we view the basic morphological signal operators as a class of nonlinear systems obeying a supremum/infimum-of-sums superposition and endow them with analytic tools that parallel the functionality of and have many conceptual similarities with ideas and tools used in linear systems. In the time/space domain, these systems are found equivalent to a max-plus or min-plus convolution with their impulse response, and a class of nonlinear difference/differential equations is introduced to describe their dynamics. The hyperplanes $< \alpha, v > + b$ are eigenfunctions of such morphological systems, which leads to developing a slope response for them, as a function of the slope α, and related slope transforms for arbitrary signals. These ideas provide a transform (slope) domain for morphological systems, where dilation and erosion in time/space corresponds to addition of slope transforms, time/space hyperplanes transform into slope impulses, time/space cones become bandpass slope-selective filters, and distance transforms correspond to ideal slope filters. The paper summarizes results for 1D signals/systems and extends them to the 2D case and to sampling.

Key words: Morphological systems, slope transforms, difference equations, sampling.

1. Morphological Systems

Morphological systems that have found applications in image analysis and nonlinear filtering are (simple or complex) parallel and/or serial interconnections of the basic morphological dilations $\oplus$ or morphological erosions $\ominus$

$$(x \oplus g)(v) \triangleq \bigvee_{u \in \mathrm{E}} x(u) + g(v-u) \quad , \quad (x \ominus g)(v) \triangleq \bigwedge_{v \in \mathrm{E}} x(u) - g(u-v)$$

where $\bigvee$ denotes supremum and $\bigwedge$ denotes infimum. We assume signals defined on a d-dimensional ($d = 1, 2, ..$) continuous ($\mathrm{E} = \mathbf{R}^d$) or discrete domain ($\mathrm{E} = \mathbf{Z}^d$) and whose range is any subset of $\overline{\mathbf{R}} = \mathbf{R} \cup \{-\infty, \infty\}$. For $d = 1$ we think of $v = t$ as time, whereas for $d \geq 2$ we view $v = (v_1, ..., v_d) \in E$ as spatial argument. In convex optimization [1] and analysis [9] the nonlinear operation $\oplus$ is called 'maximal convolution' and an operation closely related to $\ominus$ is the 'infimal convolution' $(x \Box g)(v) \triangleq \bigwedge_u x(u) + g(v-u)$. Henceforth, we refer to $\oplus$ and $\Box$ as the *max-plus* and *min-plus convolution* to distinguish them from the more abstract concept of a dilation and erosion system.

* This is an invited paper. It was written while the author was supported by the US National Science Foundation under Grant MIP–9396301.

J.Serra and P. Soille (eds.), Mathematical Morphology and Its Applications to Image Processing, 149-160

So far morphological systems have been analyzed only in the time/space domain by using their algebraic properties and lacked a transform domain. In this paper we use analogies from linear systems to endow morphological systems with various new concepts and analytic methods that enable us to determine their output and properties in time/space and in a transform domain. First, in analogy to linear systems which obey a sum-of-products superposition, we call a signal operator $\mathcal{D} : x \mapsto y = \mathcal{D}(x)$ a **dilation system** if it obeys the *supremum-of-sums superposition*

$$\mathcal{D}\left[\bigvee_i c_i + x_i(v)\right] = \bigvee_i c_i + \mathcal{D}[x_i(v)] \tag{1}$$

where $c_i \in \mathbf{R}$. Two elementary signals useful for analyzing morphological systems are the *zero impulse* μ and *zero step* λ, defined in the 1D case $v = t$ as

$$\mu(t) \triangleq \begin{cases} 0, & t = 0 \\ -\infty, & t \neq 0 \end{cases} \quad , \quad \lambda(t) \triangleq \begin{cases} 0, & t \geq 0 \\ -\infty, & t < 0 \end{cases}$$

and in the $d \geq 2$ case as $\mu(v) \triangleq \sum_{i=1}^{d} \mu(v_i)$ and $\lambda(v) \triangleq \sum_{i=1}^{d} \lambda(v_i)$. For example, a signal can be represented as a sup of weighted impulses:

$$x(v) = \bigvee_u x(u) + \mu(v - u)$$

If the system is *shift-varying*, let $g(v, u) = \mathcal{D}[\mu(v - u)]$ be its response due to an input impulse at $v = u$. Then

$$y(v) = \mathcal{D}[x(v)] = \bigvee_u x(u) + g(v, u)$$

If the system $\mathcal{D}$ is *shift-invariant*, then $g(v, u) = g(v-u, 0)$, which we write simply as $g(v-u)$; further, we call $g(v) = \mathcal{D}[\mu(v)]$ the system's **impulse response**. A *dilation shift-invariant (DSI)* system is uniquely determined in the time/spatial domain by its impulse response, which also controls its causality and stability [6, 7]. For example,

$$\mathcal{D} \text{ is DSI} \iff \mathcal{D}(x) = x \oplus g, \quad g \triangleq \mathcal{D}(\mu)$$

Thus any DSI system is equivalent to a max-plus convolution of the input with its impulse response.

Operators $\mathcal{E} : x \mapsto y = \mathcal{E}(x)$ that are shift-invariant and obey an infimum-of-sums superposition, i.e. as in (1) but with $\bigvee$ replaced by $\bigwedge$, are called herein *erosion shift-invariant (ESI)* systems. These are equivalent to a min-plus convolution, because $\mathcal{E}$ is ESI iff $\mathcal{E}[x(v)] = x(v) \ominus [-f(-v)] = x(v) \square f(v)$, where $f = \mathcal{E}(-\mu)$ is defined as their impulse response.

We also develop some nonlinear difference equations to describe the time/space dynamics of discrete DSI or ESI systems. Inspiration here comes from the linear difference equations which can describe a very large class of discrete linear shift-invariant (LSI) systems. Thus, replacing sum with maximum and multiplication with addition yields **max-plus difference equations**. The 1D case is discussed in [6, 7]; this paper focuses mainly on the following 2D case:

$$y[n,m] = \left(\bigvee_{(k,j)\in M_o} a_{kj} + y[n-k, m-j] \right) \vee \left(\bigvee_{(p,q)\in M_i} b_{pq} + x[n-p, m-q] \right) \quad (2)$$

The masks M_o, M_i are pixel coordinate sets that determine which output and input samples will be added with constants to form the current output sample. Similarly, the dynamics of ESI systems can be described by min-plus difference equations as in (2) but with $\bigvee$ replaced by $\bigwedge$. For dilation (resp. erosion) systems the useful information in a signal x exists only at points v where $x(v) > -\infty$ (resp. $x(v) < +\infty$). Thus, all coefficient sequences a_{kj}, b_{pq} in the max (resp. min) difference equation are from $\mathbf{R} \cup \{-\infty\}$ (resp. $\mathbf{R} \cup \{+\infty\}$). The vast majority of discrete max/min-plus convolutions $\oplus$,$\ominus$ used in applications employs a finite structuring element, and they can be modeled by the above max/min difference equations by ignoring the recursive part (i.e., if all $a_{kj} = \pm\infty$). The only exception has been recursive erosions whose output mask M_o is within a 3×3 or 5×5 pixel neighborhood and can generate the distance transform of binary images [10, 2]. Whenever the max/min equations have a recursive part, we show that this corresponds to max/min-plus convolution of the input signal with an infinite-support structuring function.

To create a **transform domain** for morphological systems, we first note that the affine signals $x(v) = <\alpha, v> + b$ (which are planes in the 2D and lines in the 1D case) are *eigenfunctions* of any DSI system $\mathcal{D}$ or ESI system $\mathcal{E}$ because

$$\mathcal{D}[<\alpha, v> + b] = <\alpha, v> + b + G(\alpha) \ , \ G(\alpha) \triangleq \bigvee_v g(v) - <\alpha, v>$$

$$\mathcal{E}[<\alpha, v> + b] = <\alpha, v> + b + F(\alpha) \ , \ F(\alpha) \triangleq \bigwedge_v f(v) - <\alpha, v>$$

where $\alpha = (\alpha_1, ..., \alpha_d) \in \mathbf{R}^d$ and $<\alpha, v> = \sum_{i=1}^{d} \alpha_i v_i$. We call the corresponding eigenvalues $G(\alpha)$ and $F(\alpha)$ the **slope response**[1] of the DSI and ESI system. It measures the amount of shift in the intercept of the input hyperplanes with slope vector α. It is also conceptually similar to the frequency response of LSI systems which is their multiplicative eigenvalue for input exponentials, whereas G (or F) is the additive eigenvalue of DSI (or ESI) systems for input hyperplanes. This nonlinear analysis leads to developing signal transforms called *slope transforms* whose properties and application to morphological systems has some striking conceptual similarities with Fourier transforms and their application to LSI systems.

This paper summarizes our results in [6, 7, 8] for the 1D case and provides their extensions to the 2D case and to sampling.

2. Slope Transforms

The following two slope transforms, introduced in [6, 7, 8] in the context of morphological systems, were motivated by the algebraic expression of their eigenvalues

[1] For *shift-varying* DSI systems $\mathcal{D}$ the function $G(\alpha, v) = \bigvee_u g(v, v-u) - <\alpha, u>$ with $g(v, u) = \mathcal{D}[\mu(v-u)]$ can play the role of a slope response, because $\mathcal{D}[<\alpha, v>] = G(\alpha, v) + <\alpha, v>$.

corresponding to their eigenfunctions $<\alpha,v>+b$. (Recall that the Fourier transform can be similarly inspired by the form of the eigevalues (frequency response) of LSI systems corresponding to their exponential eigenfunctions.) Thus, viewing the slope response as a signal transform with variable the slope vector α, we define for any signal $x(v)$ its **upper slope transform** as the function $X_\vee : \mathbf{R}^d \to \overline{\mathbf{R}}$ and as **lower slope transform**[2] the function $X_\wedge : \mathbf{R}^d \to \overline{\mathbf{R}}$ defined, for each $\alpha \in \mathbf{R}^d$, as

$$X_\vee(\alpha) \triangleq \bigvee_{v \in E} x(v) - <\alpha,v> \quad , \quad X_\wedge(\alpha) \triangleq \bigwedge_{v \in E} x(v) - <\alpha,v>$$

For 1D signals $x(t)$, all the hyperplanes $<\alpha,v>$ used in slope transforms become lines αt with slope $\alpha \in \mathbf{R}$. A geometrical intuition behind the slope transforms can be obtained by realizing that a hyperplane that has *slope* vector α and passes from a point $(v, x(v))$ on the graph of a signal $x(v)$ has an *intercept* equal to $X = x(v) - <\alpha,v>$. Thus the upper and lower slope transforms are the max and min intercepts of hyperplanes with varying slopes intersecting the signal's graph. These extreme intercepts occur when the hyperplane becomes tangent to the graph. In general, $x(v)$ is covered from above by all the hyperplanes $X_\vee(\alpha)+<\alpha,v>$ whose infimum creates an *upper envelope* $\hat{x}(v)$ and is covered from below by planes $X_\wedge(\alpha)+<\alpha,v>$ whose supremum creates the *lower envelope* $\check{x}(v)$:

$$\hat{x}(v) \triangleq \bigwedge_{\alpha \in \mathbf{R}^d} X_\vee(\alpha)+<\alpha,v> \quad , \quad \check{x}(v) \triangleq \bigvee_{\alpha \in \mathbf{R}^d} X_\wedge(\alpha)+<\alpha,v>$$

We view the signals $\hat{x}(v)$ and $\check{x}(v)$ as the 'inverse' upper and lower slope transform of $x(v)$, respectively.

Theorem 1. *For any signal* $x : \mathbf{R}^d \to \overline{\mathbf{R}}$,
(a) $X_\vee(\alpha)$ *and* $\check{x}(v)$ *are convex, whereas* $X_\wedge(\alpha)$ *and* $\hat{x}(v)$ *are concave. (b) For all* v, $\check{x}(v) \le x(v) \le \hat{x}(v)$. *(c) At any point* v

$$\hat{x}(v) = x(v) \iff x(v) \geq \frac{px(v-qu)+qx(v+pu)}{p+q} \quad \forall p,q>0, \quad \forall ||u||=1. \tag{3}$$

At any v, $x(v) = \check{x}(v)$ *iff the* $\geq$ *sign in* (3) *is replaced by* $\leq$.
(d) $\hat{x}(v) = x(v)$ *for all* v *if* x *is concave, and* $\check{x} = x$ *if* x *is convex. (e)* $\hat{x}$ *is the smallest concave upper envelope of* x*, and* $\check{x}$ *is the greatest convex lower envelope of* x.

Proof: Similar to the proof of the 1D case given in [8].

Thus, there is one-to-one correspondence between $X_\vee(\alpha)$ and the signal envelope $\hat{x}(v)$. However, all signals between $x(v)$ and $\hat{x}(v)$ will have the same upper slope transform.

Tables I and II list several properties and examples of the upper slope transform. Their proofs for 1D signals are in [8]. The most striking is that max-plus convolution $\oplus$ in the time/space domain corresponds to addition in the slope domain. Note the

---

[2] In convex analysis [9], given a convex function h there uniquely corresponds another convex function $h^*(\alpha) = \bigvee_v <\alpha,v> - h(v)$ called the *conjugate* of h. The lower slope transform of h and its conjugate function are closely related since $h^*(\alpha) = -H_\wedge(\alpha)$.

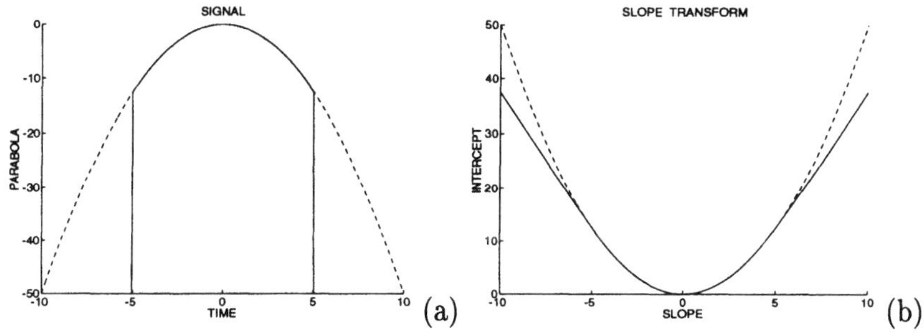

Fig. 1. (a) Original parabola signal $x(t) = -t^2/2$ (in dashed line) and a time-limited version (in solid line) resulting from adding to the signal a rectangular pulse with support $[-5, 5]$. (b) Upper slope transform of the parabola (in dashed line) and of its time-limited version (in solid line).

analogy with LSI systems where convolution of signals in time/space corresponds to multiplying their Fourier transforms. Also, consider the space pulse $w(v) = I_{rB_p}(v)$, where $I_S(v) = 0$ for $v \in S$ and $-\infty$ else denotes the *indicator function* of a set S, and $rB_p = \{v : ||v||_p = r\}$ is a ball with radius r with respect to the $||\cdot||_p$ norm defined by $||v||_p = (\sum_i |v_i|^p)^{1/p}$ if $p = 1, 2, \ldots$ and $||v||_{p=\infty} = \max_i |v_i|$. Since $W(\alpha) = \bigvee_{||v||_p \leq r} - < \alpha, v >$, from Hölder's inequality $|< \alpha, v >| \leq ||v||_p ||\alpha||_q$ where $p^{-1} + q^{-1} = 1$, we obtain $W(\alpha) = r||\alpha||_q$. Adding $w(v)$ to a signal $x(v)$ yields a space-limited signal $x(v) + w(v)$ whose upper slope transform is the min-plus convolution of the original signal's slope transform with the window's slope transform. See Fig. 1. This is a kind of nonlinear blurring. Consider the analogy with the blurring that occurs when we multiply a signal x by a time window in which case the original Fourier transform of x is convolved with the window's Fourier transform.

Whatever we discussed for upper slope transforms also applies to the lower slope transform, the only differences being the interchange of suprema with infima, concave with convex, and dilation with erosion.

For **differentiable** signals, the maximization or minimization of the intercept $x(v) - < \alpha, v >$ involved in both slope transforms can also be done, for a fixed α, by finding its value at the stationary point v^* such that $\nabla x(v^*) = \alpha$. At the point $(v^*, x(v^*))$ the hyperplane becomes tangent to the graph. This extreme value of the intercept (as a function of the slope α) is the *Legendre transform* of the signal x:

$$X_L(\alpha) \triangleq x\left((\nabla x)^{-1}(\alpha)\right) - < \alpha, (\nabla x)^{-1}(\alpha) >$$

where f^{-1} denotes the inverse of a function f. It is extensively used in mathematical physics [3]. If the signal $x(v)$ is concave or convex and has an invertible gradient, its Legendre transform is single-valued and equal (over the slope regions it is defined) to the upper or lower transform. Examples 7–12 in Table II deal with such signals x with invertible gradients.

If a differentiable signal is neither convex nor concave or if it does not have an invertible gradient, the Legendre transform is multi-valued; i.e., $X_L(\alpha)$ is a set of real numbers for each α. For example, consider the cosine $x(t) = \cos(\omega_0 t)$ over all time, which is an infinite sequence of convex and concave cosine pulses. Then

$$X_L(\alpha) = \{Y(\alpha) + \alpha kT, -Y(\alpha) + \alpha T(k - 0.5) : k = 0, \pm 1, \pm 2, ...\} \ , \ T = \frac{2\pi}{\omega_0}$$

where Y is the slope transform of a single concave cosine pulse (Example 12, Table II). In general, the number of different functions in the multivalued Legendre transform is equal to the number of consecutive convex and concave pieces making up the signal. This could be finite or infinite. This multivalued Legendre transform is defined for the 1D case in [4] as a 'slope transform' and is expressed via stationary points; i.e., $X_L(\alpha) = \{x(t^*) - \alpha t^* : \dot{x}(t^*) = \alpha\}$. Its properties in [4] seem similar to the properties of the upper/lower slope transform, but there are some important differences (see [7, 8]) stemming from the fact that operations among multivalued Legendre transforms are actually set operations.

An arbitrary signal can be analyzed using slope transforms toward at least two different goals: signal reconstruction, or envelope reconstruction. For exact signal reconstruction, we should segment the signal into consecutive convex and concave pieces and find the slope transform of each piece. The set collection of slope transforms of the signal pieces can reconstruct the signal exactly. The disadvantage here is the multivaluedness of the transform. Alternatively, for extracting information about the long-scale behavior of the signal, as manifested by its upper and lower envelope, we could compute its upper and lower slope transforms and take their inverses, which give us the two envelopes. Examples of this latter case include the impulse responses of systems described by recursive max/min difference equations and amplitude-modulated signals where we seek to estimate their envelope.

3. 1D Max-plus Difference Equations and Slope Filters

Consider the 1D causal recursive DSI system $y_1[n] = \max(y_1[n-1] + a_1, x[n])$ with $a_1 < 0$, which is a max-plus convolution of the input with the causal line $g_1[n] = a_1 n + \lambda[n]$. (Its theory is discussed in [6, 7].) The output $y_1[n]$ provides a type of upper envelope of $x[n]$; see Fig. 2a. The slope response of this system is $G_1(\alpha) = -\lambda(\alpha - a_1)$ and hence rejects all negative slopes $< a_1$. To reject some positive slopes we must pass the input through an anti-causal system $y_2[n] = \max(y_2[n+1] + a_2, x[n])$ with $a_2 > 0$, run backwards in time (see Fig. 2a). It corresponds to a max-plus convolution of the input with the anti-causal line $g_2[n] = a_2 n + \lambda[-n]$. Its slope response is $G_2(\alpha) = -\lambda(a_2 - \alpha)$ and hence it rejects all positive slopes $> a_2$. To symmetrize this process we can take the maximum $y = y_1 \vee y_2$ of the two envelopes as the final estimated upper envelope of the input. The mapping $x \mapsto y$, i.e., the maximum of two DSI systems, is another DSI system with overall impulse response $g = g_1 \vee g_2$ and overal slope response $G = G_1 \vee G_2$:

$$g[n] = \begin{cases} a_1 n, & n \geq 0 \\ a_2 n, & n \leq 0 \end{cases} \ , \quad G(\alpha) = \begin{cases} 0, & a_1 \leq \alpha \leq a_2 \\ +\infty, & \text{else} \end{cases}$$

This is an ideal-cutoff *bandpass slope-selective* filter. To design a *symmetric* slope filter we select $a_2 = -a_1 = \alpha_0 > 0$ which passes upper slopes with magnitude $\leq \alpha_0$ unchanged and rejects all other slopes. This is the case in Fig. 2a. Such bandpass slope filters have been applied to envelope detection for AM signals in [6, 7].

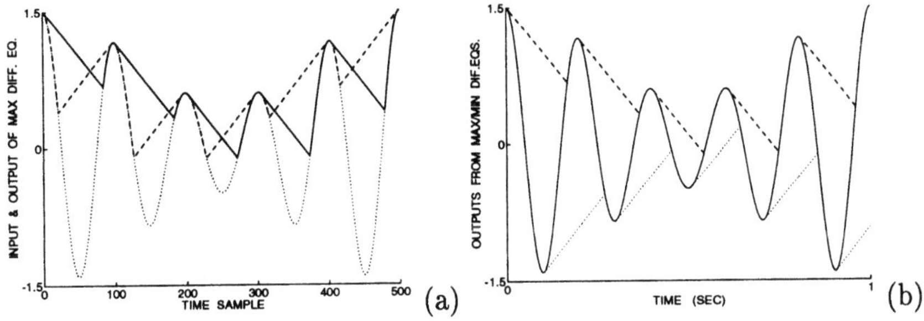

(a) (b)

Fig. 2. (a) Dotted line shows input signal $x[n] = [1 + 0.5\cos(2\pi n/500)]\cos(2\pi n/100)$. The solid (resp. dashed) line is the output of the recursive equation $y[n] = \max(y[n-1] \pm 0.01, x[n])$ run in forward (resp. backward) time. Final upper envelope is the max of the solid and dashed curves. (b) Solid line shows input $x(t) = [1 + 0.5\cos(2\pi t)]\cos(10\pi t)$. Upper dashed line is the output of a max differential equation with coefficient $\alpha_0 = 5$ whose input is the signal $x(t)$. The lower dotted line is the output of the corresponding dual min differential equation $y'(t+) = \min(x'(t+), \alpha_0)$ if $y(t) = x(t)$ and $y'(t+) = \alpha_0$ if $y(t) < x(t)$.

4. Max Differential Equation

Can we now find continuous-time systems whose slope response is an ideal-cutoff slope-selective filter as in the discrete case? The continuous-time counterpart of the causal 1st-order recursive DSI system would correspond in the time domain to a morphological dilation by a causal line $g(t) = -\alpha_0 t + \lambda(t)$, $\alpha_0 > 0$. From Fig. 2b we can imagine that dilating a signal $x(t)$ by the half-line $g(t)$ produces a type of upper envelope where, scanning toward the positive time direction, all the parts of the signal with slope larger than $-\alpha_0$ remain unchanged, whereas parts with slope smaller than $-\alpha_0$ are covered by line of slope $-\alpha_0$ which extends until a point of the signal graph with slope larger than $-\alpha_0$, after which time the same pattern repeats. The dynamics of this dilation are described by the following max differential equation:

$$y'(t+) = \left\{ \begin{array}{ll} \max(x'(t+), -\alpha_0), & \text{if } y(t) = x(t) \\ -\alpha_0, & \text{if } y(t) > x(t) \end{array} \right\}, \quad y(0) = x(0) \qquad (4)$$

where $x'(t+) = \lim_{p \downarrow 0}[x(t+p) - x(t)]/p$. We use right-sided derivatives because: (i) they are sufficient to create the forward dynamics, and (ii) the input and mostly the output signal might not possess a two-sided derivative at all points. Obviously, the solution of (4) is $y(t) = x(t) \oplus g(t)$.

The above dynamical system can be hardware-implemented with electronic circuits using analog differentiators and comparators. For sampled signals, it is interesting to note that replacing derivatives in (4) with simple one-sample differences transforms the max differential equation into the 1-st order max difference equation; compare Figs. 2a,b.

5. 2D Min-plus Difference Equations

The min version of the 2D difference equation (2), viewed as a nonlinear system $\Psi : x \mapsto y = \Psi(x)$, is assumed to be recursively computable. As explained in [5] for 2D linear difference equations, this depends on (i) the shape of the output mask $M_o = \{(k,j) : a_{kj} < +\infty\}$ determining which past output samples are involved in the recursion, (ii) the boundary conditions, i.e., the locations and values of the output samples $y[n,m]$ which are prespecified as initial conditions, and (iii) the scanning order in which the output samples should be computed. We assume boundary conditions of value $+\infty$ and of a shape (dependent on M_o and the scanning order) appropriate so that the difference equation is an ESI system recursively computable. Obviously, $(0,0) \notin M_o$. The nonrecursive part of this equation represents a min-plus convolution $\square$ of the input array $x[n,m]$ with the 2D finite-support structuring function $b[n,m] = b_{nm}$. This is well understood from the existing theory and geometric intuition about erosions by finite-support structuring functions. Thus, we henceforth focus only on the recursive min version of (2) by setting $b_{pq} = +\infty$ except from $b(0,0) = 0$. This yields the autoregressive 2D min-plus difference equation

$$y[n,m] = \left(\bigwedge_{(k,j)\in M_o} a_{kj} + y[n-k, m-j] \right) \wedge x[n,m] \tag{5}$$

If $f[n,m] = \mathcal{E}(-\mu[n,m])$ is the impulse response of the corresponding ESI system $\mathcal{E}$, then $y = x \square f$. Finding a closed-formula expression for f is generally not possible. However, we can first find the slope response F and then, via inverse lower slope transform, find the impulse response f or its envelope $\check{f}$. Applying lower slope transforms to both sides of (5) and using the fact that $Y_\wedge(\alpha) = F(\alpha) + X_\wedge(\alpha)$ yields

$$F(\alpha_1, \alpha_2) = \left(\bigwedge_{(k,j)\in M_o} F(\alpha_1,\alpha_2) + a_{kj} - k\alpha_1 - j\alpha_2 \right) \wedge (0) \tag{6}$$

A nontrivial (i.e., different than $-\infty$) solution F is

$$F(\alpha) = I_R(\alpha) = \begin{cases} 0, & \alpha \in R \\ -\infty, & \alpha \notin R \end{cases} , \quad R = \{(\alpha_1,\alpha_2) : k\alpha_1 + j\alpha_2 \leq a_{kj} \; \forall (k,j) \in M_o\}$$

Thus the system acts as an *ideal-cutoff slope filter* passing all input lower slopes α in the planar region R unchanged and rejecting the rest. R is a convex region determined by the inequalities $k\alpha_1 + j\alpha_2 \leq a_{kj}$. The inverse slope transform on F yields the lower envelope $\check{f}$ of the impulse response f. Over short-scale periods f has the shape induced by the sequence $\{a_{kj}\}$. But over scales much longer than the size of the coefficient mask M_o, f behaves like its lower envelope $\check{f}$. Together F and $\check{f}$ can describe the long-scale dynamics of the system. In addition, if f is a plane, then the above analysis is also exact for the short-scale behavior.

Example 1: Let $M_o = \{(0,1),(0,1)\}$, and

$$y_1[n,m] = \min(y_1[n-1,m] + a_{10}, y_1[n,m-1] + a_{01}, x[n,m]) \tag{7}$$

Assuming boundary conditions $y_1[n,m] = +\infty$ if $n < 0$ or $m < 0$ and a bottom-left to top-right scanning order, the impulse response (found by induction) and slope response (shown in Fig. 3a for $a_{10} = a_{01} = 1$) are

$$f_1[n,m] = a_{10}n + a_{01}m - \lambda[n,m] \quad , \quad F_1(\alpha_1,\alpha_2) = \lambda(a_{10} - \alpha_1, a_{01} - \alpha_2) \tag{8}$$

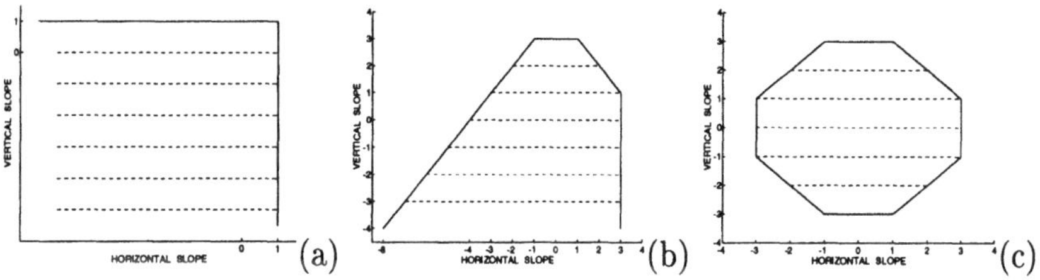

Fig. 3. Regions of support of binary slope responses of ESI systems described by 2D min-plus difference equations.

Thus this system acts as a 2D lowpass slope filter passing all input lower slopes $\alpha_1 \leq a_{10}$ and $\alpha_2 \leq a_{01}$, and rejecting the rest. In this case, $f = \check{f}$ is convex. This example demonstrates that when ESI systems described by min difference equations have a recursive part (i.e., when at least one $a_{kj} \neq +\infty$), their impulse response has infinite support. The recursion (7) with $a_{10} = a_{01} = 1$ is used to compute the first pass $y_1 = x \Box f_1$ of the distance transform for the city-block distance (using the 5-pixel diamond as the unit disk) of a binary image x [10, 2]. The distance transform y is completed via a second pass $y = y_1 \Box f_2$, where $f_2[n,m] = f_1[-n,-m]$, or equivalently as $y = y_1 \wedge y_2$ where $y_2 = x \Box f_2$. Thus the distance transform $x \mapsto y$ is an ESI system with impulse response $f = f_1 \wedge f_2$ and slope response F, where

$$f[n,m] = |n| + |m| \quad , \quad F(\alpha) = F_1(\alpha) \wedge F_1(-\alpha) = \begin{cases} 0, & |\alpha_1|, |\alpha_2| \leq 1 \\ -\infty, & \text{else} \end{cases}$$

F_1 is the indicator function of the region in Fig. 3a, and F is the indicator function of the unit square.

Example 2: Let $M_o = \{(0,1),(0,1),(1,1),(-1,1)\}$ with $a_{10} = a_{01} = 3$ and $a_{11} = a_{-11} = 4$. Then, as in Example 1, running the min difference equation in a bottom-left to top-right scan yields the first pass y_1 of the chamfer (3,4) distance algorithm [2]. The slope response F_1 of the corresponding ESI system is found from (6) and shown in Fig. 3b. The slope response of the complete distance computation system is $F(\alpha) = F_1(\alpha) \wedge F_1(-\alpha)$ and is the indicator function of the octagon shown in Fig. 3c. Thus, in general, the 2D discrete distance transforms are ESI systems whose slope responses are indicator functions of symmetric polygonal approximations to the disk in the slope plane and whose impulse responses are approximations to space cones. They are 2D ideal-cutoff bandpass slope filters.

6. Sampling

Consider sampling a 1D continuous-time signal $x_c(t)$ at time instants $t = nT$ and obtaining the *sampled* signal $x_s(t) = \bigvee_n x[n] + \mu(t - nT)$, where $x[n] = x_c(nT)$, $n = 0, \pm 1, \pm 2, \ldots$, is the *discrete-time* signal. Let $X_c(\alpha) = \bigwedge_t x_c(t) - \alpha t$ and $X_s(\alpha) = \bigwedge_n x_c(nT) - \alpha nT$ be the continuous-time upper slope transforms of the signals $x_c(t), x_s(t)$, and let $X_d(\alpha) = \bigvee_n x[n] - \alpha n$ be the upper slope transform of the discrete-time signal $x[n]$. Then

$$X_d(\alpha) = X_s(\alpha/T) \leq X_c(\alpha/T)$$

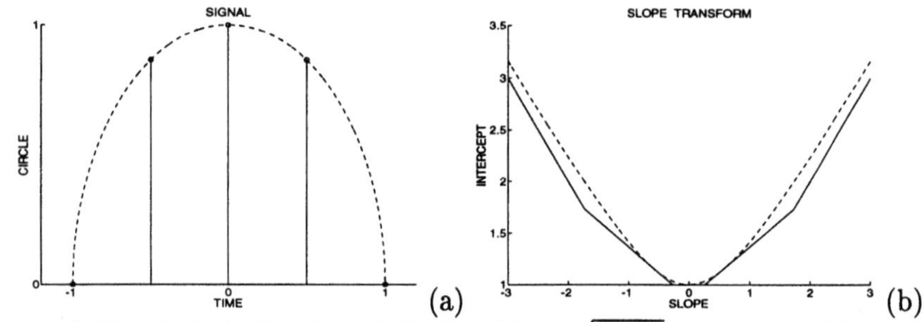

Fig. 4. (a) Signal circle (in dashed line) $x_c(t) = \sqrt{1-t^2}$, $|t| \leq 1$, and its sampled version (in solid lines) $x_s(t) = x_c(nT)$ with $T = 0.5$. (b) Upper slope transforms of original circle (in dashed line) and of its sampled version (in solid line).

Namely, the upper slope transform of the sampled signal is smaller or equal to the slope-scaled version of the transform of the original continuous-time signal, and going from the continuous to the discrete time axis simply scales the slope by T. Another effect of sampling is to replace parts of the slope transform of the continuous-time signal with supporting lines (see Fig. 4).

Reconstruction from Samples: Consider a concave *piecewise linear* signal $x_c(t)$ with corner points at the time instants $t_1 < t_2 < ... < t_N$ and corresponding values $x_1, x_2, ..., x_N$. Let $\alpha_1 > \alpha_2 > ... > \alpha_{N-1}$ be the slopes of the line pieces comprising the signal from left to right, where $\alpha_n = (x_{n+1} - x_n)/(t_{n+1} - t_n)$ for $n = 1, 2, ..., N-1$. The signal and its upper slope transform are

$$x_c(t) = \begin{cases} -\infty, & t < t_1 \\ x_n + \alpha_n t, & t_n \leq t \leq t_{n+1} \\ -\infty, & t > t_N \end{cases} \quad ; \quad X_c(\alpha) = \begin{cases} x_1 - \alpha t_1, & \alpha > \alpha_1 \\ x_n - \alpha t_n, & \alpha_{n-1} \geq \alpha \geq \alpha_n \\ x_N - \alpha t_N, & \alpha_{N-1} > \alpha \end{cases} \tag{9}$$

for $n = 2, .., N-1$. Thus, the upper slope transform of a concave piecewise-linear signal is a convex piecewise-linear function. Further, the upper slope transform of any sampled signal is always a convex piecewise-linear function. Hence, if $x_c(t)$, and hence $x_s(t)$, is a concave piecewise-linear signal and the sampling time instants $t = nT$ include all the times at which its corner points occur, then $X_s(\alpha)$ is piecewise linear with corner points at slopes $\alpha_n = (x[n+1] - x[n])/T$. By performing a continuous-time inverse slope transform on $X_s(\alpha)$ we obtain the upper envelope $\hat{x}_s(t)$ of $x_s(t)$ which by (9) is a piecewise linear interpolation of the samples $x[n]$. This linear interpolation is an aproximation to the original signal $x_c(t)$. The smaller the sampling period T, the better the approximation. Therefore, sampling followed by the composition of a slope transform and its inverse reconstructs piecewise-linear approximations to the original signal.

Another reconstruction algorithm, which applies to slope-limited signals $x_c(t)$, i.e., $|x_c'(t)| \leq \alpha_0$, is to pass the sampled signal $x_s(t)$ through the max/min differential equation in forward and bakward time, i.e., to convolve the sampled signal with a time cone $\pm\alpha_0|t|$. This will reconstruct partially piecewise-linear approximations to the original signal of the type shown in Fig. 2. It is in analogy with the standard approach of reconstructing a band-limited signal from its samples by passing its sampled version from a lowpass frequency-selective filter.

Discrete Computation: Even if the signal is defined on discrete time, its slope transform is defined on a continuous slope domain. How can we discretize slope? In discrete-time the computation of the upper slope transform $X(\alpha) = \max\{x[n] - \alpha n : n = 1,..,N\}$ for a *finite-length* signal $x[n]$, $n = 1,...,N$, requires $2N - 1$ additions and $N-1$ comparisons for each slope α. $X(\alpha)$ is always convex and piecewise-linear; hence we only need to know its values at its corner points occuring at slopes α_k, $k = 1,..,N-1$. If $x[n]$ is concave, then these slopes are known: $\alpha_k = x[k+1] - x[k]$, assuming $T = 1$. The inverse slope transform $\hat{x}[n] = \bigwedge_\alpha X(\alpha) + \alpha n$ involves minimization of a convex function. Its minima will occur at the corner points α_k. Hence, to reconstruct $x[n]$ or its envelope from its slope transform we only need to compute $\hat{x}[n] = \bigwedge_k X(\alpha_k) + \alpha_k n$. We refer to the finite sequence $X(\alpha_k)$ as a *discrete slope transform*, where for both the forward and the inverse transform we only need values at a finite set of slopes α_k. For arbitrary signals, we can a priori know all these possible corner point slopes if the signals are quantized. Thus, assuming that $x[n]$ is uniformly quantized to $L = 2^B$ levels (with a B-bit quantizer) and Δ is the quantization step size, then all corner point slopes will be $\alpha_k = k\Delta$, $|k| \leq 2L$. Hence for the slope transform and its inverse we only need values at these uniformly-spaced slopes. Then the computation of the discrete slope transform and its inverse has complexity about $O(LN)$. Since L is independent of N, if $N \gg L$ (e.g. in images), the total complexity is linear.

7. Envelope Filters

The mapping between a signal x and its upper (resp. lower) envelope $\hat{x} = \phi(x)$ (resp. $\check{x} = \gamma(x)$), equal to the composition of the upper (resp. lower) slope transform and its inverse, is actually a lattice closing ϕ (resp. opening γ) because it is increasing, idempotent, and extensive (resp. anti-extensive) [7]. We call such morphological filters *envelope closing and opening*, respectively.

Upper (resp. lower) envelopes of signals x are also obtained by passing x through max (resp. min) difference or differential equations; see Fig. 2. These envelopes are actually max/min-plus convolutions of the input with conical structuring functions. The infinite extent of these cones makes the mapping idempotent. The map is also increasing and extensive (resp. anti-extensive) for the max (resp. min) equations. Thus, the max/min recursive equations create closing/openings and can be viewed as another class of envelope filters. It is interesting that a single morphological dilation $\oplus$ or erosion $\ominus$ can generate a closing or opening.

References

1. R. Bellman and W. Karush, "On the Maximum Transform", *J. Math. Anal. Appl.*, 6, pp. 67–74, 1963.
2. G. Borgefors, "Distance Transformations in Digital Images", *Comp. Vision, Graphics, Image Process.*, 34, 344–371, 1986.
3. R. Courant and D. Hilbert, *Methods of Mathematical Physics*, Wiley, NY, 1962.
4. L. Dorst and R. van den Boomgaard, "An Analytical Theory of Mathematical Morphology", *Proc. Int'l Work. Math. Morphology & Applic. to Signal Processing*, Barcelona, May 1993.
5. D. E. Dudgeon and R. M. Mersereau, *Multidimensional Digital Signal Processing*, Prentice Hall, NJ, 1984.

TABLE I: Properties of Upper Slope Transform

No.	Signal: $x(v)$	Transform: $X_\vee(\alpha)$
1.	$\bigvee_i c_i + x_i(v)$	$\bigvee_i c_i + X_i(\alpha)$
2.	$x(v - v_0)$	$X(\alpha) - < \alpha, v_0 >$
3.	$x(v) + < \alpha_0, v >$	$X(\alpha - \alpha_0)$
4.	$x(rv), \quad r \in \mathbf{R}$	$X(\alpha/r)$
5.	$rx(v) \ , r > 0$	$rX(\alpha/r)$
6.	$x(v) \oplus y(v)$	$X(\alpha) + Y(\alpha)$
7.	$\bigvee_u x(u) + y(v+u)$	$X(-\alpha) + Y(\alpha)$
8.	$x(v) \leq y(v) \ \forall v$	$X(\alpha) \leq Y(\alpha) \ \forall \alpha$
9.	$y(v) = \begin{cases} x(v), & \lvert\lvert v \rvert\rvert_p \leq r \\ -\infty, & \lvert\lvert v \rvert\rvert_p > r \end{cases}$	$Y(\alpha) = X(\alpha) \Box r \lvert\lvert \alpha \rvert\rvert_q$

TABLE II: Examples of Upper Slope Transforms

No.	Signal: $x(v)$	Transform: $X_\vee(\alpha)$
1.	$< \alpha_0, v >$	$-\mu(\alpha - \alpha_0)$
2.	$< \alpha_0, v > + \lambda(v)$	$-\lambda(\alpha - \alpha_0)$
3.	$\mu(v - v_0)$	$-< \alpha, v_0 >$
4.	$\lambda(v - v_0)$	$-< \alpha, v_0 > - \lambda(\alpha)$
5.	$\begin{cases} 0, & \lvert\lvert v \rvert\rvert_p \leq r \\ -\infty, & \lvert\lvert v \rvert\rvert_p > r \end{cases}$	$r\lvert\lvert \alpha \rvert\rvert_q, \quad \frac{1}{p} + \frac{1}{q} = 1, \ p \geq 1$
6.	$-\alpha_0 \lvert\lvert v \rvert\rvert_p, \quad \alpha_0 > 0$	$\begin{cases} 0, & \lvert\lvert \alpha \rvert\rvert_q \leq \alpha_0 \\ +\infty, & \lvert\lvert \alpha \rvert\rvert_q > \alpha_0 \end{cases}$
7.	$\sqrt{1 - t^2}, \quad \lvert t \rvert \leq 1$	$\sqrt{1 + \alpha^2}$
8.	$-t^2/2$	$\alpha^2/2$
9.	$-\lvert\lvert v \rvert\rvert_p^p / p \ , \ p > 1$	$\lvert\lvert \alpha \rvert\rvert_q^q / q \ , \ 1/p + 1/q = 1$
10.	$\exp(v)$	$\alpha[1 - \log(\alpha)]$
11.	$\tanh(t), \quad t \geq 0$	$\sqrt{1 - \alpha} - \alpha \log \left(\frac{1 + \sqrt{1 - \alpha}}{\sqrt{\alpha}} \right)$
12.	$\cos(\omega_0 t), \quad \lvert t \rvert \leq \frac{\pi}{2\omega_0}$	$\sqrt{1 - \frac{\alpha^2}{\omega_0^2}} + \left(\frac{\alpha}{\omega_0} \right) \sin^{-1} \left(\frac{\alpha}{\omega_0} \right)$

6. P. Maragos, "Max-Min Difference Equations and Recursive Morphological Systems", *Proc. Int'l Work. Math. Morphology & Applic. to Signal Processing*, Barcelona, May 1993.
7. P. Maragos, "Morphological Systems: Slope Transforms and Max–Min Difference and Differential Equations", *Signal Processing*, Sep. 1994.
8. P. Maragos, "Slope Transforms: Theory and Application to Nonlinear Signal Processing", submitted to IEEE Trans. on Signal Processing.
9. R. T. Rockafellar, *Convex Analysis*, Princeton Univ. Press, Princeton, 1972.
10. A. Rosenfeld and J. L. Pfaltz, "Sequential Operations in Digital Picture Processing", *J. ACM*, 13, pp. 471-494, Oct. 1966.
11. J. Serra, "Equicontinuous Functions: A Model for Mathematical Morphology", *Proc. SPIE vol.1769: Image Algebra and Morphological Image Processing III*, pp. 252–263, 1992.

TWO DUAL REPRESENTATIONS OF MORPHOLOGY BASED ON THE PARALLEL NORMAL TRANSPORT PROPERTY

LEO DORST and REIN VAN DEN BOOMGAARD*
Dept. of Mathematics and Computer Science,
University of Amsterdam, The Netherlands
leo@fwi.uva.nl and rein@fwi.uva.nl

This paper is an extended and improved version of the paper [1] in the 2nd International Workshop on Visual Form, Capri, 1994.

Abstract. A familiar way to describe shapes is through their behavior under the operations of mathematical morphology. In this paper we provide a quantitative analysis of the basic operation of mathematical morphology: *dilation.* This operation has the important property that it transports points such that normals to surfaces are preserved. As a consequence, straight lines are *eigenfunctions of morphology.* A representation of the objects on a basis of these eigenfunctions should clarify the basic operation (remember how the Fourier transform illuminates linear filtering!), and finding such representations is the subject of this paper.

We present two ways to convert the parallel normal transport property into a computational representation of *tangential dilation,* which is a suitably defined generalization of the dilation of object boundaries. One is the *slope transform,* designed for the dilation of functions, the other is the *normal transform* designed for the dilation of geometrical objects. For both transforms, we show how tangential dilation in the spatial domain becomes *addition* in the transformed domain (plain addition for the slope transform, radial harmonic addition for the normal transform). Though both representations are complete, there are applications in which one is preferable over the other - we give some recommendations for the selection.

Key words: mathematical morphology, eigenfunction, tangential dilation, slope transform, Legendre transform, Gauss map

1. Introduction

Mathematical morphology describes the contact of *sets*, and does so typically in an algebraic and set-theoretic notation. If one would like to use it for the description and analysis of the contact of *physical rigid bodies*, a more quantitative description is required. Such a representation can be based on the eigen-objects of morphology: the planes.

In previous papers [2][3], we have presented the *slope transform* of a function for precisely this purpose. The graph of any function can be represented as the caustic of its tangent planes, and these tangent planes can be characterized by their intercept with the value axis as a function of their slope. This representation is additive under dilation. It is closely related to the Legendre transform of theoretical physics [4], the Young-Fenchel conjugate of convex analysis [5][6] and to the $\mathcal{A}$-transform [7].

* Work done under NWO/SION project 612-322-205: Model-controlled Image Processing.

J.Serra and P. Soille (eds.), Mathematical Morphology and Its Applications to Image Processing, 161-170

Application of the slope transform to the contact of geometrical *object surfaces* (rather than to the morphology of *signals*) requires their representation by *functions.* This can be done locally in the standard way of differential geometry [8] as a height function in some chosen direction (Monge patches). It can be done globally if one permits set-valued functions, and this appears to present no essential problems [3]. However, it is unsatisfying to have to introduce a preferential axis to describe objects that are free to roam through space.

In this paper, we introduce a dual representation of morphology that is *isotropic*, and hence more suited for the description of the contacts of rigid objects. Just like the slope transform, it is based on the representation of object surfaces by their tangent planes, since planes are the morphological eigenfunctions. The new element is that we characterize these tangent planes by projective covectors rather than by their slopes relative to some fiducial direction. The resulting transform we propose to call the *normal transform*; it is related to the Gauss map, but invertible (which the Gauss map is not). Under this normal transform, dilation of object surfaces becomes radial harmonic addition of their transforms.

2. Surfaces in Contact

Consider two objects A and $\breve{B}$, with oriented surfaces ∂A and $\partial\breve{B}$, both assumed to be smooth (but at whatever scale, so they can approximate sharp-cornered object surfaces arbitrarily precisely). Let A and $\breve{B}$ each be given a reference point, to keep track of their translations - we will not permit rotations. Bring ∂A and $\partial\breve{B}$ into touching contact by some translation, such that the normals at the point of contact are opposite. The loci of all positions of the reference point of $\partial\breve{B}$, relative to that of ∂A, in such touching contact forms an object surface which we will call the *tangential dilation result* of ∂A and ∂B, denoted $\partial A \breve{\oplus} \partial B$. (Here $\breve{B}$ is the point-mirrored image of B relative to its reference point, and so B is the point-mirrored image of $\breve{B}$ - we need this mirroring to correspond to the conventional notation of dilation based on Minkowski sums of sets.)

To find the correspondence of this tangential dilation of object boundaries to the classical dilation of the objects themselves, consider the operation locally, on a small patch where A and B are convex. If we assign local coordinate systems to A and B which permit us to describe part of the surface as a function (with the object below the graph, free-space above) , then we can describe the operation for convex A and B as a *dilation of functions* (see e.g. [9]):

$$(f \oplus g)(x) = \sup_u [f(u) + g(x - u)]. \tag{1}$$

Here f and g are height functions on a domain X, such that $(x, f(x))$, for $x \in X$, is a patch of ∂A, $(x, g(x))$, for $x \in X$, is a patch of ∂B, and $(x, (f \oplus g)(x))$ is a patch of the dilation result. Note that the result is symmetrical in ∂A and ∂B: it is invariant under the coordinate transformation $u \mapsto x - u$.

Let $\bar{u}$ be the value of u for which the supremum is reached; it is the abscissa of the contact point in the coordinate system of the ∂B-patch. At the once-differentiable

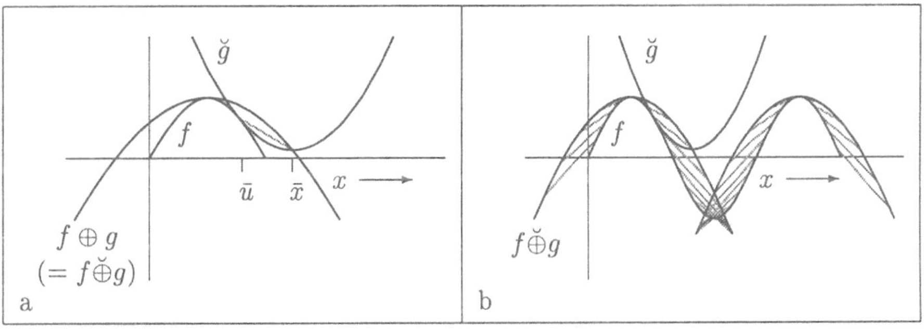

Fig. 1. Dilation and the slope theorem. (a) parallel transport of slope for convex functions; (b) tangential dilation: parallel transport everywhere.

parts of $f \oplus g$, we have an equality of derivatives noted in [10] and proved in [11]:

$$\nabla(f \oplus g)(x) = \nabla g(x - \bar{u}) = \nabla f(\bar{u}) \tag{2}$$

Derivation: Immediate from differentiation of eq.(1) to x and $\bar{u}$. ■

Geometrically, this means that dilation of two surface patches is a parallel transport of the tangent planes to that surface: the slopes of f at $\bar{u}$, of g at $\bar{x} - \bar{u}$ and of $f \oplus g$ at $\bar{x}$ are all equal (Fig. 1a). For this reason we refer to eq.(2) as the *slope theorem.* Obviously, when the slopes in coordinate directions of the Monge patches are preserved, then so are the normals to the surfaces ∂A, ∂B and $\partial(A \oplus B)$.

It is this property which may be used to define the tangential dilation most clearly, and that is how we introduced it in [2]:

> Given smooth surfaces ∂A and ∂B with reference points o_A and o_B. Construct a surface $\partial A \breve{\oplus} \partial B$ by the following procedure: for any point p of ∂A (relative to o_A), determine the normal n_p to A at p. Find all points q relative to o_B such that the normal to ∂B at q equals n_p (or equivalently, the points $-q$ such that the normal to $\partial \breve{B}$ equals $-n_p$). Construct all points of $\partial A \breve{\oplus} \partial B$ corresponding to this contact as: $p + q$, for all q.

The tangential dilation is *not* identical to the boundary of the dilation of A and B, but contains it:

$$\partial(A \oplus B) \subseteq \partial A \breve{\oplus} \partial B, \tag{3}$$

since the condition is satisfied at all differentiable points of the classical dilation by the slope theorem[1]. The tangential dilation includes points that represent a contact in which ∂A and $\partial \breve{B}$ touch locally, but intersect somewhere else (Fig. 1b). By not excluding those points, the tangential dilation is a purely local operation, and this makes its analysis much more tractable. The operation is *not* closed on the set of surfaces that are the boundaries of objects, since that woudl exclude self-intersections

[1] Note that $p+q$ is indeed the correct result for the classical dilation of eq.(1): both the function values and their abscissae add up: $x = \bar{u} + (x - \bar{u})$ and $(f \breve{\oplus} g)(x) = f(\bar{u}) + g(x - \bar{u})$.

like Fig. 1b. Tangential dilation *is* closed on the set of smooth differentiable surfaces – and these include surfaces with self-intersections and cusps, as in Fig. 1b. In the following, α and β will be used to denote such surfaces.

Such a generalization of the dilation operation to contours is not wholly new to morphology: for polytopes, Ghosh [12] has introduced an analogous generalization to create an algebra based on the dilation operation.

3. Eigenobjects of (Tangential) Dilation

A plane $n-1$ dimensional surface α has the same normal ν at any point. Under tangential dilation by a surface β, each point p of α therefore translates by the same amount, namely by q such that the normal of β at q equals ν. Therefore, the dilation result is also a plane (in general, a set of planes), with the same normal ν. We have found:

> An $n-1$ dimensional plane surface is an eigenfunction of the tangential dilation in dimension n.

Taking our cue from representation theory, we look for a representation of arbitrary surfaces in terms of these eigenfunctions. That should then form a representation in which the dilation operation is simple. We present two such representations: the *slope transform* (a generalization of the Legendre transform, introduced before in [2]) and the *normal transform* (which is related to the Gauss map).

4. The Slope Transform

The results in this section are taken from [2] and [3].

Let a differentiable function $f: X \to \mathbf{R}$ be given. At a point $(x, f(x))$, the tangent plane is given by all points $(u, \nabla f(x)\cdot(u-x)+f(x))$, for $u \in X$. We can characterize this plane by the slope $\nabla f(x)$ and the intercept $f(x) - \nabla f(x)\cdot x$. Indeed, we may move to a dual representation in which $\omega = \nabla f(x)$ is the independent variable, and consider the intercept of the tangent plane as a function of ω. This is the *slope transform* of f. We introduce the notation:

$$stat_x[f(x)] = \{f(u) \mid \nabla f(u) = 0, u \in X\} \tag{4}$$

for the stationary values of a differentiable real-valued function f. Then we can compute the slope transform $\mathcal{S}[f]$ of f as:

$$\mathcal{S}[f](\omega) = stat_x[f(x) - \omega\cdot x]. \tag{5}$$

Note that the analytical evaluation of the slope transform involves inverse functions. If ∇f is invertible, then the slope transform can be written as:

$$\mathcal{S}[f](\omega) = f((\nabla f)^{-1}(\omega)) - \omega\cdot(\nabla f)^{-1}(\omega). \tag{6}$$

In that case, the slope transform is identical to the Legendre-transform of f. The original function f can be reconstructed from its slope transform by:

$$f(x) = stat_\omega[\mathcal{S}[f](\omega) + \omega\cdot x] \tag{7}$$

for a wide class of functions. Since the 'functions' are to represent the class of differentiable surfaces (not just object boundaries), an extension to a more global representation of the surfaces leads to a description in which their graphs are naturally considered as parametrizable curves. The derivation of the slope transform, and the relationship to the Legendre transform [4], the Young-Fenchel conjugate of convex analysis [5][6], and the $\mathcal{A}$-transform of [7] can be found in [3].

The tangential dilation introduced above can be formulated using the 'stat' operator as:

$$(f\breve{\oplus}g)(x) = stat_u[f(u) + g(x-u)]. \tag{8}$$

Note that this result contains the classical dilation result of eq.(1): $(f \oplus g)(x) \subseteq (f\breve{\oplus}g)(x)$.

It is now straightforward to show that *tangential dilation of functions becomes addition of their slope transforms* [2] [3]:

$$\mathcal{S}[f\breve{\oplus}g] = \mathcal{S}[f] + \mathcal{S}[g]. \tag{9}$$

The slope transform thus indeed provides a simple representation of the tangential dilation operation, namely as *addition.* There is a nice analogy to the way in which the Fourier transform represents convolution as multiplication [3]. Using the relationship of tangential dilation of boundaries to the dilation of the sets themselves, this simple representation can be made useful to 'classical' morphology as well.

5. The Normal Transform

The function representation of the slope transform is convenient for morphological processing of *signals*, but *not* the most natural representation for morphology on geometrical *objects.* The preferential treatment of the function direction, and with it the use of the slope itself, will have to be replaced by an isotropic treatment of directions based on normals.

At any point p of a differentiable surface α, we can set up a tangent plane to the surface. It is the best linear approximation to the surface at p. The orientation of this tangent plane can be specified by a 1-form (or co-vector) ν_p at p; a tangent vector v in the plane is then characterized by $\nu_p(v) = 0$. Thus our use of the 1-form ν_p permits an undetermined scalar factor: $c\nu_p$ denotes the same tangent plane. (For readers unfamiliar with covectors: ν_p is like a vector n_p normal to the surface at p, and $\nu_p(v)$ is like $n_p.v$, the inner product of n_p and v).

For the construction of the tangential dilation, we need to be able to find all points at which a certain tangent plane occurs; therefore we want a representation in which a covector yields a position vector. The object surface determines a relationship between position vectors and covectors, and is therefore an object in the cotangent bundle $T^*(X)$ of the base space X, a typical point being (p, ν_p). The cotangent bundle object is not unique, however, due to the projective freedom in the covectors indicating the same tangent plane: (p, ν_p) should be the same as $(p, c\nu_p)$. We can make it unique by the following procedure: we represent the pair (p, ν_p) by a covector (p, ω_p) such that $\omega_p = c\nu_p$ and $\omega_p(p) = 1$. (This is called a projectivization of the cotangent bundle, and it leads to a *contact manifold*, see [4].) Thus we have:

$$\omega_p = \frac{\nu_p}{\nu_p(p)}. \tag{10}$$

To obtain the desired map, we now consider the section (p, ω_p) for all p not as providing ω_p given p, but as providing p given ω_p. (There is no problem switching to this dual point of view for Euclidean $X = E^n$; we will restrict ourselves to such spaces in this paper.) We call ω_p the *normal transform* of p. By performing the normal transform at all points of an object surface α, we obtain the normal transform $\mathcal{N}[\alpha]$ of the object surface.

The surface $\mathcal{N}[\alpha]$ constructed in this way has the interesting property that its normal at a point ω_p is proportional to p. Indeed, if we perform the normal transform on $\mathcal{N}[\alpha]$, we obtain α again. This means that the *normal transform is an involution* (an operation that is its own inverse). Notationally we have to be a bit careful, since the normal transform was only defined on X. Let us denote by I the operation that converts covectors of the dual space into vectors of the base space X, and vice versa, so that we can indeed do the normal transform again (if we denote a point p by an $n \times 1$ column vector, then Ip is the $1 \times n$ row covector with corresponding coefficients). Then we can write the involution property as:

$$I\mathcal{N}[I\mathcal{N}[\alpha]] = \alpha. \tag{11}$$

Derivation: Let p_i denote the i-th component of p, ω_i the i-th component of ω_p. The identity $\omega_p(p) = 1$ is then written as $\omega_i p_i = 1$ (Einstein convention). Then $\dot{\omega}_i p_i + \omega_i \dot{p}_i = 0$. Since w_p represents a tangent plane to the surface at p, we have $\omega_i \dot{p}_i = 0$, and it follows that $\dot{\omega}_i p_i = 0$. Therefore, Icp represents a tangent plane to the dual surface point at $I\omega_p$ (c any non-zero real). The transform of the dual surface point is hence $Icp_i/(cp_j\omega_j) = Ip_i$, and hence $I\mathcal{N}[\alpha]$ transforms to $I\alpha$. ∎

It is instructive to verify this for a parametrized curve $p(t) = (p_1(t), p_2(t))^T$ in E^2. The (right-handed) normal to the curve at p is the cotangent vector $(\nu_1, \nu_2)(t) = (-\dot{p}_2, \dot{p}_1)(t)$, so the transform at p is

$$\begin{pmatrix} p_1 \\ p_2 \end{pmatrix}(t) \rightarrow (\omega_1, \omega_2)(t) = \frac{(-\dot{p}_2, \dot{p}_1)}{\dot{p}_1 p_2 - \dot{p}_2 p_1}(t). \tag{12}$$

Some algebraic manipulation demonstrates that the formula is invariant under the exchange of $p \leftrightarrow I\omega$. Therefore the transformation (including I) is an involution.

As a representation of the normals on the original surface, the normal transform is related to the Gauss-map. The Gauss-map image of a point p with normal n_p is the point $n_p/||n_p||$ on the unit sphere. Therefore the Gauss map contains directional information only, the position information is lost, and inversion has become impossible. A generalized Gauss-map has been used by Ghosh [12] to describe a dilation of polytope contours (similar to our tangential dilation of differentiable curves). Other mappings from differential geometry related to the normal transform are the *pedal* curve, $n_p(n_p.p)$, which is invertible but does not scale well, and the *dual curve* $(n_p, n_p.p)$ which is overdetermined [13]. To the best of our knowledge, the normal transform is new.

Tangential dilation has a simple representation in the normal transform. Let $p+q$ be a point of the surface $\alpha\breve{\oplus}\beta$, obtained by tangential dilation of α at p and β at q. Let the normal covector at the considered points be ν (so $\nu = \nu_p = \nu_q = \nu_{p+q}$). Then the transform is:

$$\begin{aligned}\mathcal{N}[\alpha\breve{\oplus}\beta]: \quad \omega_{p+q} &= \frac{\nu_{p+q}}{\nu_{p+q}(p+q)} = \frac{\nu}{\nu(p+q)} \\ &= \frac{\nu}{\nu(p)+\nu(q)} \end{aligned} \tag{13}$$

since covectors are linear. Thus the direction of ω_{p+q} is the same as that of ω_p and of ω_q (namely the direction of ν), and the magnitude of w_{p+q} is the harmonic sum of the magnitudes of ω_p and ω_q:

$$\frac{1}{||\omega_{p+q}||} = \frac{1}{||\omega_p||} + \frac{1}{||\omega_q||}. \tag{14}$$

We will denote this by $\omega_{p+q} = \omega_p \,//\, \omega_q$, or for the object surfaces α and β by:

$$\mathcal{N}[\alpha\breve{\oplus}\beta] = \mathcal{N}[\alpha] \,//\, \mathcal{N}[\beta]. \tag{15}$$

Compare this to eq.(9) for the the slope transform.

6. Symmetries: Signals versus Objects

The input objects to morphology, be they functions or object surfaces, may be subjected to certain symmetry transmations, and these have an effect on their transforms. We have noted these effects in Table I for some common symmetries. One should choose a representation in which symmetries of the input objects are most easily represented; thus the (desired or observed) symmetries help in the selection of the dual transform. General remarks can be made in terms of *signals* and *objects*.

- *Signals: Slope Transform*
  If a surface is obtained as a *signal*, namely as a real-valued function on some n-dimensional space X, then one should use the slope transform to describe the morphology. This is especially so when there are symmetries in X (such as translation invariance) that are not symmetries of $X \times \mathbf{R}$. In that case, the slope transform is the most natural representation of dilation.
  Such is the case in the processing of grey-valued images: the intensity dimension has properties rather different from the spatial dimensions. Thus in *grey-value morphology*, the *slope transform* should be used to analyze the effect of morphology on the images, and as a tool for filter design.
- *Objects: Normal Transform*
  If a surface is obtained as the boundary of an *object*, with all directions in space being equivalent in their permitted symmetries, then the normal transform should be used to describe the morphology.
  When considering the shape of objects in images, only the symmetries of the spatial dimensions matter. Thus in morphological processing on *binary images*, one should use the *normal transform* for the analysis and design of filters.

TABLE I

Properties of the two dual transforms. f and g denote functions, α and β denote surfaces.

property	original signal	slope transform	original object	normal transform
transform	$f(x)$	$stat_x[f(x) - \omega x]$	$p \in \alpha$	$\frac{\nu_p}{\nu_p(p)} \in \mathcal{N}[\alpha]$
inverse transform	$stat_\omega[\mathcal{S}[f](\omega) + \omega x]$	$\mathcal{S}[f](\omega)$	$I\frac{\nu_q}{\nu_q(q)} \in \alpha$	$q \in I\mathcal{N}[\alpha]$
translation	$a + f(x)$ $f(x - a)$	$a + \mathcal{S}[f](\omega)$ $-a\omega + \mathcal{S}[f](\omega)$	$\alpha + a$	$\mathcal{N}[\alpha]//\mathcal{N}[a]$
rotation	$ax + f(x)$	$\mathcal{S}[f](\omega - a)$	$R\alpha$	$R\mathcal{N}[\alpha]$
scaling	$f(ax)$ $af(x)$ $af(\frac{x}{a})$	$\mathcal{S}[f](\frac{\omega}{a})$ $a\mathcal{S}[f](\frac{\omega}{a})$ $a\mathcal{S}[f](\omega)$	 $a\alpha$	 $\mathcal{N}[\alpha]/a$
point inversion	$\check{f}(x) \equiv -f(-x)$	$-\mathcal{S}[f](\omega)$	$\check{\alpha} = -\alpha$	$-\mathcal{N}[\alpha]$
affine transform			$\mathcal{A}\alpha$	$(\mathcal{A}^T)^{-1}\mathcal{N}[\alpha]$
dilation	$(f\breve{\oplus}g)(x)$	$(\mathcal{S}[f] + \mathcal{S}[g])(\omega)$	$\alpha\breve{\oplus}\beta$	$\mathcal{N}[\alpha] \,//\, \mathcal{N}[\beta]$
addition	$(f + g)(x)$	$(\mathcal{S}[f]\breve{\oplus}\mathcal{S}[g])(\omega)$	$\alpha \,//\, \beta$	$\mathcal{N}[\alpha]\breve{\oplus}\mathcal{N}[\beta]$

There are of course situations that are ambiguous. One occurs in the scanning tunneling microscope, a morphological measurement instrument for atomic surfaces [10]. Here an atomic probe moves scanning in contact with an atomic surface, and the probe's height is measured as a *signal.* Thus one might use the slope transform; but since the signal is a height function, one may also view the result as an isotropic *object boundary* representation and use the normal transform.

7. An Example of the Two Dual Transforms

As an example of the use of the transformations, we describe the dilation of a parabola $y = \frac{1}{2a}x^2$ and the circle $x^2 + y^2 = r^2$, in both representations.

– *The Slope Transform View*
  The slope transform of $f(x) = \frac{1}{2a}x^2$ is $\mathcal{S}[f](\omega) = -\frac{a}{2}\omega^2$ (see [2]). A circle is represented by the set-valued function $g(x) = \pm\sqrt{r^2 - x^2}$, of which the slope transform is the two-sheeted hyperbola $\mathcal{S}[g](\omega) = \pm r\sqrt{1 + \omega^2}$. The upper half circle corresponds to the upper sheet of the hyperbola.

  These slope transforms are drawn in Fig. 2b for $a = 1$, $r = 2$, as is their sum. The inverse slope transform of the sum gives the tangential dilation of the two functions. The result is indicated in Fig. 2a as the thickly drawn curve.

– *The Normal Transform View*
  The normal transform of the parabola $p_2 - \frac{1}{2a}p_1^2 = 0$ is $\omega_p = (\omega_1, \omega_2) = (2/p_1, -2a/p_1^2)$, so $a\omega_1^2/2 + \omega_2 = 0$. The normal transform of the circle $p_1^2 + p_2^2 = r^2$ is the circle $\omega_1^2 + \omega_2^2 = \frac{1}{r^2}$. Introduce polar coordinates: the circle has

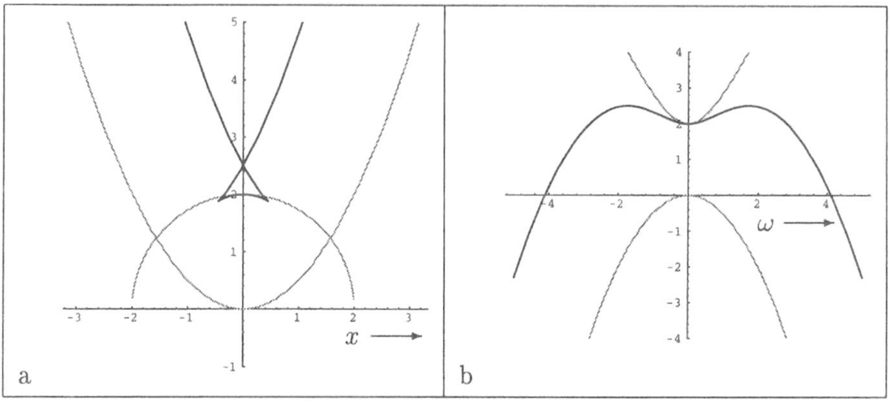

Fig. 2. The tangential dilation of a parabola $y = x^2/2$ and a circle with radius 2, in spatial domain (a) and slope domain (b), where it is addition.

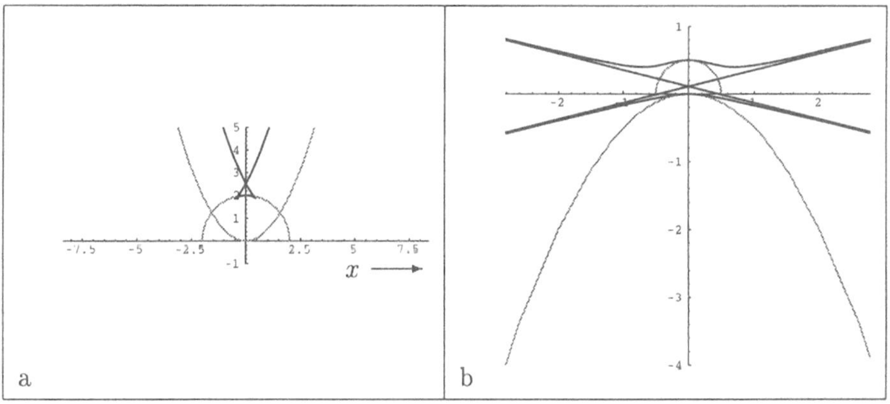

Fig. 3. The tangential dilation of a parabola $y = x^2/2$ and a circle with radius 2, in spatial domain (a) and normal domain (b), where it is harmonic addition (dark curve).

$\rho(\phi) = \frac{1}{r}$, the parabola $\rho(\phi) = -\frac{2\sin\phi}{a\cos^2\phi}$. Thus the harmonic sum is:

$$\frac{1}{r - \frac{a\cos^2\phi}{2\sin\phi}}(\cos\phi, \sin\phi), \tag{16}$$

and the inverse normal transform yields:

$$(\cot\phi(r\sin\phi - a), \frac{2a\cos^2\phi + 3r\sin\phi - r\sin 3\phi}{4\sin^2\phi})^T. \tag{17}$$

Fig. 3 shows the plot of this solution.

The plots for the dilation results Figs.2a,3a are indeed identical, even though the computation of the dilation is performed in different dual domains. This example illustrates the fact that there is no fundamental reason why one should use one transform or the other. We have found that the normal transform is easier to do analytically: it does not require the computation of inverse functions, while the slope transform does.[2]

8. Towards Morphological Systems

To conclude, both transforms convert the basic operation of tangential dilation into a simple addition operation in the transformed domain. As such, they both are counterpart of the Fourier transform in linear filtering, which transforms the involved operation of convolution into the simple operation of multiplication. We believe that the morphological transforms provide the analytical apparatus to develop a *morphological systems theory* with a power and rigor fully comparable to linear systems theory. We will then have two equally consistent theories of signal processing, each applicable to the analysis and control of different aspects of the natural world.

References

1. L. Dorst and R. van den Boomgaard. Two dual representations of morphology based on the parallel normal transport property. To appear in proceedings of 2nd International Workshop on Visual Form, Capri, 1994.
2. L. Dorst and R. van den Boomgaard. An analyical theory of mathematical morphology. In J. Serra and P. Salembier, editors, *Mathematical Morphology and its Applications to Signal Processing*, pages 245—250, Barcelona, Spain, May 1993. Universitat Politècnica de Catalunya.
3. L. Dorst and R. van den Boomgaard. Morphological signal processing and the slope transform. invited paper for Signal Processing, to appear 1994.
4. V.I. Arnold. *Mathematical Methods of Classical Mechanics*. Springer Verlag New York, 1989.
5. A.D. Ioffe and V.M. Tihomirov. *Theory of Extremal Problems*. North-Holland, Amsterdam, 1979.
6. J. Mattioli. Differential equations of morphological operators. In J. Serra and P. Salembier, editors, *Mathematical Morphology and its Applications to Signal Processing*, pages 162—167, Barcelona, Spain, May 1993. Universitat Politècnica de Catalunya.
7. P. Maragos. Max-min difference equations and recursive morphological systems. In J. Serra and P. Salembier, editors, *Mathematical Morphology and its Applications to Signal Processing*, pages 128—133, Barcelona, Spain, May 1993. Universitat Politècnica de Catalunya.
8. B. O'Neill. *Elementary Differential Geometry*. Academic Press, New York, 1966.
9. H.J.A.M. Heijmans. Mathematical morphology: a geometrical approach in image processing. *Nieuw Archief voor Wiskunde*, 10:237–276, 1992.
10. D. Keller. Reconstruction of STM and AFM images distorted by finite-sized tips. *Surface Science*, 253:353—364, 1991.
11. R. van den Boomgaard. *Mathematical Morphology: Extensions towards Computer Vision*. PhD thesis, University of Amsterdam, March 1992.
12. P.K. Ghosh. An algebra of polygons through the notion of negative shapes. *CVGIP: Image Understanding*, 54(1):119—144, 1991.
13. J.W. Bruce and P.J. Giblin. *Curves and Singularities*. Cambridge University Press, 1984.

[2] Although the parametric slope transform introduced in [3] meets this objection, for the addition of slope transforms an inversion is still necessary.

DOMINANCE AND INCIDENCE STRUCTURES WITH APPLICATIONS TO STOCHASTIC GEOMETRY AND MATHEMATICAL MORPHOLOGY

HENK J.A.M. HEIJMANS
CWI
P.O. Box 94079, 1090 GB Amsterdam, The Netherlands

and

ADRIAN J. BADDELEY
Department of Mathematics
University of Western Australia, Nedlands WA 6009, Australia

Abstract. Mathematical morphology is based on set-theoretic notions such as inclusion and intersection. In this paper it is shown how such notions can be extended to complete lattices. This results in so-called dominance and incidence structures. Such structures can be regarded as the geometric counterpart of adjunctions, which play an important role in morphology. This paper discusses the theoretical foundations, some applications from mathematical morphology, and an application to the Buffon-Sylvester problem in stochastic geometry.

Key words: dominance structure, incidence structure, complete lattice, adjunction, Buffon-Sylvester problem, distance transform, opening, slope transform, conditional closing

1. Introduction

One of the most elementary concepts from the theory of morphological operators is the adjunction, a pair of operators consisting of a dilation and an erosion [5, 6]. Although, in general, adjunctions are defined in an algebraic manner, they have a geometric interpretation, namely in terms of dominance and incidence. The notion of dominance corresponds to the inclusion relation in set theory. The notion of incidence can also be illustrated by means of sets: two sets X, Y are incident if they have non-empty intersection.

In this paper, we define general dominance and incidence structures between two complete lattices. We show that there is a unique relation between adjunctions on the one hand, and dominance and incidence structures on the other. We illustrate our abstract theory with applications to mathematical morphology (Minkowski operations, openings, slope transform) and stochastic geometry (the Buffon-Sylvester problem).

2. Buffon-Sylvester problem: formulation

For a closed set $A \subseteq \mathbb{R}^2$, we denote by $[A]$ the collection of all straight lines which intersect A, i.e., $[A] = \{\ell \in \Lambda \mid \ell \cap A \neq \varnothing\}$, where Λ consists of all straight lines. The Buffon-Sylvester problem [1, 2, 8, 10] concerns the probabilities of events $[A]$

J.Serra and P. Soille (eds.), Mathematical Morphology and Its Applications to Image Processing, 171-178

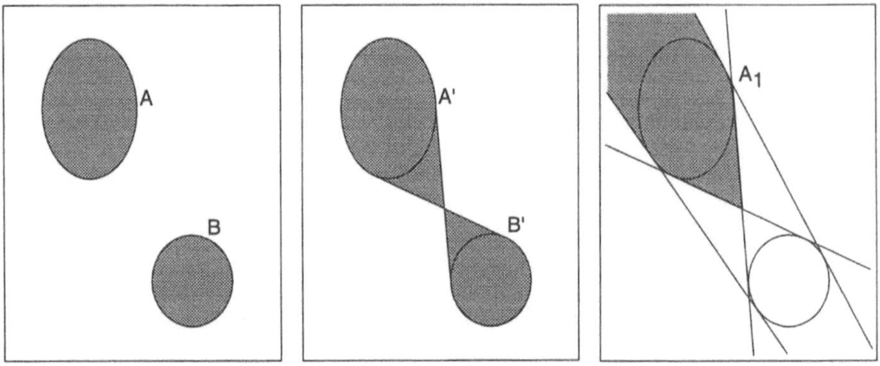

Fig. 1. Two disjoint compact convex sets A, B (left), the constructed sets A', B' (middle), and the set A_1. This last set is defined in §7.

and finite unions and intersections of such events, given a probability distribution on Λ. The probability $P([A])$ of a compact convex set A can be computed relatively easy, given a probability distribution on Λ. The classical example is the 'isotropic uniform random' distribution [1, 8], in which case $P([A])$ is proportional to $L(\partial A)$, the length of the boundary of A.

The following three principles, introduced by Sylvester [10], can be used to compute $P([A])$ for compact sets A other than convex sets. Denote by $\text{co}(X)$ the convex hull of a set X, and by $1_{[X]}$ the characteristic function on Λ corresponding with the event $[X]$.

(P1) If A is compact and path-connected, then $[A] = [\text{co}(A)]$.

(P2) If A, B are compact, convex, and $A \cap B \neq \varnothing$, then

$$1_{[A]\cap[B]} = 1_{[A]} + 1_{[B]} - 1_{[A\cup B]} = 1_{[A]} + 1_{[B]} - 1_{[\text{co}(A\cup B)]},$$

which yields that

$$P([A] \cap [B]) = P([A]) + P([B]) - P([\text{co}(A \cup B)]). \tag{1}$$

(P3) If A, B are compact, convex, and $A \cap B = \varnothing$ then

$$[A] \cap [B] = [A'] \cap [B'],$$

where A', B' are the sets indicated in Figure 1.

In the final case, formula (1) applies to A', B' yielding an expression for $P([A] \cap [B])$ in the case that $A \cap B = \varnothing$:

$$P([A] \cap [B]) = P([A']) + P([B']) - P([\text{co}(A \cup B)]).$$

Here we have used that (see §7)

$$\text{co}(A \cup B) = \text{co}(A' \cup B'). \tag{2}$$

Sylvester [10] described the construction in Figure 1 as drawing a tight string around A, B with a single crossover. In §7 we show that this construction can be formalized in terms of incidence structures and conditional closings.

3. Adjunctions

Before we come to the main theme of this paper we present a brief reminder on the theory of adjunctions. A comprehensive discussion can be found in [5]; see also [6].

Let $\mathcal{L}, \mathcal{M}$ be complete lattices. Denote the least and greatest element of $\mathcal{L}$ by $O_{\mathcal{L}}$ and $I_{\mathcal{L}}$, respectively. The pair of operators $\varepsilon : \mathcal{L} \to \mathcal{M}$, $\delta : \mathcal{M} \to \mathcal{L}$ is called an *adjunction* between $\mathcal{L}$ and $\mathcal{M}$ if

$$\delta(Y) \leq X \iff Y \leq \varepsilon(X), \quad X \in \mathcal{L},\, Y \in \mathcal{M}.$$

Then ε distributes over infima ($\varepsilon(\bigwedge_{i\in I} X_i) = \bigwedge_{i\in I} \varepsilon(X_i)$), and ε is called an *erosion*; δ distributes over suprema ($\delta(\bigvee_{i\in I} X_i) = \bigvee_{i\in I} \delta(X_i)$), and δ is called a *dilation*. With every dilation there corresponds a unique erosion, and vice versa. If (ε, δ) is an adjunction between $\mathcal{L}$ and $\mathcal{M}$, then

$$\varepsilon\delta\varepsilon = \varepsilon, \quad \delta\varepsilon\delta = \delta, \quad \varepsilon\delta \geq \mathsf{id}_{\mathcal{M}}, \quad \delta\varepsilon \leq \mathsf{id}_{\mathcal{L}}.$$

Here $\mathsf{id}_{\mathcal{L}}$ denotes the identity operator on $\mathcal{L}$. In particular, $\varepsilon\delta$ is a *closing* on $\mathcal{M}$ and $\varepsilon\delta$ is an *opening* on $\mathcal{L}$. This yields in particular that

$$\varepsilon\delta(M) \text{ is the largest solution } Y \in \mathcal{M} \text{ of } \delta(Y) = \delta(M). \tag{3}$$

4. Dominance and incidence structures

Two mathematical notions which form the basis for the morphological approach in image processing are set inclusion (or dominance) and set intersection. The second notion can be used to define an incidence relation as follows: two sets X and Y are incident if $X \cap Y \neq \varnothing$. We generalize these two notions to arbitrary complete lattices and show that they provide an alternative route towards the definition of adjunctions.

Definition 1 *Let $\mathcal{L}, \mathcal{M}$ be arbitrary complete lattices; the binary relation $\Subset$ on $\mathcal{M} \times \mathcal{L}$ is called a* dominance relation *if for two families $\{X_i \mid i \in I\} \subseteq \mathcal{L}$ and $\{Y_j \mid j \in J\} \subseteq \mathcal{M}$ the following is true:*

$$\bigvee_{j\in J} Y_j \Subset \bigwedge_{i\in I} X_i \iff \forall i,j \ : Y_j \Subset X_i. \tag{4}$$

Taking for I and J the empty set, one gets respectively $Y \Subset I_{\mathcal{L}}$ for $Y \in \mathcal{M}$ and $O_{\mathcal{M}} \Subset X$ for $X \in \mathcal{L}$. The dominance relation is compatible with the partial orderings of $\mathcal{L}$ and $\mathcal{M}$ in the following sense: if $Y \Subset X$, $Y' \leq Y$, and $X \leq X'$, then $Y' \Subset X'$.

In the following section we present a number of examples.

Proposition 1 *Given a dominance relation $\Subset$ on $\mathcal{M} \times \mathcal{L}$, define the operators $\varepsilon : \mathcal{L} \to \mathcal{M}$ and $\delta : \mathcal{M} \to \mathcal{L}$ by*

$$\varepsilon(X) = \bigvee\{Y \in \mathcal{M} \mid Y \Subset X\} \ \text{ and } \ \delta(Y) = \bigwedge\{X \in \mathcal{L} \mid Y \Subset X\}. \tag{5}$$

The pair (ε, δ) defines an adjunction between $\mathcal{L}$ and $\mathcal{M}$. Furthermore,

$$Y \Subset X \iff Y \leq \varepsilon(X) \iff \delta(Y) \leq X, \tag{6}$$

for every $X \in \mathcal{L}, Y \in \mathcal{M}$.

Conversely, if (ε, δ) *is an adjunction between* $\mathcal{L}$ *and* $\mathcal{M}$*, then the relation* $\Subset$ *on* $\mathcal{M} \times \mathcal{L}$ *given by (6) forms a dominance relation and (5) holds.*

A proof is given in [3] and [5].

Suppose that the mapping $X \mapsto X^*$ defines a negation on $\mathcal{L}$, and that $\Subset$ is a dominance relation on $\mathcal{M} \times \mathcal{L}$. Define another relation $\sim$ on $\mathcal{M} \times \mathcal{L}$ as follows:

$$Y \sim X \iff Y \not\Subset X^*. \tag{7}$$

The following property follows immediately from (4):

$$\bigvee_{j \in J} Y_j \sim \bigvee_{i \in I} X_i \iff \exists i, j \, : \, Y_j \sim X_i. \tag{8}$$

A relation $\sim$ with this property is called an *incidence relation*. This terminology is based on the following observation: set inclusion $\subseteq$ is a dominance on $\mathcal{P}(E) \times \mathcal{P}(E)$. The associated incidence relation is: $Y \sim X \iff Y \not\subseteq X^c \iff Y \cap X \neq \varnothing$.

The adjunction in (6) can also be expressed in terms of incidence:

$$\varepsilon(X) = \bigvee \{Y \in \mathcal{M} \mid Y \not\sim X^*\} \text{ and } \delta(Y) = \left[\bigvee \{X \in \mathcal{L} \mid Y \not\sim X\}\right]^*. \tag{9}$$

In fact, dominance relations provide a more general tool for the construction of adjunctions than incidence relations, as the latter presuppose the existence of a negation on $\mathcal{L}$. Note, however, that with every dominance relation $\Subset$ on $\mathcal{M} \times \mathcal{L}$ one can associate an incidence relation $\sim$ on $\mathcal{M} \times \mathcal{L}'$ by putting $Y \sim X \iff Y \not\Subset X$. Here $\mathcal{L}'$ denotes the opposite lattice of $\mathcal{L}$, i.e., the set $\mathcal{L}$ with the opposite ordering $X \leq' Y$ iff $X \geq Y$.

5. Examples from mathematical morphology

In this section we discuss a number of examples which emerge in the context of mathematical morphology [9]. These examples illustrate the general occurrence of dominance and incidence structures, and hence adjunctions, in morphology. In [3] we have treated in less or greater detail, applications to Kendall's random set theory, microscopy, and robot motion planning.

5.1. Minkowski addition and subtraction

Let A be a given subset of $\mathbb{R}^d$. Define, for $X, Y \subseteq \mathbb{R}^d$,

$$Y \sim X \iff A_y \cap X \neq \varnothing \text{ for some } y \in Y.$$

It is easy to verify that this defines an incidence relation on $\mathcal{P}(\mathbb{R}^d) \times \mathcal{P}(\mathbb{R}^d)$. The corresponding dominance relation is

$$Y \Subset X \iff A_y \subseteq X \text{ for all } y \in Y.$$

The associated adjunction (ε, δ) on $\mathcal{P}(\mathbb{R}^d)$ consists of a Minkowski addition and subtraction:

$$\varepsilon(X) = X \ominus A, \; \delta(Y) = Y \oplus A.$$

Note that $Y \sim X$ iff $(Y \oplus A) \cap X \neq \varnothing$ iff $Y \cap (X \oplus \check{A}) \neq \varnothing$; as such it generalizes the incidence relation defined by $Y \cap X \neq \varnothing$.

5.2. Distance transform

Let (E,d) be a metric space. For $h \in E$ and $r > 0$, denote by $B^\circ(h,r)$ the open ball with radius r centred at h. If $h \in E$ and $X \subseteq E$, then we denote by $d(h,X)$ the distance between h and X, i.e., $d(h,X) = \inf\{d(h,x) \mid x \in X\}$. Let $\mathcal{L}$ be the complete lattice consisting of all functions $F : E \to \overline{\mathbb{R}}_+$ ordered by (nota bene) $F \leq G$ iff $F(h) \geq G(h)$ for every $h \in E$.

Let the relation $\Subset$ on $\mathcal{P}(E) \times \mathcal{L}$ be given by

$$X \Subset F \iff d(h,X) \geq F(h), \quad \text{for all } h \in E.$$

Note that this is equivalent to $X \cap B^\circ(h,F(h)) = \varnothing$ for every $h \in E$. It is easy to verify that this relation defines a dominance structure. The corresponding adjunction $(\mathbf{\Delta}^\leftarrow, \mathbf{\Delta})$ between $\mathcal{L}$ and $\mathcal{P}(E)$ is given by

$$\begin{aligned} \mathbf{\Delta}(X)(h) &= d(h,X), \quad \text{for } h \in E, X \subseteq E \\ \mathbf{\Delta}^\leftarrow(F) &= \Big[\bigcup_{h \in E} B^\circ(h,F(h))\Big]^c, \; F \in \mathcal{L}. \end{aligned}$$

$\mathbf{\Delta}(X)$ is called the *distance transform* of X, and $\mathbf{\Delta}^\leftarrow(F)$ is called the *inverse distance transform* of F; see e.g. [5].

The mapping $F \mapsto F^*$, where $F^*(x) = 1/F(x)$, defines a negation on $\mathcal{L}$; here $1/0 = \infty$ and $1/\infty = 0$. This yields the incidence relation

$$X \sim F \iff d(h,X) \leq 1/F(h), \quad \text{for some } h \in E.$$

5.3. Opening

Let $\mathcal{L}$ be an arbitrary complete lattice; denote by $\mathcal{O}^+(\mathcal{L})$ the complete lattice of increasing operators on $\mathcal{L}$. For $\mathcal{B} \subseteq \mathcal{L}$ and $\psi \in \mathcal{O}^+(\mathcal{L})$ we define

$$\mathcal{B} \Subset \psi \iff B \leq \psi(B), \quad \text{for every } B \in \mathcal{B}.$$

The reader can readily verify that this defines a dominance relation. The corresponding adjunction between $\mathcal{O}^+(\mathcal{L})$ and $\mathcal{P}(\mathcal{L})$ is the pair (Inv_+, α), where $\mathrm{Inv}_+(\psi) = \{X \in \mathcal{L} \mid \psi(X) \geq X\}$ is the *extensivity domain of* ψ, and $\alpha(\mathcal{B})$ is the opening on $\mathcal{L}$ given by

$$\alpha(\mathcal{B})(X) = \bigvee\{B \in \mathcal{B} \mid B \leq X\};$$

see also [5, §6.1].

The mapping $\psi \mapsto \psi^*$ defines a negation on $\mathcal{O}^+(\mathcal{L})$. We leave it as an exercise to the reader to compute the corresponding incidence relation.

5.4. Slope transform

Let E be a topological vector space with adjoint E^*. Elements of E and E^* are denoted by x and x^*, respectively. The value of x^* at x (inner product) is denoted by $\langle x, x^* \rangle$. Let $\mathcal{M} = \mathrm{Fun}(E, \overline{\mathbb{R}})$ and $\mathcal{L} = \mathrm{Fun}(E^*, \overline{\mathbb{R}})$. Define a binary relation on $\mathcal{M} \times \mathcal{L}$ in the following way:

$$f \Subset f^* \iff f(x) \leq f^*(x^*) + \langle x, x^* \rangle, \quad \text{for every } x \in E, x^* \in E^*.$$

This is a dominance relation. Note that $f \Subset f^*$ can be interpreted as follows: the function f^* corresponds with a one-parameter family of straight lines $\ell_v(x) = \langle x, v\rangle + f^*(v)$, which lie above f, i.e., $f \le \ell_v$ for every parameter value $v \in E^*$.

The associated adjunction (ε, δ) between $\mathcal{L}$ and $\mathcal{M}$ is given by

$$\delta(f)(x^*) = \bigvee_{x \in E} (f(x) - \langle x, x^*\rangle) \quad \text{and} \quad \varepsilon(f^*)(x) = \bigwedge_{x^* \in E^*} (f^*(x^*) + \langle x, x^*\rangle).$$

Recently, it has been recognised independently by Maragos [7] and Dorst and van den Boomgaard [4] that this transform δ plays a role in morphological signal processing which is quite analogous to the role of the Fourier transform in linear signal processing. It is called the *A-transform* or *slope transform*, and is very closely related to the *Young-Fenchel conjugate* in convex analysis.

6. Conditional closing

Throughout this section we assume that $\mathcal{L}$ is a complete Boolean lattice with complement operation $X \mapsto X^*$. Assume further that $\sim$ is an incidence relation on $\mathcal{M} \times \mathcal{L}$ with corresponding adjunction (ε, δ) between $\mathcal{L}$ and $\mathcal{M}$. Define, for fixed $B \in \mathcal{L}$, the set $\mathcal{L}_{(\le B)} = \{X \in \mathcal{L} \mid X \le B\}$. Then $\mathcal{L}_{(\le B)}$ is a complete Boolean lattice with complement $X \mapsto X^* \wedge B$.

The restriction of $\sim$ to $\mathcal{M} \times \mathcal{L}_{(\le B)}$ is an incidence relation too, and the corresponding adjunction $(\varepsilon_B, \delta_B)$ between $\mathcal{L}_{(\le B)}$ and $\mathcal{M}$ is given by

$$\begin{aligned} \varepsilon_B(X) &= \varepsilon(X \vee B^*), \quad X \in \mathcal{L}_{(\le B)}, \\ \delta_B(X) &= \delta(Y) \wedge B, \quad Y \in \mathcal{M}; \end{aligned}$$

see [3] as well as [5, §3.4]. Of special interest here is the closing $\varepsilon_B\delta_B$, which will be used in the following section. We call this closing a *conditional closing*, expressing the fact that elements X in $\mathcal{L}$ are subject to the condition $X \le B$.

Proposition 2 *If $M \in \mathcal{M}$, then the largest solution $Y \in \mathcal{M}$ which satisfies*

$$\delta(Y) \wedge B = \delta(M) \wedge B \tag{10}$$

is $Y = \varepsilon(\delta(M) \vee B^*)$.

Proof: We can write (10) as $\delta_B(Y) = \delta_B(M)$. The largest solution is given by

$$Y = \varepsilon_B\delta_B(M) = \varepsilon((\delta(M) \wedge B) \vee B^*) = \varepsilon(\delta(M) \vee B^*);$$

see (3). This concludes the proof. □

7. Buffon-Sylvester problem: formal solution

We apply the abstract theory developed in the previous section to the Buffon-Sylvester problem introduced in §2. In particular, we shall be concerned with the proof of principles (P1)–(P3).

Let $\mathcal{L} = \mathcal{P}(\Lambda)$ and $\mathcal{M} = \mathcal{P}(\mathbb{R}^2)$. We denote elements of $\mathcal{L}$ by Ξ rather than by X. The relation

$$Y \sim \Xi \iff \exists \ell \in \Xi : \ell \cap Y \neq \varnothing,$$

defines an incidence relation on $\mathcal{M} \times \mathcal{L}$. We compute the associated adjunction (ε, δ) by using relation (9). It is easy to verify that

$$\delta(Y) = [Y], \quad Y \subseteq \mathbb{R}^2. \tag{11}$$

To compute ε we use that

$$\varepsilon(\Xi) = \bigcup \{Y \subseteq \mathbb{R}^2 \mid Y \not\sim \Xi^{\mathrm{c}}\}.$$

Evidently,

$$\begin{aligned} Y \not\sim \Xi^{\mathrm{c}} &\iff \forall \ell \in \Xi^{\mathrm{c}} : \ell \cap Y = \varnothing \\ &\iff \forall \ell \in \Lambda : \ell \notin \Xi \Rightarrow Y \subseteq \ell^{\mathrm{c}}. \end{aligned}$$

This implies that

$$\varepsilon(\Xi) = \bigcap \{\ell^{\mathrm{c}} \mid \ell \notin \Xi\} = \Big[\bigcup \{\ell \mid \ell \notin \Xi\}\Big]^{\mathrm{c}}. \tag{12}$$

The closing $\varepsilon\delta$ is given by

$$\varepsilon\delta(Y) = \bigcap \{\ell^{\mathrm{c}} \mid \ell \in \Lambda \text{ and } \ell \cap Y = \varnothing\}.$$

The reader may readily verify that $\varepsilon\delta(Y) = \mathrm{co}(Y)$ if Y is compact and path-connected. As $\delta\varepsilon\delta = \delta$ this gives immediately that $[Y] = [\mathrm{co}(Y)]$ if Y is compact and path-connected. Therefore, (P1) is proved. As (P2) is obvious, it remains to consider (P3).

If we apply Proposition 2 with $[B] = \delta(B)$ instead of B, and A instead of M, we find that the largest set A_1 which satisfies

$$[A_1] \cap [B] = [A] \cap [B]$$

is given by a conditional closing

$$A_1 = \varepsilon([A] \cup [B]^{\mathrm{c}}). \tag{13}$$

Note that the adjective 'conditional' refers to the condition that the lines in Λ being considered should intersect B. In combination with (12) this gives

$$A_1 = \Big[\bigcup \{\ell \mid \ell \notin [A] \text{ and } \ell \in [B]\}\Big]^{\mathrm{c}}.$$

The set A_1 has been depicted in Figure 1. In a similar way we construct a set B_1, and we get that

$$[A_1] \cap [B_1] = [A] \cap [B]. \tag{14}$$

To arrive at the sets A', B' in (P3) we put

$$A' = A_1 \cap \mathrm{co}(A \cup B), \quad B' = B_1 \cap \mathrm{co}(A \cup B).$$

Since $A \subseteq A_1$ and $B \subseteq B_1$, we have $A \subseteq A' \subseteq A_1$ and $B \subseteq B' \subseteq B_1$. In combination with (14) this gives

$$[A] \cap [B] = [A'] \cap [B'].$$

Thus (P3) is proved.

To prove e.g. (2) in §2 we use that

$$\begin{aligned} A' &= A_1 \cap \mathrm{co}(A \cup B) = \varepsilon([A] \cup [B]^c) \cap \varepsilon\delta(A \cup B) \\ &= \varepsilon\Big(([A] \cup [B]^c) \cap [A \cup B]\Big). \end{aligned}$$

The inclusion '$\subseteq$' in (2) is trivial. We prove '$\supseteq$'. Note that

$$\mathrm{co}(A' \cup B') = \varepsilon\delta(A' \cup B') = \varepsilon(\delta(A') \cup \delta(B')).$$

Now

$$\begin{aligned} \delta(A') &= \delta\varepsilon\Big(([A] \cup [B]^c) \cap [A \cup B]\Big) \\ &\subseteq ([A] \cup [B]^c) \cap [A \cup B] \\ &\subseteq [A \cup B] = \delta(A \cup B). \end{aligned}$$

This yields the result.

References

1. R. V. Ambartzumian. *Combinatorial Integral Geometry, with applications to mathematical stereology.* John Wiley and Sons, Chichester, 1982.
2. A. J. Baddeley. Appendix A. In *R. V. Ambartzumian, Combinatorial Integral Geometry,* pages 194–214. John Wiley and Sons, New York and Chichester, 1982.
3. A. J. Baddeley and H. J. A. M. Heijmans. Incidence and lattice calculus with applications to stochastic geometry and image analysis. Research report BS-R9213, CWI, 1992.
4. L. Dorst and R. van den Boomgaard. Morphological signal processing and the slope transform. *Signal Processing,* to appear.
5. H. J. A. M. Heijmans. *Morphological Image Operators.* Academic Press, Boston, 1994.
6. H. J. A. M. Heijmans and C. Ronse. The algebraic basis of mathematical morphology – part I: Dilations and erosions. *Computer Vision, Graphics and Image Processing,* 50:245–295, 1990.
7. P. Maragos. Morphological systems: slope transforms and max-min difference and differential equations. *Signal Processing,* to appear.
8. L. A. Santaló. *Integral Geometry and Geometric Probability.* Encyclopedia of Mathematics and Its Applications, vol. 1. Addison-Wesley, 1976.
9. J. Serra. *Image Analysis and Mathematical Morphology.* Academic Press, London, 1982.
10. J. J. Sylvester. On a funicular solution of buffon's 'problem of the needle' in its most general form. *Acta Mathematica,* 14:185–205, 1890.

THE MULTISCALE MORPHOLOGY DECOMPOSITION THEOREM

J. ANDREW BANGHAM, PIERRE CHARDAIRE and PAUL LING
School Of Information Systems, University Of East Anglia, Norwich, NR4 7TJ, U.K.

Abstract. Sieves decompose one dimensional bounded functions, e.g. f to a set of increasing scale granule functions $\{d_r\}_{r=1}^{R}$, that represent the information in a manner that is analogous to the pyramid of wavelets obtained by linear decomposition. Sieves based on sequences of increasing scale open-closings with flat structuring elements (M and N filters) map f to $\{d_r\}$ and the inverse process maps $\{d_r\}$ to f. Experiments show that a more general inverse exists such that $\{\hat{d}_r\}$ maps to $\hat{f}$ and back to $\{\hat{d}_r\}$, where the granule functions $\{\hat{d}_r\}$ are a subset of $\{d_r\}$ in which granules may have changed amplitudes, that may include zero but not a change of sign. An analytical proof of this inverse has been obtained. This key property could prove important for feature recognition and opens the way for an analysis of the noise resistance of these sieves. The resulting theorems do not apply to parallel open-closing filters.

Key words: Mathematical Morphology, Median Filters, Ordinal Filters, Rank, Granularity, Granulometry.

1. Introduction

The decompositions described here are related to 'skeletons' obtained by repeated erosions [3], multiscale openings (resp. closings [5, 6]) and to alternating sequential filters [8], however, they yield results that are quantitatively sufficiently different as to warrant a new name. We call the multiscale decompositions in this paper, sieves.

In this paper, one dimensional (1D) sieves are constructed from alternating sequential filters with flat structuring elements (N and M filters [7]). An N-sieve is a set of increasing scale alternating closing and opening operations operating sequentially on a signal. The scale or mesh, r, at each stage of the filter is determined by the length of the structuring element (window). For a complete decomposition the window increases from 2 to $R+1$, where the signal is a bounded function of length R samples. Although some of the ideas can be extended from 1D to 2D, it is not yet clear how this should be achieved in detail.

Sieves have a number of advantages over linear decomposition for image segmentation [7], for noise reduction and for pattern recognition [1]. In particular they preserve edges, they are not 'blinded' by impulsive noise [1], and they operate independently of frequency. They also have a number of advantages over pyramids of openings (respectively closings), [5, 4], in particular they are substantially more resistant to noise and signals do not rapidly 'bleach out' as the maxima (resp. minima) are consistently selected by the filtering stages. It has also been shown experimentally that complete decomposition using one dimensional M- and N-sieves is, at most an $n \log n$, problem and analysis suggests that it is an order n problem. In practice the complete decomposition takes about the same time to compute as an

J.Serra and P. Soille (eds.), Mathematical Morphology and Its Applications to Image Processing, 179-184

FFT.

We developed this self contained theory [2] in the contex of filtering of one dimensional signals with flat structuring elements. In this particular case, much stronger properties can be proved than in the more general case of two or more dimensional signals. For instance, by using a generalization of the concepts of unimodal functions, each stage of the sieve can be proved to be idempotent, a property that does not hold in the more general case.

2. Outline of the Decomposition

An outline of the decomposition is given that includes the important results but does not include the intermediate steps. Definition 3 concisely defines the non-zero intervals of a function. Definition 4 defines granules in terms of these intervals and Definition 5 defines a set of functions that are compatible with granules of scale r in that certain key properties do not change on adding the granules to that function.

Theorem 6 states that an N-sieve yields a set of granule functions. The next step is to show that functions obtained by summing the granule functions are r-$\mathcal{N}$compatible with each other at each scale. The final theorem affirms the experimental results obtained earlier.

Throughout we shall let F denote the set of functions from $\mathbf{Z}$ to $\mathbf{Z}$. The elements of F are to represent digitalized signals.

We let[1]

$$\mathcal{C}_r = \{\, [x, x+r-1] \mid x \in \mathbf{Z} \,\}.$$

So $\mathcal{C}_r$ is the set of intervals of $\mathbf{Z}$ with r elements.

Definition 1 *For each integer, $r \geq 1$, the functions, $\gamma_r, \psi_r, \mathcal{N}^r, \mathcal{M}^r : F \to F$ are defined by*

$$\gamma_r f(x) = \min_{\xi \in \mathcal{C}_r : \xi \ni x} \max_{u \in \xi} f(u),$$
$$\psi_r f(x) = \max_{\xi \in \mathcal{C}_r : \xi \ni x} \min_{u \in \xi} f(u).$$

and

$$\mathcal{N}^r = \psi_r \gamma_r, \qquad \mathcal{M}^r = \gamma_r \psi_r.$$

γ_r and ψ_r are known as the opening operator and the closing operator respectively. $\mathcal{N}^r$ and $\mathcal{M}^r$ are known as the rth stage of the N-sieve and the M-sieve respectively.

Definition 2 *We say that f is* r-monotonic *if and only if for each interval, $[x, y]$, with $0 \leq y - x \leq r$, f is monotonic on $[x, y]$.*

Definition 3 *Suppose that $f \in F$ and $x \in \mathbf{Z}$. We define $R_f(x)$ to be the maximum $z \in \mathbf{Z}$ such that f is constant on $[x, z]$ (with $R_f(x) = \infty$ if this maximum is unbounded) and and we define $L_f(x)$ to be the minimum $y \in \mathbf{Z}$ such that f is constant on $[y, x]$ (again with $L_f(x) = -\infty$ if this minimum is unbounded). We define*

$$\mathcal{I}_f^+(x) = [x, R_f(x)], \qquad \mathcal{I}_f^-(x) = [L_f(x), x],$$

[1] Throughout intervals such as $[a, b]$, $[a, b)$ etc. will be subsets of $\mathbf{Z}$ rather than the more usual $\mathbf{R}$.

and

$$\mathcal{I}_f(x) = [L_f(x), R_f(x)] = \mathcal{I}_f^+(x) \cup \mathcal{I}_f^-(x).$$

So $\mathcal{I}_f(x)$ is the largest interval about x on which f is constant. We shall call $\mathcal{I}_f(x)$ the interval of f at x.

Definition 4 *For $r \geq 1$, a function, $d \in F$, is said to be a r-$\mathcal{N}$*granule function *if and only if for all $x \in \mathbf{Z}$,*

$$d(x) \neq 0 \implies |\mathcal{I}_d(x)| = r,$$

and for all $x, y \in \mathbf{Z}$ with $x < y$ and $\mathcal{I}_d(x) \neq \mathcal{I}_d(y)$,

$$\begin{aligned} d(x), d(y) > 0 &\implies L_d(y) - R_d(x) \geq r + 2, \\ d(x), d(y) < 0 &\implies L_d(y) - R_d(x) \geq r + 1. \end{aligned}$$

Any interval, $\mathcal{I}_d(x)$, of an r-$\mathcal{N}$granule function is known as a granule *and $d(x)$ is called the value of the granule, $\mathcal{I}_d(x)$.*

Definition 5 *For each r-$\mathcal{N}$granule function, d, we let $\mathcal{N}Comp_r(d)$ denote the set of all $f \in F$ such that*

$$d(x) > 0 \implies \begin{cases} f \text{ is increasing on } [L_d(x) - r - 1, L_d(x)], \\ f \text{ is constant on } \mathcal{I}_d(x), \\ f \text{ is decreasing on } [R_d(x), R_d(x) + r + 1], \end{cases}$$

and

$$d(x) < 0 \implies \begin{cases} f \text{ is decreasing on } [L_d(x) - r, L_d(x)], \\ f \text{ is constant on } \mathcal{I}_d(x), \\ f \text{ is increasing on } [R_d(x), R_d(x) + r]. \end{cases}$$

Clearly $\mathcal{N}Comp_r(d)$ is closed under summation and under $f \mapsto \chi \circ f$ for any increasing function $\chi: \mathbf{Z} \to \mathbf{Z}$ (e.g. $t \mapsto t^+$).

Theorem 6 *Suppose that $f \in F$, we define $(f_r)_{r \geq 1} \subseteq F$ inductively by*

$$f_1 = f, \qquad \text{and} \qquad f_{r+1} = \mathcal{N}^{r+1} f_r, \quad \text{for } r \geq 1,$$

and we define $(d_r)_{r \geq 1} \subseteq F$ by

$$d_r = f_r - f_{r+1}, \qquad \text{for } r \geq 1.$$

Then

$$f = d_1 + \cdots + d_r + f_{r+1}, \qquad \text{for } r \geq 1,$$

and the following hold:

(i) f_r is r-monotonic, for each $r \geq 1$.
(ii) d_r is an r-$\mathcal{N}$granule function, for each $r \geq 1$.
(iii) $s > r \geq 1 \implies f_s \in \mathcal{N}Comp_r(d_r)$.
(iv) $s > r \geq 1 \implies d_s \in \mathcal{N}Comp_r(d_r)$.

This theorem gives a precise characterization of the set of functions produced by the decomposition algorithm. Let us notice that if f is a function with bounded support then $f_r = 0$, for all $r > R$, for some $R \geq 1$.

Theorem 7 *Suppose that for some $R \geq 1$, $d_1, \ldots, d_R$, $\tilde{f} \in F$ are such that*
(i) d_r is an r-$\mathcal{N}$granule function, for $r = 1, \ldots, R$;
(ii) $\tilde{f}$ is $(R+1)$-monotonic;
(iii) $1 \leq r < s \leq R \implies d_s \in \mathcal{N}Comp_r(d_r)$;
(iv) $\tilde{f} \in \mathcal{N}Comp_r(d_r)$, for $r = 1, \ldots, R$;
and we let

$$f = d_1 + \cdots + d_R + \tilde{f}.$$

Then, on defining $(f_r)_{r \geq 1} \subseteq F$ inductively by

$$f_1 = f, \qquad \text{and} \qquad f_{r+1} = \mathcal{N}^{r+1} f_r, \quad \text{for } r \geq 1,$$

we have

$$f_r - f_{r+1} = d_r, \qquad \text{for } r = 1, \ldots, R,$$

and

$$f_{R+1} = \tilde{f}.$$

This states that a function mainly obtained as a sum of increasing scale granule functions such that any larger granule function is r-$\mathcal{N}$compatible at scale r with any smaller granule function d_r precisely decomposes into this set of granules.

Theorem 8 *Consider a function f such that $f = d_1 + \cdots + d_R$ where d_i are the N-granule functions obtained by applying the decomposition algorithm. Consider any $\hat{f}$ obtained from f by replacing function d_i by $\hat{d}_i$, such that $\hat{d}_i(x) = 0$ when $d_r(x) = 0$, $\hat{d}_r$ is constant and non-negative on each $\mathcal{I}_{d_r}(x)$ with $d_r(x) > 0$ and $\hat{d}_r$ is constant and non-positive on each $\mathcal{I}_{d_r}(x)$ with $d_r(x) < 0$.*

If we define

$$\hat{f}_1 = \hat{f}, \qquad \text{and} \qquad \hat{f}_{r+1} = \mathcal{N}^{r+1} \hat{f}_r \quad \text{for } r \geq 1$$

then since the decomposition of $\hat{f}$ to $\hat{d}$ clearly satisfies (i) and (iii) of Theorem 7, we have by Theorem 7, with, $\tilde{f} = 0$

$$\hat{f}_r - \hat{f}_{r+1} = \hat{d}_r, \qquad \text{for } r = 1, \ldots, R,$$

and

$$\hat{f}_r = 0, \qquad \text{for all } r \geq R+1.$$

This theorem states that if we modify the amplitude (but not the sign) of some granules obtained by the N-sieve algorithm then the application of this algorithm to the re-composed signal will produce the same set of r-$\mathcal{N}$granule functions.

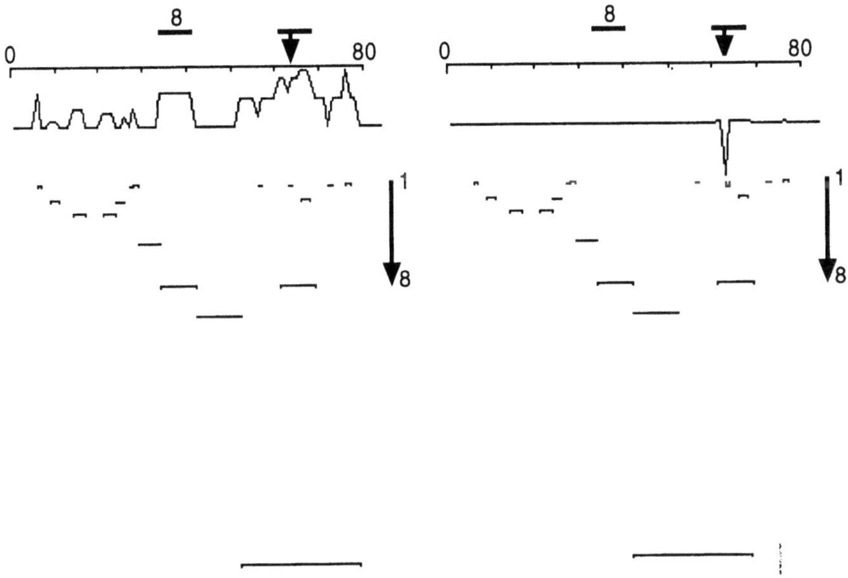

Fig. 1. Left panel shows the decomposition of a signal that includes two 8 sample pulses the second with a noise impulse, arrowed. The right panel shows the effect of increasing the amplitude of this impulse to -500. Notice that auto-scaling has been used.

3. Results Using this Property

It is important to notice that, to a certain extent, Theorem 8 implies that the granules are independent of each other. It is obvious in the simple case of a signal containing two well separated pulses of different widths that either could become infinitely large without affecting the ability of the multiscale sieve to resolve the scale and position of the other. Figure 1 shows a less extreme example. The signal, top trace, contains two eight sample long pulses that are indicated. Decomposition using an N-sieve (shown in Fig. 1) yields two granules at scale 8 as expected. Notice that the second pulse is corrupted by noise, in particular that there is a small downward facing impulse, arrowed. If this impulse were of infinite-negative amplitude then Theorem 8 indicates that the scale 8 granules would be unchanged. The right panel of Fig. 1 confirms the result (for display purposes the impulse is changed to amplitude -500). This is quite different from linear multiscale decomposition such as an FFT, or a wavelet decomposition, both of which would be 'blinded' by an infinitely large impulse.

References

1. J.A. Bangham, T. Campbell, and R. Aldridge. Multiscale median and morphological filters used for 2D pattern recognition. *Signal Processing*, 1994 (in press).
2. J.A. Bangham, P. Chardaire, C. Pye, and D. Ling. Multiscale nonlinear decomposition: the sieve decomposition theorem. *IEEE Transactions on Pattern Analysis and Machine Intelligence*, 1994 (submitted).

3. H. Blum. Biological shape and visual science (part 1). *Journal of Theoretical Biology*, 38:205–287, 1973.
4. M. Chen and P. Yan. A multiscale approach based upon morphological filtering. *IEEE Transactions on Pattern Analysis and Machine Intelligence*, 11(7):694–701, July 1989.
5. P. Maragos. Pattern spectrum and multiscale shape representation. *IEEE Transactions on Pattern Analysis and Machine Intelligence*, 11(7):701–716, July 1989.
6. G. Matheron. *Random sets and integral geometry.* Wiley, 1975.
7. P. Salembier and M. Kunt. Size sensitive mutliresolution decomposition of images with rank order based filters. *Signal Processing*, 27(2):205–241, May 1992.
8. S. Sternberg. Grayscale morphology. *Computer Graphics and Image Processing*, 35:333–355, 1986.

STATISTICAL PATTERN SPECTRUM FOR BINARY PATTERN RECOGNITION

C.S. REGAZZONI and G.L. FORESTI
Department of Biophysical and Electronic Engineering (DIBE)
University of Genova, Via all'Opera Pia 11A, I-16145 Genova, Italy
Ph. +39 10 3532792, Fax: +39 10 3532134, E-mail: carlo@dibe.unige.it

and

A.N. VENETSANOPOULOS
Department of Electrical and Computer Engineering,
University of Toronto,
10 King 's College Road, Toronto, Canada

Abstract.
A new shape descriptor based on Statistical Morphology is presented. The descriptor, called specstrum, is a statistical extension of pattern spectrum, (i.e., pecstrum) useful to represent shape information related to binary patterns in noisy conditions. The major features of the specstrum are an increased stability under varying noisy conditions and a more regular shape description capability. Results are presented for a parking surveillance application.

Key words: Binary Statistical Morphology, Shape descriptor, Pattern spectrum, Parking surveillance

1. Introduction

Shape is one of the main descriptive feature to characterize objects of interest in many applications. In this paper, a shape descriptor of binary patterns based on Binary Statistical Morphology (BSM) operators [1, 6] is proposed. The analysis is carried on starting from a vectorial shape descriptor based on Mathematical Morphology, i.e., the pattern spectrum ("pecstrum") [2, 3].

The pecstrum provides information on the way the area of an object is distributed from its details to the coarse structure. Extracted information depends on two main parameters: the type of morphological filter [4] employed to transform the image through different levels of detail and the shape of the set used to investigate the image itself (i.e., the structuring element). The pecstrum is a information non-preserving descriptor [3] for it provides an integral evaluation (i.e., non-spatially distributed) about the area distribution of objects at different detail levels.

The goal of this paper is to describe a new shape descriptor, the Statistical Pecstrum, here defined as "specstrum". Specstrum provides different information with respect to the pecstrum in that the distribution of the area is adaptively evaluated at different resolution levels by means of BSM operators instead of morphological ones. BSM operators [1] are a generalization of morphological ones in that they allow one to take into account of noise effects. This is possible by selecting a real-valued parameter, the β parameter, which is associated to the type of filter employed. Spec-

J.Serra and P. Soille (eds.), Mathematical Morphology and Its Applications to Image Processing, 185-192

strum extraction is performed by selecting different BSM operators (i.e., choosing different β values) when analyzing object shape at different degrees of resolution.

An appropriate scheduling of β values through iterations allows one to obtain an increased stability to noise. Besides this, a further advantage of using specstrum with respect to object recognition applications, is the different resolution in size distribution which can be obtained by choosing β values. Depending on this choice, the object shape can be inspected at different "speed", i.e., information on shape details at a certain level can be either expanded or compressed depending on classification requirements.

In Section 2 a brief background on BSM operators is presented, while in Section 3 specstrum is described. In Section 4 results are presented concerning with a parking surveillance application.

2. Binary Statistical Morphology

Erosion and dilation are the elementary set-based operators (or, in functional terms, Morphological Filters, MFs [4]) of Mathematical Morphology [11]. If the set of elements in a binary image and the structuring element (i.e., a subset of image points), are denoted by X and B, respectively, erosion and dilation can be defined as:

$$X \ominus B = \{z : B + z \subseteq X\} \tag{1}$$
$$X \oplus B = \{z : B + z \cap X \neq \emptyset\} \tag{2}$$

where + indicates a translation of B to an image location z. Statistical Morphological Filters (SMFs) recently introduced by Yuille et al. [5] provide a model for including a-priori knowledge about the noise level as an additional parameter of an MF. Elementary operators of Statistical Morphology, i.e., Statistical Dilation (SD) and Statistical Erosion (SE), are obtained from a probabilistic definitions of set-based operators. In [1, 6], we described a computationally efficient implementation of SD and SE for the case of binary images by defining Binary Statistical Morphological Filters. BSMFs can be obtained from SMFs by quantization and thresholding. A generalized version of Binary Statistical Dilation (BSD) is provided by the following expression:

$$X \oplus_\beta B = \{j : H_j^* = 1\}$$
$$H_m^* = \begin{cases} 1 \text{ if } \beta \geq ln\left[\frac{\theta}{1-\theta}\frac{N-M_B^1(m)}{M_B^1(m)}\right] \\ 0 \text{ if } \beta < ln\left[\frac{\theta}{1-\theta}\frac{N-M_B^1(m)}{M_B^1(m)}\right] \end{cases} \tag{3}$$

where H_m^* is the output of the SD filter at the image location m, thresholded at level θ, B_m is the structuring element at m, with a cardinality equal to N, and β is a parameter taking into account the noise level. The dependence on an image X is provided by the term $M_B^1(m) = card\{x \in (B + z \cap X)\}$, which is the number of elements in the binary image X in the area intersected by B_m. In the limit $\beta \to \infty$, BSD becomes Mathematical Dilation: in that case an element m does not belong to the statistically dilated set only if all elements of B_m are not elements of X. For $\beta = 0$, BSD corresponds to a thresholded linear average. The threshold is fixed at

$\theta = 0.5$ if equally probable outputs are assumed. For intermediate β values, BSD behaves like a rank-order filter [7], i.e., the rank decreases for increasing β values. Continuous β ranges can be established over which BSD has the same behaviour, i.e., the same rank number. A similar reasoning applies to Binary Statistical Erosion (BSE), denoted as $X \ominus_\beta B$, for which the expression holds:

$$X \ominus_\beta B = \{j : K_j^* = 1\}$$
$$K_m^* = \begin{cases} 1 \text{ if } \beta \leq -ln\left[\frac{\theta}{1-\theta}\frac{N-M_B^1(m)}{M_B^1(m)}\right] \\ 0 \text{ if } \beta > -ln\left[\frac{\theta}{1-\theta}\frac{N-M_B^1(m)}{M_B^1(m)}\right] \end{cases} \tag{4}$$

The definition (3) of BSD is obtained as a binarized approximation of the maximum a-posteriori (MAP) probability configuration of the output set of variables. β plays the role of the noise-model parameter within the probabilities involved in such a computation. Binary statistical opening (BSO), $\gamma_\beta(X)$, can be defined as the composition of erosion and aperture applied with the same β value, i.e.:

$$\gamma_\beta(X) = (X \ominus_\beta B) \oplus_\beta B \tag{5}$$

It is also possible to provide a definition of Binary statistical opening directly from the probabilistic formulation, as in [1]. However, expression (5) has been considered also in [1] an acceptable approximation for statistical opening. From these definitions we are now able to specify an algorithm to extract specstrum

3. Specstrum extraction

The definition of specstrum is obtained from the one given for pecstrum in [3].

In a way similar to the pecstrum in [7], we can use Statistical Morphological Filters (SMFs) to obtain shape information. We define $\psi_\beta^1(X)$ and $\psi_\beta^2(X)$ as two SMFs operating on the binary set X. A measure $m()$ can be associated with such filters to describe the modifications that they provide to X. The two filters have the characteristic that $\psi_\beta^1(X) \supseteq \psi_\beta^2(X)$. It is also required that $X \supseteq \psi_\beta^2(X)$, but this does not necessary hold for $\psi_\beta^1(X)$. Shape description can be described as a mapping from X into a function f obtained by comparing the characteristics of $\psi_\beta^1(X)$ and $\psi_\beta^2(X)$, i.e., $X \rightarrow (\psi_\beta^1(X)), \psi_\beta^2(X)) \rightarrow m[f(\psi_\beta^1(X), \psi_\beta^2(X)]$.

If $m(X)$ is a measure of the area of X, and f is chosen as the set difference $f(x,y) = x - y$, then $m[f(\psi_\beta^1(X), \psi_\beta^2(X))] > 0$ by definition. Moreover, let us define the r-th statistical opening of a set X in a recursive way as:

$$\begin{aligned} &\gamma_{0,\beta(0)}(X) = X; \\ &\gamma_{1,\beta(1)}(X) = (X \ominus_{\beta(1)} B) \oplus_{\beta(1)} B \\ &\gamma_{r,\beta(r)}(X) = [(\gamma_{r-1,\beta(r-1)}(X)) \ominus_{\beta(r)} B] \oplus_{\beta(r)} B \end{aligned} \tag{6}$$

$\beta(r)$ is the noise-model parameter associated with the r-th filter of the sequence.

If we consider $\psi_\beta^1(X) = \gamma_{\beta(X)}$, and $\psi_\beta^2(X) = \gamma_{\beta(X)} \cap X$, i.e if we take statistical opening with β and the intersection of such set with X as SMFs, then we are ensured that the two condition hold, i.e., $\gamma_{\beta(X)} \supseteq (\gamma_{\beta(X)} \cap X)$, and $X \supseteq \gamma_\beta(X) \cap X$. The statistical counterpart of deterministic granulometry can be defined as the difference between the two sets: $r \in R \rightarrow X_r = [\gamma_{r-1,\beta(r-1)}(X) - [\gamma_{r,\beta(r)}(X) \cap \gamma_{r-1,\beta(r-1)}(X)]$.

The set associated with r excludes those points of $\gamma_{r-1,\beta(r-1)}(X)$, which are not contained in $\gamma_{r,\beta(r)}(X)$. These points are not significant from the point of view of shape description at step r, as they add information which is not present in the original pattern. However, the set of such points should be of limited cardinality for introduced information has influence for the granulometry at step $r+1$.

In the case of pecstrum a real-valued function $u(r)$ is obtained by applying a measuring function $m()$ to the granulometry; the cardinality of the difference set is chosen for the spectrum, i.e., $u(r)$ is given by: $r \in R \rightarrow u(r) = m([\gamma_{r-1,\beta(r-1)}(X) - [\gamma_{r,\beta(r)}(X) \cap \gamma_{r-1,\beta(r-1)}(X)]) \in R$

$u(r)$ is a descriptor of size distribution of the object X.

If $\beta(r) = \beta(r-1) = \beta \rightarrow \infty$, i.e., β constant, the specstrum becomes the pecstrum and $u(r)$ is a strictly positive function which becomes null for $r \rightarrow \infty$; in fact we have that $\gamma_{r-1,\beta(r-1)}(X) \supseteq \gamma_{r,\beta(r)}(X)$, being BSO equal to morphological opening. Moreover, $\gamma_{r,\beta(r)}(X)$ becomes the empty set for $r \rightarrow \infty$. In other cases, $u(r)$ remains strictly positive and still converges to zero, but this situation may correspond to a fixed point of $\psi^1_\beta(X)$, i.e., a not null configuration such that $\psi^1_\beta(\psi^1_\beta(X)) = X$.

If we define $u(0)$ as $m(X)$, the continuous specstrum can be defined as:

$$sp(r) = \frac{u(r)}{u(0)} \tag{7}$$

The digitized version of continuous specstrum is defined as:

$$sp(n) = \frac{m\left(\gamma_{n-1,\beta(n-1)}(X)\right) - m\left(\gamma_{n,\beta(n)}(X) \cap \gamma_{n-1,\beta(n-1)}(X)\right)}{m(X)} \tag{8}$$

A consequence of this definition is that we are not granted that $\int_0^\infty sp(r)dr \neq 1$. A scheduling of β values must be adopted, to be ensured that $u(r)$ is limited when increasing r values increase. In this case, the area of specstrum is also limited, i.e.

$$\int_0^\infty sp(r)dr < a < +\infty \tag{9}$$

In particular, we propose to select a scheduling for which $\beta(r) \rightarrow \infty$ (i.e., $\beta > k_\beta$, see) for $r > r^* > 0$ to obtain the above condition. In this case, $u(r)$ becomes null for $r > r^* > 0$ and the integral is upper bounded. To prove this it is sufficient to note that, for $r > r^*$, the specstrum becomes the pecstrum. Let us suppose that a strategy for which $\beta(r) > k_\beta$ for $r > r^* > 0$ is chosen. Let us suppose $X^*(r^*)$ be the set obtained at that step and n^* be the maximum not-null value of the pecstrum of $X^*(r^*)$. Then, the maximum value of r for which the specstrum of X is not null is $n^* + r^*$.

Specstrum properties mainly depend on the scheduling used to select $\beta(r)$ values. An increasing logarithmic scheduling is here proposed for Logarithmic Specstrum (LS). The scheduling is based on statistic optimization strategies adopted for Markov Random Fields (i.e., Gibbs sampler [8] using Simulated Annealing [9]). The analogy arises from the observation that in all such methods the estimation of the filter output is obtained by maximizing a conditional probability of a function where an additional degree of freedom has been included, i.e., β parameter. In the case of MRFs, selecting β values can be considered as a mean of adapting the model by which noise is eliminated and information is extracted to the amount of processing already performed. For example, in the case of [8], edge points are extracted during first steps by using less restrictive models. Such models provide less certain solutions characterized by a lower noise level. Solutions obtained at first steps are then refined by increasing edge certainty: to this end, filters with a more selective response are used.

The LS follows a similar reasoning with the exception that the target of the method is to extract global, instead of local, shape information. Models used at first iterations provide a more uncertain shape information, contributing to eliminate noise, whereas further iterations provide more informative shape details thanks to decreased noise conditions. This approach can be considered acceptable when the object specificity, (i.e. salient features necessary to recognize it), are not associated with the exact boundary shape of the object itself. On the other hand, when noise is present in large percentage details over image boundaries are usually lost and cannot represent a discriminant feature. Therefore, LS seems to be a good trade-off as shape descriptor in noisy situations.

Logarithmic scheduling of β is equivalent to apply linear smoothing operators in the first steps, and to successively apply rank-order filter of decreasing rank until pure winner takes all rules are applied (i.e. dilation or erosion) in the limit conditions as $\beta(r) > TH$. This allows the extracted image descriptor to be more robust to binary noise i.e., to provide a more stable shape descriptor under varying ambient noise. Thanks to the generalizing capability provided by BSMFs a high computational efficiency can be reached.

The algorithm used to compute the Specstrum is similar to the one proposed for a skeleton extraction in [10]:

a) Initialization: $n = 0, S_{-1}(X) = X$.

b) Iteration of the following steps:

1) $S_n(X) = [S_{n-1}(X) \ominus_{\beta(n)} B]$

2) $\gamma_{n,\beta(n)}(X) = S_n(X) \oplus_{\beta(n)} B$

3) $sp(n) = [m(S_{n-1}(X)) - m(\gamma_{n,\beta(n)}(X) \cap S_{n-1}(X))] \setminus m(X)$;

4) if $S_n(X) = \emptyset$ then
   $n^* = n$; Stop;

5) $n = n + 1$; $\beta(n) = SCH(n)$; goto 1.

SCH() is a scheduling function which provides a different β value at each iteration.

4. Results and conclusion

Tests to prove the effectiveness of the method were made on patterns extracted from an attention focusing mechanism of a car surveillance system. The system is based on a preliminary change detection phase, where binary patterns which should correspond to cars are individuated. In Fig. 1, an original image, the related background and the result of the change detection method are shown.

In Fig. 2 granulometries obtained by choosing a scheduling function providing a constant value are shown. In Fig. 3 corresponding specstrum are plotted. As one can see, an increasing convergence speed towards the empty set is shown for increasing β values. In the case of null β value, the process converge to a not-null set, corresponding to a fixed point of the linear average filter; many small oscillations in the specstrum indicate the slow progressive convergence towards that fixed point. However, a too high speed can provide a not sufficiently descriptive specstrum, i.e., few features for further classification stages. Therefore, such histograms show the necessity of a different scheduling.

In Fig. 4 the granulometry obtained by applying LS is shown, i.e., an increasing logarithmic scheduling function. A trade-off is obtained between convergence speed and the degree of significance with respect to shape of the granulometries. The successive shapes at increasing r values correspond in a smooth way to the profile of the car. Our conjecture is that this is due to the slow increasing of the β parameter, corresponding to slow cooling of temperature in Simulated Annealing.

Specstrum stability to noisy conditions is tested by using corrupted images shown in Fig. 5. Noise points are chosen randomly up to a percentage of 50%. In Fig. 6 specstrum is shown up to 25% of noise. LS is used. In this conditions, specstrum is relatively stable, indicating that noise does not affect to a great extent shape information.

These results confirm that the proposed shape descriptor has good characteristics for being used on pattern detected in noisy conditions. Specstrum can be very useful for those situations where it is not possible to apply computationally heavy methods for completely eliminating noise from binary patterns to be recognized. For example, in the considered application, simpler approaches (e.g., simple differences) can be used to perform real-time change detection, before characterizing extracted noisy patterns by using specstrum.

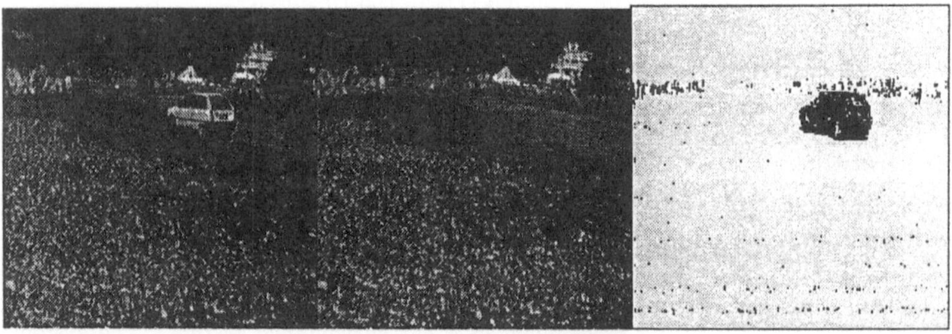

Fig. 1. Original (left), background (center), and result of change-detection (right)

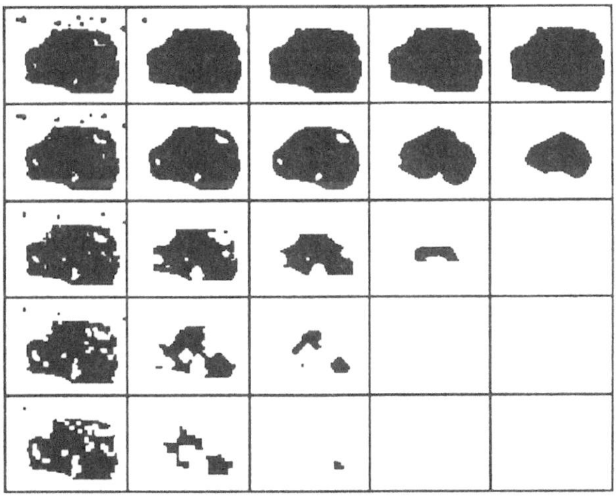

Fig. 2. Statistical granulometries for fixed values of β at different iterations r: β varies from top to bottom, by assuming values 0.4, 0.8, 1.4, and 50. r increases from left to right. r values equal to 1, 4, 7, 15, 23 are plotted.

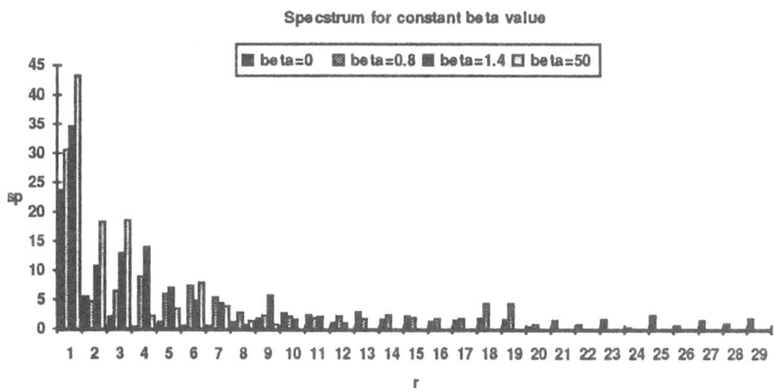

Fig. 3. Specstrum for a constant scheduling, $\beta(r) = \beta$. Each column for a given r indicates specstrum value for a different, constant β value.

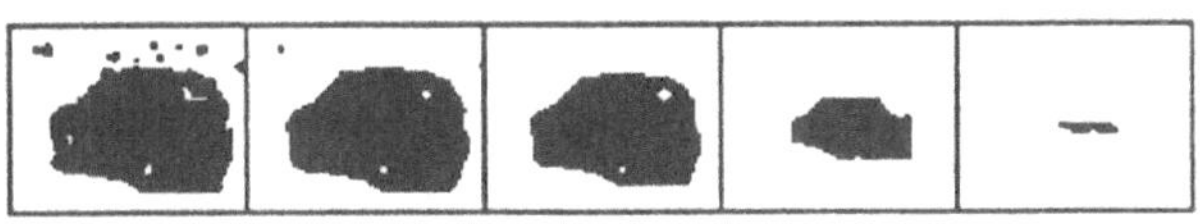

Fig. 4. Granulometries obtained for Logarithmic Specstrum. Representation values r are the same used for Fig. 2.

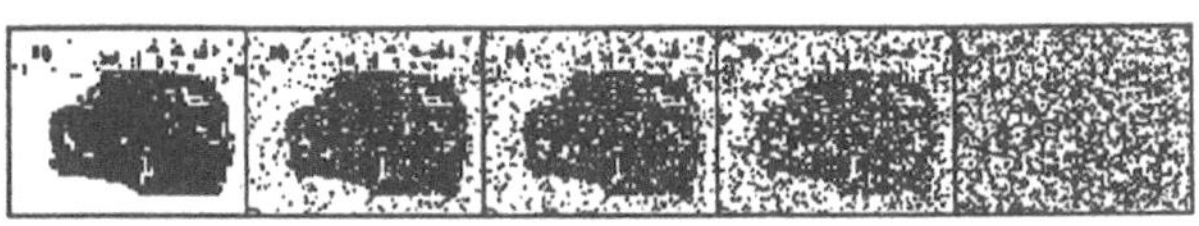

Fig. 5. Binary car image affected by increasing noise levels. From left to right, images are shown with 0%, 10%, 15%, 25%, 50% percentage of noisy points.

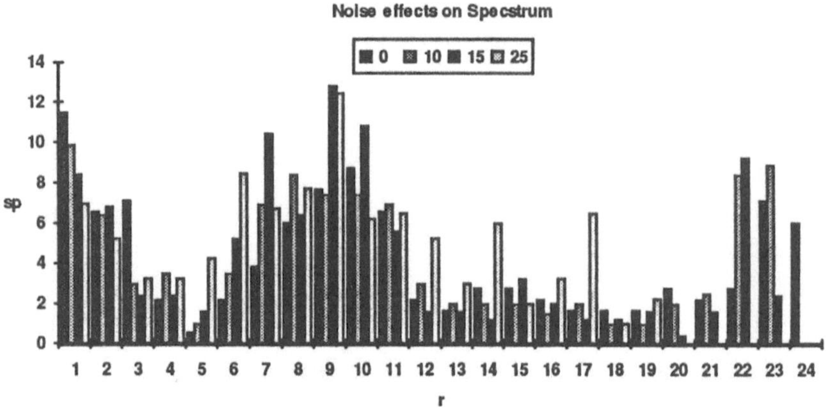

Fig. 6. Noise effects on specstrum. The specstrum of the first four images in Fig. 5 is computed. Each column at a given r value show the corresponding specstrum value for images corrupted by 0%, 10%, 15%, 25%, percentage of noisy points.

References

1. C.S. Regazzoni, A.N. Venetsanopoulos, G.L. Foresti, and G. Vernazza, "Statistical Morphological Filters for Binary Image Processing", Proc. Int Conf. Acoustics Speech and Signal Processing ICASSP '94, Adelaide, Australia, 1994 (in press).
2. J.F. Bronskill and A.N. Venetsanopoulos, "Multidimensional shape description and recognition using mathematical morphology", Journal of Intelligent and Robotic Systems, Vol. 1, pp. 117-143, 1988.
3. V. Anastassopoulos and A.N. Venetsanopoulos, "The classification properties of the Pecstrum and its use for Pattern Identification", Circuit Systems Signal Processing, Vol. 10, N. 3, pp. 294-326, 1991.
4. P. Maragos and R.W. Schafer, "Morphological Filters-Part II: Their relations to Median, Order Statistic, and Stack Filters", IEEE Transactions on ASSP, Vol. ASSP-35, N. 8, pp. 1170-1184, August 1987.
5. A. Yuille, L. Vincent, and D. Geiger, "Statistical Morphology and Bayesian Reconstruction", Journal of Mathematical Imaging and Vision, Vol. 1, N. 3, pp. 223-238, 1992.
6. C.S. Regazzoni, G.L. Foresti, and A.N. Venetsanopoulos, "Binary Statistical Morphological Filters", submitted to IEEE Transactions on Image Processing, 1994.
7. I. Pitas and A.N. Venetsanopoulos, Non-linear Digital Filters: Principles and Applications, Kluwer Academic, Boston, 1990.
8. S. Geman and D. Geman, "Stochastic relaxation, Gibbs distribution and the Bayesian restoration of images", IEEE Transactions on PAMI, Vol. PAMI-6, No.6, pp. 721-741, 1984.
9. S. Kirkpatrick, C.D. Gelatt, and M.P. Vecchi, "Optimization by Simulated Annealing", Science, Vol. 220, No.4598, pp. 671-680, 1982 .
10. D. Schonfeld and J. Goutsias, "Optimal Morphological Pattern Restoration from Noisy Binary Images, ", IEEE Transactions on PAMI, Vol.PAMI-13, pp. 14-29, 1991.
11. J. Serra, Image Analysis and Mathematical Morphology, Academic Press, New York, 1982.

GENERALIZED GEODESIC DISTANCES APPLIED TO INTERPOLATION AND SHAPE DESCRIPTION

PIERRE SOILLE
Ecole des Mines de Paris, Centre de Morphologie Mathématique,
35, rue Saint-Honoré, F-77305 Fontainebleau Cedex, France

Abstract.
The time necessary to follow a path defined on a grey scale image is defined as the sum of the image values along the path. The geodesic time associated with two points of the image is nothing but the smallest amount of time necessary to link these two points. Starting from this notion, we define a new geodesic metric on the image plane: the generalized geodesic distance. The generalized geodesic distance betweeen two points is the length of the shortest path(s) linking these points in a minimum amount of time. This distance is used for defining a propagation function. Applications to shape description and interpolation from contour data are provided.

Key words: image analysis, mathematical morphology, geodesic transformations, distance, propagation function, interpolation, shape

1. Introduction

The geodesic distance (Lantuéjoul & Beucher, 1980 and 1981) between two points p and q of a connected set X is the length of the shortest path(s) linking these two points *and* included in X. The geodesic distance is denoted by $d_X(p,q)$. It is sometimes referred to as a distance in non-convex domains (Piper & Granum, 1987) or a constrained distance (Verwer, Verbeek & Dekker, 1989).

Lantuéjoul & Maisonneuve (1984) define the propagation function in terms of geodesic distances. The value of the propagation function P at a given pixel x of a connected compact set X is the supremum of the lengths of the geodesic arcs (i.e., the shortest paths) starting from x and included in X:

$$P_X(x) = \sup_{y \in X}\{d_X(x,y)\}.$$

The propagation function is at the basis of the definition of several morphological features of simply connected sets: length, ends, geodesic centre, and stretching factor (Maisonneuve & Lantuéjoul, 1984). Figure 1 shows the propagation function of a connected set together with its longest geodesic arc. Efficient algorithms for computing the hexagonal and dodecagonal propagation functions are detailed in (Maisonneuve & Schmitt, 1989). Here, we obtained an Euclidean propagation function by using the Euclidean geodesic distance algorithm described in (Soille, 1991) and by processing only a restricted set of boundary pixels as detailed in Schmitt (1989).

From Fig. 1c, it can be seen that the longest geodesic arc tends to stick to the object boundary. It follows that using the length of this arc as the length of

J.Serra and P. Soille (eds.), Mathematical Morphology and Its Applications to Image Processing, 193-200

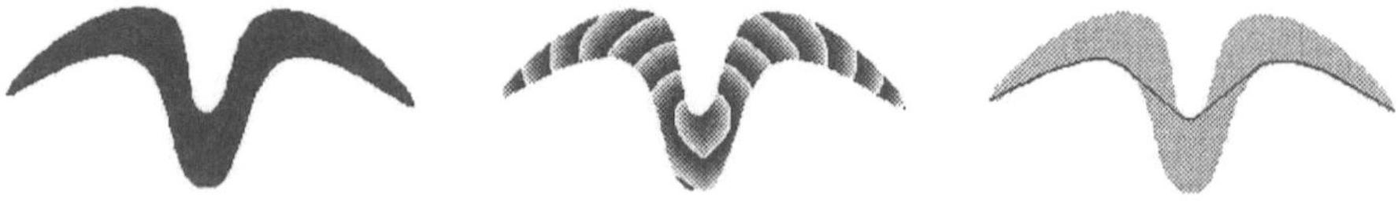

(a) Simply connected set X (b) Propagation function on X (the distances are shown modulo 16) (c) Longest geodesic arc in X

Fig. 1. Propagation function of a simply connected set and its longest geodesic arc.

the object is somewhat arbitrary. For instance, measured lengths before and after bending an object are not identical. Similarly, the geodesic centre tends to lie close to the object boundary rather than on its medial axis.

The scope of this paper is to present a generalization of the propagation function alleviating these problems. It is based on the notion of geodesic time (Soille, 1992, 1993a, and 1993b).

The paper is organized as follows. Section 2 recalls the notion of geodesic time. It is shown that it can be used to define a new metric: the generalized geodesic distance. The propagation function based on this new metric is defined in section 3. Applications to shape characterization and interpolation of contour data are detailed in section 4.

2. Geodesic Time and Generalized Geodesic Distance

Let f be a discrete grey scale image, i.e., a mapping of a subset $\mathcal{D}_f$ of $\mathbf{Z}^n$ called the definition domain of f into the set of nonnegative real numbers $\mathbf{R}_0^+$ union $+\infty$. The *time* $t_f(\mathcal{P})$ necessary to cover a discrete path $\mathcal{P}$ of length l defined on a discrete grey scale image f equals the mean of the values of f taken two at a time along $\mathcal{P}$:

$$t_f(\mathcal{P}) = \sum_{i=1}^{l} \frac{f(p_{i-1}) + f(p_i)}{2} = \frac{f(p_0)}{2} + \frac{f(p_l)}{2} + \sum_{i=1}^{l-1} f(p_i). \qquad (1)$$

$t_f(\mathcal{P})$ is therefore independent of the direction used to cover the path. An example is given in Fig. 2a.

The geodesic time $t_f(p,q)$ separating two points p and q in a grey scale image f is the smallest amount of time needed to link p to q in f:

$$t_f(p,q) = \inf\{t_f(\mathcal{P}) \mid \mathcal{P} \text{ links } p \text{ to } q\}.$$

The idea of grey-weighted distance transform introduced by Rutovitz (1968, p. 128) is closely related to the concept of geodesic time. Grey-weighted distances have been used by Beucher (1990, pp. 92–104) for investigating geodesic operators over a refringence graph, Verbeek & Verwer (1990) for solving the Eikonal equation and Meyer (1992) for integrating images. Kimmel & Bruckstein (1993) proposed an implementation of the grey-weighted distance transform using an implicit representation of a curve evolution process (Osher & Sethian, 1988) (Sapiro *et al.*, 1993). The initial curve corresponds to the contours of the input set and it is embedded in a higher

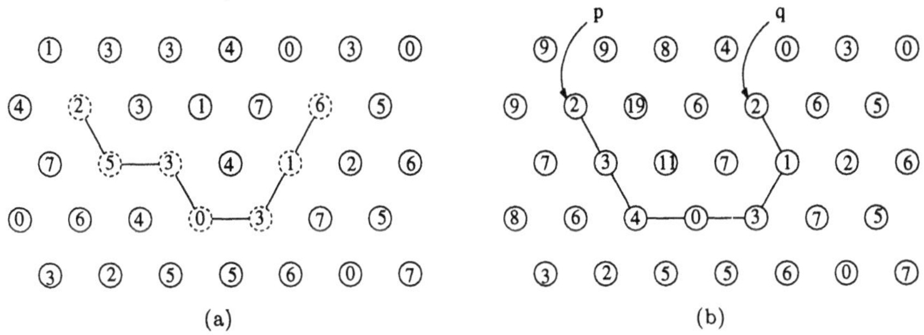

Fig. 2. *(a)* Discrete path $\mathcal{P}$ on a grey scale image defined in the hexagonal grid: the time necessary to cover this path equals 16 (refer to Eq. 1). *(b)* Geodesic or shortest path between two points p and q on a grey scale image. It is a geodesic since there exists no other path linking p to q in a smaller amount of time.

dimensional function. The curve is then propagated as a level set of a bivariate function, the equations of motion being solved using sophisticated numerical techniques derived from hyperbolic conservation laws. The simplicity of our approach makes it more appealing for practical applications.

The geodesic time does not define a metric for the domain of definition of f. Indeed, two different points are separated by a null geodesic time if there exists a path with zero values linking the points. We call the geodesics of f the paths linking any pair of points in a minimal amount of time and different from $+\infty$. An example of geodesic based on geodesic time caculations is shown in Fig. 2b.

A new and interesting geodesic metric[1] is defined by considering the actual length of the geodesics defined in a grey scale image. The generalized geodesic distance $d_f^\star(p,q)$ between two points p and q of a grey scale image f is the shortest length L of the path(s) linking p to q in a minimum amount of time if it is different from $+\infty$, and is $+\infty$ otherwise:

$$d_f^\star(p,q) = \begin{cases} \inf\{L(\mathcal{P}) \mid \mathcal{P} \text{ links } p \text{ to } q \text{ and } t_f(\mathcal{P}) = t_f(p,q)\} & \text{if } t_f(p,q) \neq +\infty \\ +\infty & \text{otherwise.} \end{cases}$$

For instance, the generalized geodesic distance separating the points p and q of Fig. 2b equals 6. The generalized geodesic distance defines a geodesic metric for $\mathcal{D}_f$:

$$\begin{array}{rl} 0) & d_f^\star(p,q) \in \mathbf{R}_0^+ \cup \infty, \\ i) & d_f^\star(p,q) = 0 \Leftrightarrow p = q, \\ ii) & d_f^\star(p,q) = d_f^\star(q,p), \\ iii) & d_f^\star(p,q) \leq d_f^\star(p,r) + d_f^\star(r,q). \end{array}$$

The geodesic distance as defined in the binary case (Lantuéjoul & Beucher, 1980) is a particular case of the generalized geodesic distance where f has only two values: 1 inside the geodesic mask and $+\infty$ outside.

A geodesic dilation can be defined in terms of generalized geodesic distances. The geodesic dilation of size n of a set X with respect to a grey scale image f is the set

[1] We refer to a geodesic metric for a function satisfying the three axioms of a metric but taking values in $\mathbf{R}_0^+ \cup +\infty$ rather than $\mathbf{R}_0^+$.

of points of the domain of definition of f whose generalized geodesic distance to X is lower or equal to n and it is denoted by $\delta_f^{(n)}(X)$:

$$\delta_f^{(n)}(X) = \{x \in \mathcal{D}_f \mid d_f^\star(x, X) \leq n\},$$

where $d_f^\star(x, X) = \inf_{y \in X} d_f^\star(x, y)$. The geodesic erosion of size n a set X in a grey scale image f is the set of points of X whose distance to the complement of X, denoted by X^c, is strictly greater than n:

$$\varepsilon_f^{(n)}(X) = \{x \in X \mid d_f^\star(x, X^c) > n\}.$$

Note that the proposed geodesic dilations and erosions are dual with respect to set complementation: $\varepsilon_f^{(n)}(X) = [\delta_f^{(n)}(X^c)]^c$.

3. Generalized Propagation Function

Starting from a simply connected set X, we want to define a propagation function alleviating the problems mentioned in section 1. In other words, we would like the geodesic arcs follow the medial axis of the set rather than its concavities. This can be achieved using generalized geodesic distance calculations on the complemented distance transform of X.

We first transform X into its Euclidean distance mapping ED (Danielsson, 1980)(Vincent, 1991*b*). This distance function is then complemented as follows:

$$[ED(X)]^c(x) = \max_{y \in X}\{[ED(X)](y)\} - [ED(X)](x).$$

The value of the propagation function P at a given pixel x of a set X is now defined as the largest generalized geodesic distance of the geodesics starting from x, included in X, and considering the complement of the Euclidean distance mapping on X:

$$P_X^\star(x) = \sup_{y \in X}\{d^\star_{[ED(X)]^c}(x, y)\}. \tag{2}$$

In the following, this latter propagation function is referred to as the 'generalized propagation function'. For a simply connected set X, it can be shown that it is enough to consider the points y of the internal boundary of X rather than $y \in X$ in Eq. 2. An example of time propagation function[2] is shown in Fig. 3.

This latter figure should be compared with Fig. 1. The longest geodesic arc (Fig. 3c) follows now the medial axis of the object. Morphological features defined for the usual propagation function (Maisonneuve & Lantuéjoul, 1984) can be adapted to the generalized propagation function:

- The geodesic diameter or length of X is the maximal value of the generalized propagation function on X.
- The geodesic center is the connected set of points where the generalized propagation function reaches its minimal value. This value is referred to as the geodesic radius.

[2] The time propagation function is defined by replacing the generalized geodesic distance $d^\star$ with the geodesic time t in Eq. 2.

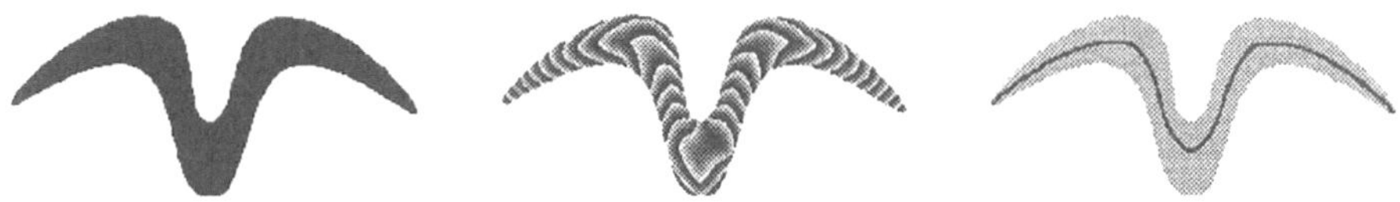

(a) Simply connected set X (b) Time propagation function on X (time values are shown modulo 16) (c) Longest geodesic arc in X

Fig. 3. Propagation function based on generalized geodesic distance calculations and corresponding longest geodesic arc.

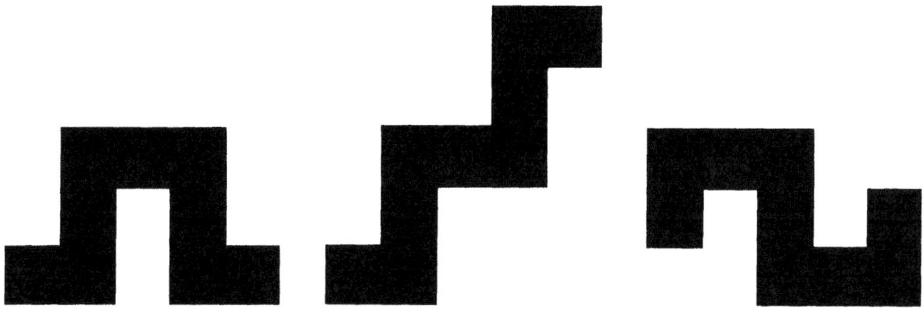

(a) Test shape 1 (b) Test shape 2 (c) Test shape 3

Fig. 4. Three shapes used for length measurements.

- A length index is defined by considering the ratio between $\pi L^2(X)$ and $4A(X)$ where $L(X)$ is the length of X and $A(X)$ the surface area of X.
- The ends of the set are defined as the regional maxima of the generalized propagation function on X.

4. Applications

We demonstrate the usefulness of our developments for shape characterization and interpolation of contour elevation data.

4.1. Shape characterization

Fig. 4 shows 3 test shapes used for our experiment. Intuitively, these 3 shapes should output identical length measurements. The length of the longest geodesic arc for a constant value within the shape varies however from one shape to another: $4\sqrt{2}+1$ for the first, $5\sqrt{2}$ for the second, and $3\sqrt{2}+2$ for the third. Using the generalized propagation function, the length of the longest geodesic arcs are almost identical as shown in Fig. 5.

4.2. Interpolation of Contour Data

A contour data representation of a digital elevation model or an image consists in a set of contour lines of constant intensity value. Such data are obtained either from topographic maps or by compressing an original image with smooth variations (lossy

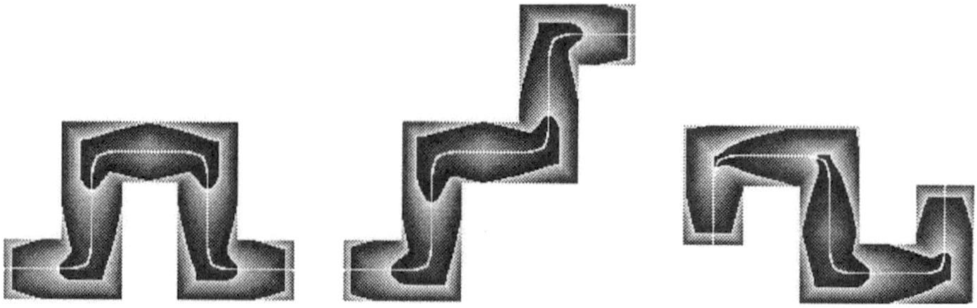

(a) Test shape 1 (b) Test shape 2 (c) Test shape 3

Fig. 5. Longest geodesic arcs superimposed on the time propagation function for the 3 shapes shown in Fig. 4 (the values of the time propagation function are shown modulo 256).

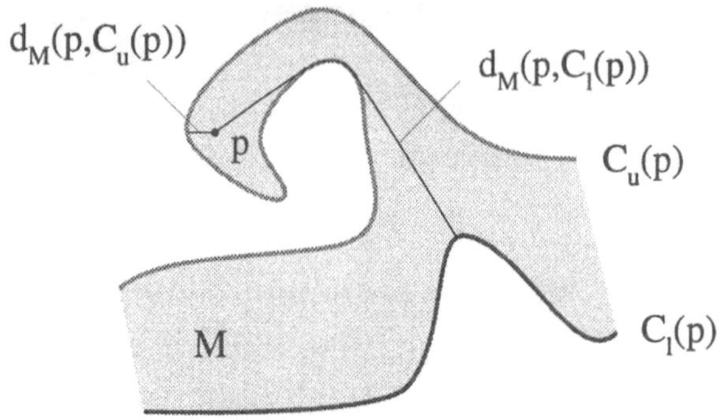

Fig. 6. Magnified section of an image of iso-intensity contour lines with a pixel p lying within the in between contour line space M, and geodesics from p to its lower $C_l(p)$ and upper $C_u(p)$ contour line within M.

compression technique). In both cases, there is a need for interpolating the values that are located in between successive contour lines. The interpolated value of a pixel located in between two successive contour lines can be calculated from a linear interpolation along the geodesics going from its high contour line to its low contour line and passing through the pixel itself (Soille, 1991). This is illustrated in Fig. 6

Starting from an image of iso-intensity contour lines I, the interpolated value of a pixel p located in the space M in between two successive contour lines is equal to the weighed mean of $h_{C_l(p)}$ and $h_{C_l(p)}$ by the geodesic distances from p to $C_u(p)$ and to $C_l(p)$ respectively:

$$H(p) = \frac{h_{C_l(p)} * d_M[p, C_u(p)] + h_{C_u(p)} * d_M[p, C_l(p)]}{d_M[p, C_l(p)] + d_M[p, C_u(p)]}. \tag{3}$$

In (Soille, 1991 and 1992), it has been shown that this methodology performs better than all existing interpolation algorithms. However, the steepest slope path resulting from classical geodesic calculations tends to stick to the concavities of the

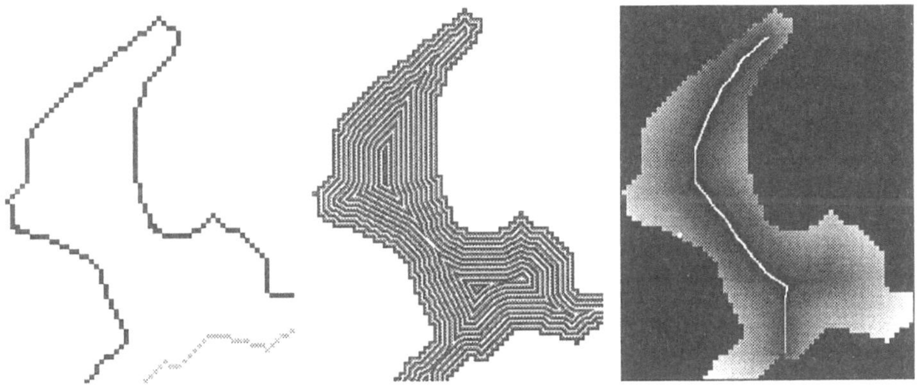

(a) Two contour lines

(b) Complement of the Euclidean distance function

(c) Shortest path from a point to the low contour line

Fig. 7. Interpolation from contour data using generalized geodesic distance calculations.

contour lines rather than following valley lines (see Fig. 6). We propose to alleviate this problem by using generalized geodesic distances rather than usual geodesic distances. By doing so, Eq. 3 becomes:

$$H(p) = \frac{h_{\mathcal{C}_l(p)} * d^{\star}{}_{[ED(M)]^c}[p, \mathcal{C}_u(p)] + h_{\mathcal{C}_u(p)} * d^{\star}{}_{[ED(M)]^c}[p, \mathcal{C}_l(p)]}{d^{\star}{}_{[ED(M)]^c}[p, \mathcal{C}_l(p)] + d^{\star}{}_{[ED(M)]^c}[p, \mathcal{C}_u(p)]}, \quad (4)$$

where $[ED(M)]^c$ is the complement of the Euclidean distance of the in between contour line space.

The methodology is illustrated in Fig. 7.

The interpolation technique with the use of generalized geodesic distances can be adapted for 3-dimensional reconstruction from planar cross-sections. This leads to a similar to that proposed by Usson & Montanvert (1993) but using generalized geodesic rather than Euclidean distances.

5. Conclusion

A new metric based on grey-weighted distance calculations has been presented and is at the basis of a generalization of the binary geodesic transformations for grey scale geodesic masks. We showed that the geodesics based on this metric are of interest for both shape characterization and interpolation from contour data. The notions of skeleton and skeleton via anchor points (Vincent, 1991*a*) are closely related to concepts presented in this paper. This issue will be addressed in future work. Finally, it is expected that the simulation of physical processes such as those studied in (Jeulin, Vincent & Serpe, 1992) will benefit of our developments.

References

Beucher, S. (1990), Segmentation d'images et morphologie mathématique, PhD thesis, Ecole des Mines de Paris.

Danielsson, P.-E. (1980), 'Euclidean distance mapping', *Computer Graphics and Image Processing* **14**, 227–248.

Jeulin, D., Vincent, L. & Serpe, G. (1992), 'Propagation algorithms on graphs for physical applications', *Journal of Visual Communication and Image Representation* **3**(2), 161–181.

Kimmel, R. & Bruckstein, A. (1993), Sub–pixel distance maps and weighted distance transforms, *in* 'Geometric methods in computer vision II', Vol. SPIE–2031, pp. 259–268.

Lantuéjoul, C. & Beucher, S. (1980), 'Geodesic distance and image analysis', *Mikroskopie* **37**, 138–142.

Lantuéjoul, C. & Beucher, S. (1981), 'On the use of the geodesic metric in image analysis', *Journal of Microscopy* **121**, 39–49.

Lantuéjoul, C. & Maisonneuve, F. (1984), 'Geodesic methods in image analysis', *Pattern Recognition* **17**(2), 177–187.

Maisonneuve, F. & Lantuéjoul, C. (1984), 'Geodesic convexity', *ACM Transactions on Graphics* **3**(2), 169–174.

Maisonneuve, F. & Schmitt, M. (1989), 'An efficient algorithm to compute the hexagonal and dodecagonal propagation function', *ACM Transactions on Graphics* **8**(2), 515–520.

Meyer, F. (1992), Integrals and gradients of images, *in* P. Gader, E. Dougherty & J. Serra, eds, 'Image Algebra and Morphological Image Processing III', Vol. Proc. SPIE 1769, pp. 200–211.

Osher, S. & Sethian, J. (1988), 'Fronts propagating with curvature speed: algorithms based on Hamilton–Jacobi formulations', *Journal of Computational Physics* **79**, 12–49.

Piper, J. & Granum, E. (1987), 'Computing distance transformations in convex and non-convex domains', *Pattern Recognition* **20**(6), 599–615.

Rutovitz, D. (1968), Data structures for operations on digital images, *in* G. Cheng, R. Ledley, D. Kollock & A. Rosenfeld, eds, 'Pictorial pattern recognition', pp. 105–133.

Sapiro, G., Kimmel, R., Shaked, D., Kimia, B. & Bruckstein, A. (1993), 'Implementing continuous-scale morphology via curve evolution', *Pattern Recognition* **26**(9), 1363–1372.

Schmitt, M. (1989), 'Geodesic arcs in non-Euclidean metrics, application to the propagation function', *Revue d'intelligence artificielle* **3**(2), 43–76.

Soille, P. (1991), 'Spatial distributions from contour lines: an efficient methodology based on distance transformations', *Journal of Visual Communication and Image Representation* **2**(2), 138–150.

Soille, P. (1992), Morphologie mathématique : du relief à la dimensionalité—Algorithmes et méthodes—, PhD thesis, Université Catholique de Louvain, Louvain-la-Neuve, Belgium.

Soille, P. (1993*a*), Generalized geodesy via geodesic time, Submitted to Pattern Recognition Letter.

Soille, P. (1993*b*), The geodesic time function: principles and applications, *in* 'The 1993 International Conference on Confocal Microscopy & 3D Image Processing', Sydney, p. 107.

Usson, Y. & Montanvert, A. (1993), Reconstruction tridimensionnelle à partir des distances discrètes, *in* 'Colloque géométrie discrète en imagerie : fondements et applications', Strasbourg, pp. 20–21.

Verbeek, P. & Verwer, B. (1990), 'Shading from shape, the eikonal equation solved by grey-weighted distance transform', *Pattern Recognition Letters* **11**, 681–690.

Verwer, B., Verbeek, P. & Dekker, S. (1989), 'An efficient cost algorithm applied to distance transforms', *IEEE Transactions on Pattern Analysis and Machine Intelligence* **11**(4), 425–429.

Vincent, L. (1991*a*), Efficient computation of various types of skeletons, *in* 'Medical Imaging V', Vol. Proc. SPIE 1445.

Vincent, L. (1991*b*), Exact Euclidean distance function by chain propagations, *in* 'Proc. IEEE Computer Vision and Pattern Recognition', pp. 520–525.

PERFORMANCE ANALYSIS OF A MORPHOLOGICAL VORONOI TESSELLATION ALGORITHM

E.G. KALAITZIS and I. PITAS
Department of Electrical Engineering,
University of Thessaloniki,
Thessaloniki 540 06, GREECE

Abstract. The goal of the following analysis is to estimate the computational complexity of the Voronoi tessellation of an image performed with an algorithm based on mathematical morphology. The morphological dilation operation is used to implement a set of distance functions (distance transformations) with a variety of structuring elements that approximate distance metrics, such as the Euclidean, city block and chessboard distances. The analysis has been performed for 2-D morphological Voronoi tessellation.

Key words: Voronoi tessellation, mathematical morphology, dilation, distance transformations, distance metrics, Euclidean distance, city block distance, chessboard distance

1. Introduction

Voronoi tessellation is a basic problem in computational geometry [1]. It is also a tool used in image analysis, such as object recognition [2] and texture analysis [9]. Several important problems can be solved by employing Voronoi tessellation, for example Delaunay triangulation, convex hull, object decomposition into simple components (triangles). The input to the tessellation procedure is an image containing a set of classified points (seeds). The goal is to classify the rest image points to the nearest seed (in the geometrical sense). The nearest neighbor criterion is implemented by using a distance metric. The mathematical morphology dilation operation is used to perform Voronoi tessellation. A set of structuring elements can be used to implement the various distance metrics on the discrete grid of a digitized image. The use of dilation in order to tessellate an image is discussed in [5, 6] and methods that approach the Euclidean disk growing are discussed in [7, 10]. An efficient approach to the Euclidean disk growing can be found in [8]. The novel contribution of this paper is the theoretical analysis of the computational complexity of the morphological algorithm.

2. Notations and definitions

The geometrical concepts of mathematical morphology are essentially the basis of the discussed Voronoi tessellation approach. The corresponding morphological operators rely on set theory. In order to define the symbols and tools we further use, the following assumptions are made:

Let $I \subset \mathcal{W}$ (where $\mathcal{W} \equiv \mathcal{R}^2$ *or* $\mathcal{W} \equiv \mathcal{Z}^2$) be an image domain. Let $X = \{x_1, x_2, \ldots, x_m \in I \ , \ m \in \mathcal{Z}\}$ be a set of m points in I called *seeds*. The set

J.Serra and P. Soille (eds.), Mathematical Morphology and Its Applications to Image Processing, 201-208

of all points $p \in I$ that are closer to a given seed $x_i \in X$ than any other seed $x_j \in X$, $j \neq i$ is called *Voronoi region* of x_i. Each seed corresponds to the center of a region (class). Let $d(.)$ be a distance function used to implement the above mentioned nearest neighbor criterion. The Voronoi region is then defined as:

$$V(i) \;=\; \{p \in I \;:\; d(p,x_i) < d(p,x_j)\;,\; j \neq i\,\}$$

The union of Voronoi regions for all $x_i \in X$ is called *Voronoi diagram* of X:

$$Vor(X) = \bigcup_{i=1}^{N} V(i)$$

In order to find the corresponding Voronoi diagram of a set X we introduce the Minkowski addition and furthermore the morphological dilation of two sets as follows. The Minkowski addition of two sets X and B is defined as:

$$X \oplus B \;=\; \bigcup_{b \in B} X_b$$

where X_b is the translated set X centered at b. The dilation of a set X by another set B (also called structuring element) is defined as the Minkowski set addition of X with B^s:

$$X \oplus B^s \;=\; \bigcup_{b \in B} X_{-b}$$

where B^s is the symmetric of the structuring element B with respect to its origin. Another expression for dilation is the following:

$$X \oplus B^s \;=\; \{\, x \in \mathcal{Z}^2 \;:\; B_x \cap X \neq \emptyset \,\} = \;\{x \in \mathcal{Z}^2 : B_x \uparrow X\}$$

The symbol $\uparrow$ states that the set B_x hits X.

3. Stochastic analysis

In the following we shall estimate theoretically the average number of dilation steps performed in a continuous image domain I that contains m random seeds $x_1, x_2, \ldots, x_m \in X$ uniformly distributed on the two-dimensional $n \times n$ grid embedded within I.

For every point p in the image I we denote the distance from its nearest seed as the classification distance $r_{cl}(p)$ of the point.

$$r_{cl}(p) \;=\; inf\{\; d(p,x_i)\;,\; x_i \in X\;,\; i = 1,2,\ldots,m\;\}$$

Let $dil(i)$ be the number of dilations associated with the i-th seed class; $dil(i)$ is proportional to the maximum of the classification distances among the points of the class. The maximal number of dilations performed is:

$$dil \;=\; max\{\; dil(1), dil(2), \ldots, dil(m)\;\} = \;max\{\; r_{max}(1), r_{max}(2), \ldots, r_{max}(m)\;\}$$

where $r_{max}(i)$, $i = 1, 2, \ldots, m$ is the maximal classification distance associated with the i-th seed class:

$$r_{max}(i) \;=\; sup\{\; r_{cl}(p) \;,\; p \in V(i) \;\}$$

We estimate the average number of dilation steps by calculating the corresponding discrete cumulative distribution function (*cdf*). The latter is a discrete approximation based on the continuous *cdf* of the maximal classification distance, which in turn is based on the *cdfs* of the classification distances that correspond on every image point. Finally, the *cdf* of the distance between a particular image point and another random one is used to calculate the classification distance for every point in I.

In a first approach we calculate for every point $p_0 = (x_0, y_0) \in I$ the probability that its distance from another random point $p = (x, y) \in I$ is less or equal to r. Let $F(r)$ be the cumulative distribution function (*cdf*) of the random variable r, defined as:

$$F(r, p_0) = P\{d(p_0, p) \leq r\}$$

The former probability is proportional to the area of the intersection of the domain I and its subdomain $D(p_0, r)$, where $D(p_0, r)$ consists of the points of I that their distance from the point p_0 is less or equal to r:

$$D(p_0, r) = \{p \in I \;,\; d(p, p_0) \leq r\}$$

In particular the probability P is equal to the ratio of the areas $I \cap D(p_0, r)$ and I.

$$P(d(p_0, p) \leq r) \;=\; \frac{A(I \cap D(p_0, r))}{A(I)} \tag{1}$$

Its calculation for various distance measures is described in Section 4.

The classification distance $r_{cl}(p_0)$ of the point $p_0 = (x_0, y_0)$ is its minimal distance from the m seeds. Therefore the *cdf* of the classification distance of the point p_0 is determined as:

$$F_m(r_{cl}(p_0)) = P\{\; min(r_1, r_2, \ldots, r_m) \leq r_{cl}(p_0) \;\} \tag{2}$$

where $r_i = d(p_0, x_i)$, $x_i \in X$, $i = 1, 2, \ldots, m$. The former relationship becomes:

$$F_m(r_{cl}(p_0)) = 1-(1-F(r_1, p_0))(1-F(r_2, p_0)) \ldots (1-F(r_m, p_0)) = 1-(1-F(r, p_0))^m$$

where $F(r_i, p_0) = F(r, p_0)$, $i = 1, 2, \ldots, m$ (based on the familiar formula for the *cdf* of a minimum variable).

The final number of the performed dilations in the entire image is equal to the maximum among all the classification distances $dil = r_{max} = max\{r_{cl}(p) p \in I\}$ corresponding to every point of the image. Therefore the *cdf* of the variable r_{max} is defined as:

$$F_m^{n^2}(r_{max}) = P\{\; max\{r_{cl}(p_1), r_{cl}(p_2), \ldots, r_{cl}(p_{n^2})\} \leq r_{max} \;\} \tag{3}$$

and consequently

$$F_m^{n^2}(r_{max}) = F_m(r_{cl}(p_1)) F_m(r_{cl}(p_2)) \ldots F_m(r_{cl}(p_{n^2})) = \prod_{i=1}^{n^2} F_m(r_{cl}(p_i)) \tag{4}$$

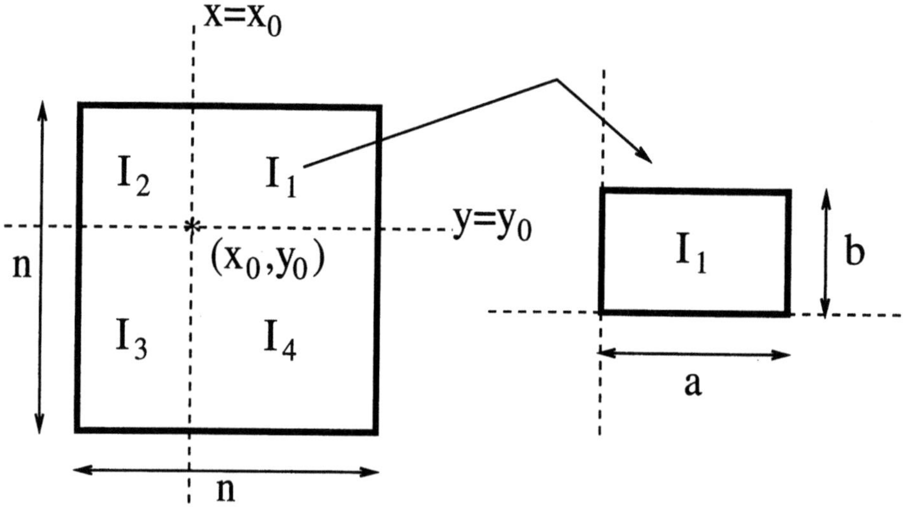

Fig. 1. Subdivision of I into 4 areas I_1, I_2, I_3, I_4 by the lines $x = x_0$ and $y = y_0$

where $F_m(r_{cl}(p_1)), F_m(r_{cl}(p_2)), \ldots, F_m(r_{cl}(p_{n^2}))$ are the *cdfs* corresponding to each one of the n^2 points of the discretized I.

The above analysis involves continuous distance metrics, in opposition to the experimental conditions that involve discrete ones on a $n \times n$ image grid. Therefore we define a discrete *cdf* based on (3), with the following rule:

$$F'(k) = F_m^{n^2}(k + 0.5) \ , \ k \in \mathcal{Z}$$

This means that we assume the probability $P(d_i \leq k + 0.5)$ being the probability of performing k dilations. If we use the associated *pdfs*, the above equation is translated into:

$$f'(k) = f_m^{n^2}(k + 0.5) - f_m^{n^2}(k - 0.5) \ , \ k \in \mathcal{Z} \tag{5}$$

With the above definition we assign to each integer k the probability density function of the space $(k - 0.5, k + 0.5)$. We can use (4) or (5) to find the expected maximal number of dilations for the morphological Voronoi tessellation algorithm. This figure is proportionally related to the speed of the algorithm.

4. Computation of the cumulative distribution functions

In this section we evaluate the probability function (1) for various distance metrics and situations. The resulting functions are used consequently as input functions to the subsequent computation steps (2 - 4) in order to calculate the average dilation number for a given number of seeds.

First we consider the case of using the square structuring element to perform dilation with respect to the chessboard distance function, defined as:

$$d(p_0, p) \ = \ max(| \ x - x_0 \ |, | \ y - y_0 \ |) \ , \ p_0 = (x_0, y_0) \in I \ , \ p = (x, y) \in I$$

The successive use of the square structuring element in order to dilate a seed point $p = (x_0, y_0) \in I$ leads to a continuously growing square that is centered at the point p with sides of length $2r$ at the r-th growing step. As defined in (1) the probability $P(d(p_0, p) \leq r)$ is equal to the intersection area of the growing square region $D(r, p_0)$ and the I domain divided by the area of the whole I. The intersection area of the I and $D(r, p_0)$ regions can be computed for various growing steps by splitting the I domain into four areas $I_i, i = 1,2,3,4$ (Fig. 1). For each one of these subdomains we assume a being the smaller and b the bigger of the two sides of their rectangular shape. The growing region in such a subdomain is one quarter of the growing square having a corner at point p_0 and sides of length r at the r-th growing step. When $0 \leq r < a$, the above mentioned intersection is a square with area r^2. When $a \leq r < b$, the intersection is a rectangle with sides a and r as the growing square overlaps the subdomain at the direction of the small side a. Finally, when $r > b$, the growing square overlaps the whole subdomain I_i and therefore the intersection area is equal to ab. These cases are displayed in Fig. 2a. For a given chessboard distance r we have to compute the four intersection areas corresponding to the four subdomains, sum them and divide with the area of I.

$$P(d(p_0, p) \leq r) = \frac{A(I \cap D(p_0, r))}{A(I)} = \sum_{i=1}^{i=4} A(I_i \cap D)/A(I)$$

We perform a similar analysis for the use of the rhombus structuring element to perform dilation with respect to the city-block distance function, defined as:

$$d(p_0, p) = | x - x_0 | + | y - y_0 | \leq r \ , \ p_0 = (x_0, y_0) \in I \ , \ p = (x, y) \in I$$

In this case the dilation of a seed point p leads to a continuously growing rhombus centered at the point p with diagonals of length $2r$ at the r-th growing step. We consider again the four subdomains I_i. As can be seen the growing region in such a subdomain is an orthogonal triangle with equal perpendicular sides of length r at the r-th dilation step (Fig. 2b.). When $0 \leq r < a$, the intersection area between the triangle and the subdomain I_i is $\frac{1}{2}r^2$ (triangle with side of length r). When $a \leq r < b$, the intersection area is $\frac{1}{2}r^2 - \frac{1}{2}(r-a)^2$ computed as the area of a triangle with sides of length r overlapping the rectangular subdomain I_i minus the area of the small triangle with sides of length $r - a$ that is outside the subdomain. When $b \leq r < a + b$, the intersection area is $\frac{1}{2}r^2 - \frac{1}{2}(r-a)^2 - \frac{1}{2}(r-b)^2$ representing the area of the triangles previously described minus the area of a second triangle with sides of length $r - b$ that is outside the subdomain. Finally, when $r > a + b$, the growing triangle overlaps the whole subdomain I_i and therefore the intersection area is equal to ab. As described previously the sum of the areas and its division by the area of I results to the cumulative distribution function corresponding to the point p_0.

Finally we consider the case of the Euclidean disc growing as a result of recursive dilations performed with a unitary circle used as a structuring element. The growing area satisfies the Euclidean distance metric definition

$$d(p_0, p) = \sqrt{(x - x_0)^2 + (y - y_0)^2} \ , \ p_0 = (x_0, y_0) \in I \ , \ p = (x, y) \in I$$

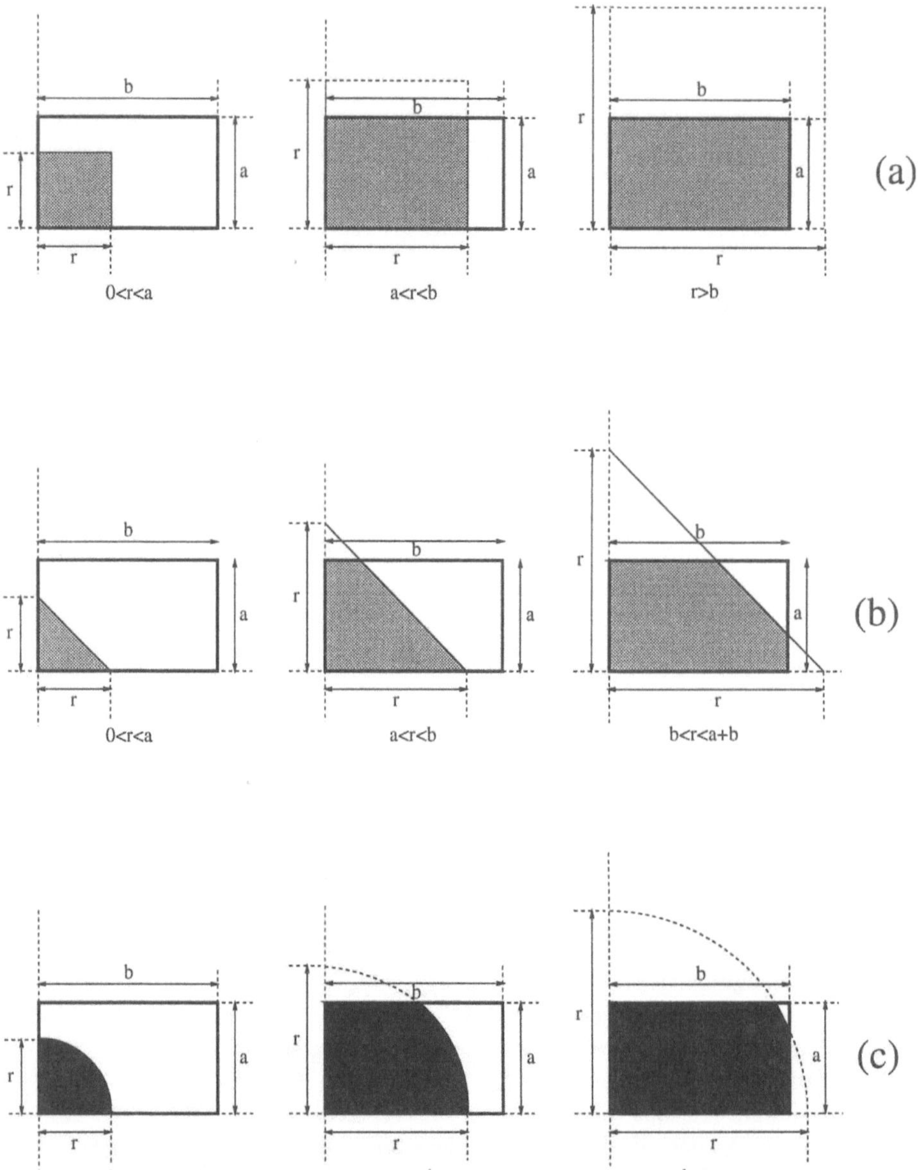

Fig. 2. Region growing in subdomain I_i with structuring elements: a)square b)rhombus c)circle

TABLE I
Theoretical and experimental average number of dilation steps in Morphological Voronoi tessellation

256 × 256 image		Euclidean		City-block		Chessboard	
seeds	density(%)	Exper.	Theor.	Exper.	Theor.	Exper.	Theor.
655	1	24.292	24.291	30.268	30.269	21.653	21.652
1310	2	16.261	16.265	20.393	20.391	14.453	14.443
1966	3	12.829	12.837	16.162	16.167	11.371	11.365
2621	4	10.874	10.844	13.717	13.708	9.5550	9.5768
3276	5	9.4834	9.5051	12.040	12.055	8.3503	8.3765
5242	8	7.2444	7.1771	9.1637	9.1757	6.2138	6.2980
6553	10	6.1901	6.2755	8.0399	8.0479	5.4908	5.4686
9830	15	4.8007	4.8767	6.2431	6.3351	4.4009	4.2385
13107	20	4.2773	4.0929	5.3038	5.3210	3.3778	3.4492
16384	25	3.3908	3.4567	4.6011	4.6029	2.8222	3.0640
19660	30	2.8834	3.1256	4.3371	4.1536	2.7020	2.6460
22937	35	2.7315	2.8514	3.8222	3.7406	2.5841	2.2746
26214	40	2.6803	2.4898	3.2607	3.3723	2.2098	2.1057
32768	50	2.2435	2.1120	2.7885	3.0225	1.5773	1.9480
39321	60	1.6793	2.0032	2.6922	2.5848	1.3938	1.5328

In this case the growing area $D(r, p_0)$ is a circle centered at point p, with radius r at the r-th growing step. The growing region in a subdomain I_i is a quadrant of the growing circle and the region of our interest is its intersection with the subdomain. In particular we assume the following cases (Fig. 2c):
When $0 \le r < a$, the intersection area is $\frac{\pi}{4}r^2$. When $a \le r < b$, the intersection area is a quadrant of the growing circle minus the circular section that is outside the subdomain. Its area is $r^2(\frac{\pi}{4} - \frac{1}{2}arctan\sqrt{(\frac{r}{a})^2 - 1}) + \frac{1}{2}a^2\sqrt{(\frac{r}{a})^2 - 1}$. When $b \le r \le c = \sqrt{a^2 + b^2})$, the intersection area is a quadrant of the growing circle minus two circular sections that are outside the subdomain. In this case its area is $r^2(\frac{\pi}{4} - \frac{1}{2}(arctan\sqrt{(\frac{r}{a})^2 - 1} + arctan\sqrt{(\frac{r}{b})^2 - 1})) + \frac{1}{2}(a^2\sqrt{(\frac{r}{a})^2 - 1} + b^2\sqrt{(\frac{r}{b})^2 - 1})$. Finally, when $r > c$, the quadrant of the growing circle overlaps the subdomain I_i and the intersection area is equal to ab. In this case the sum of the four intersection areas and its division by the area of I results to the *cdf* that corresponds to the point p.

5. Results

The *cdf* of r_{max} was evaluated above for 3 distance metrics as a function of n and m. The theoretical expected average number of dilations was determined and it was compared with the experimental average number of dilations obtained by simulations. The simulations have been performed for different seed densities on a large set of images of size 256 × 256 (approximately 1000 for each case). The results are shown in Table 1. There is a very good agreement between the theoretical analysis and the experimental results. It must be noted that the speed of morphological Voronoi tessellation is inversely proportional to the number of seeds.

References

1. F.P. Preparata and M.I. Shamos, Computational Geometry, New York: Springer-Verlag, 1985.
2. N. Ahujia and B.J. Schachter, Pattern Models. New York: J. Wiley, 1983.
3. I. Pitas and A.N. Venetsanopoulos, Nonlinear Digital Filters: Principles and Applications. Boston: Kluwer Academic, 1990.
4. R.C. Gonzalez and R.E. Wintz, Digital Image Processing: An Introduction. Addison Wesley, 1992.
5. G. Borgefors, "Distance Transformations in Digital Images," Comput. Vision, Graphics, Image Proc., vol. 34, pp. 344-371, 1986.
6. J.E. Mazille, "Mathematical Morphology and Convolutions," Journal of Microscopy, vol. 156, pp. 3-13, 1989.
7. Q.Z. Ye, "The Signed Euclidean Distance Transform and Its Applications," Proc. 9th Intern. Conf. on Pattern Recognition, pp. 495-499, Rome, Italy 1988.
8. C. Kotropoulos I. Pitas and A. Maglara, "Voronoi Tessellation and Delaunay Triangulation Using Euclidean Disk Growing in $\mathcal{Z}^2$," Int. Conf. on Acoust. Speech and Signal Processing, Mineapolis, 1993.
9. I. Pitas and C. Kotropoulos, "Texture Analysis and Segmentation of Seismic Images," IEEE Proc. Int. Conf. on Acoust. Speech and Signal Processing, Glasgow, 1989.
10. F.Y.C Shin and O.R. Mitchell, "A Mathematical Morphology Approach to Euclidean Distance Transformation," IEEE Trans. on Image Processing, vol. 1, no. 2, pp. 197-204, April 1992.

OPTIMIZATION IN VORONOI DIAGRAMS

E. BERTIN, S. MARCHAND-MAILLET and J.-M. CHASSERY
Laboratoire TIMC-IMAG, GDR TDSI CNRS, Université Joseph Fourier, Bâtiment CERMO, BP 53, F-38041 Grenoble Cedex 9, France

Abstract. In this paper, we present an algorithm for optimal image segmentation using the Voronoi diagram and the Delaunay graph. The Voronoi diagram is a powerful tool for shape description and image segmentation. The Delaunay graph is used to describe the neighborhood of each Voronoi region. This graph is used to optimize the image segmentation. The validity of our approach is demonstrated by examples.

Key words: Voronoi, Delaunay, Optimization, Segmentation.

1. Introduction

The Voronoi diagram is well known in modelization of natural phenomena. An overview of applications is given in (Okabe *et al.*, 1992). The Voronoi diagram is used in many fields such as image analysis (Ahuja *et al.*, 1985; Chassery *et al.*, 1991; Bertin *et al.*, 1993), mathematical morphology (Vincent, 1990), shape representation (Brandt *et al.*, 1992), cellular sociology (description of the relationships existing between cellular functions, and spatial positions) (Marcelpoil *et al.*, 1992), etc.

In this paper we use the Voronoi diagram and the Delaunay graph for optimal image segmentation. The goal of segmentation is to partition the image into non overlapping regions, where each region satisfies a property (homogeneous grey value).

The Voronoi diagram is used for image representation model and the Delaunay graph is involved to perform data structure coding.

The originality of this approach is to find a partition of the image into Voronoi regions according an optimal criterion based on an energy measurement using a Markov approach.

In section 2 the Voronoi partition and the Delaunay graph are presented. The section 3 presents some results concerning irregular graphs using mathematical morphology and optimization. The local computation of the Voronoi partition, involves a Markov model and we present in section 4 a new algorithm to access to an optimal partition in Voronoi regions for image segmentation.

2. Voronoi diagram and Delaunay triangulation

2.1. Definitions

Let S be a set of N planar points called seeds, extracted from a regular grid. For each seed p in S, the subset of points m closer to p than to any other seed of S

J.Serra and P. Soille (eds.), Mathematical Morphology and Its Applications to Image Processing, 209-216

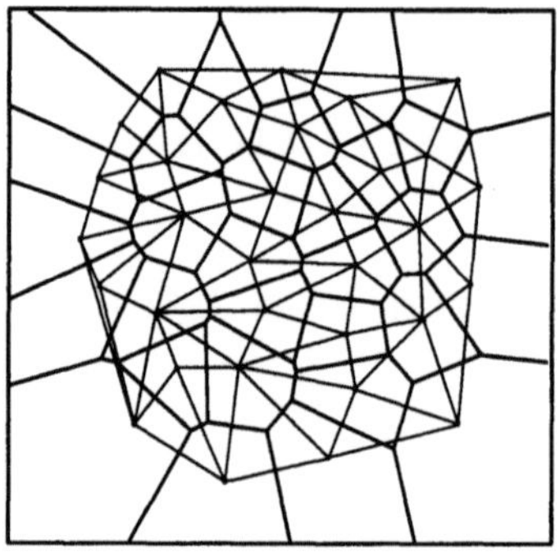

Fig. 1. Voronoi polygons (bolded straight line) and Delaunay triangulation (unbolded straight line).

defines the Voronoi region $Vor_S(p)$ associated with p:

$$Vor_S(p) = \{m \in \mathbf{R}^2, d(m,p) \leq d(m,q), \forall q \in S - p\},$$

where d is the Euclidean distance. Each Voronoi region is polygonal and convex. The set $VOR(S)$ of all the Voronoi regions is called Voronoi diagram of S:

$$VOR(S) = \bigcup_{p \in S} Vor_S(p).$$

The Delaunay graph is obtained from Voronoi diagram by duality and defined as:

$$DEL(S) = \langle S, E \rangle,$$

where S is called as the set of vertices and E is the set of edges defined as: $E = \{(p,q) \in S^2, Vor_S(p) \cap Vor_S(q) \neq \emptyset\}$.

If four seeds are not co-circular and three seeds are not on the same straight line then, the Delaunay graph is a triangulation. Figure 1 illustrates the Voronoi diagram and the Delaunay graph attached to a set of about 40 seeds.

2.2. Algorithm

To compute the Voronoi diagram we have implemented the incremental method (Bowyer, 1981) instead of divide and conquer approach. An example of the incremental method is presented in Fig. 2.

The reason of this choice is to benefit of addition or removing a seed only by local considerations. This is a fundamental property for our optimization concept. More precisely, the modification of a seed (addition, removing or displacement) is only seen as a local modification of the graph. Such property opens to the domain of Markovian approaches.

In practice 40 seconds of CPU time on a Silicon Graphics Indigo R4000 workstation are needed to generate 600000 Voronoi polygons (Bertin, 1994). The seeds can be randomly introduced or with in split and merge approach (Chassery *et al.*, 1991; Bertin *et al.*, 1993).

The incremental algorithm presents two main advantages: the run time optimality and the dynamic management of the Voronoi structure.

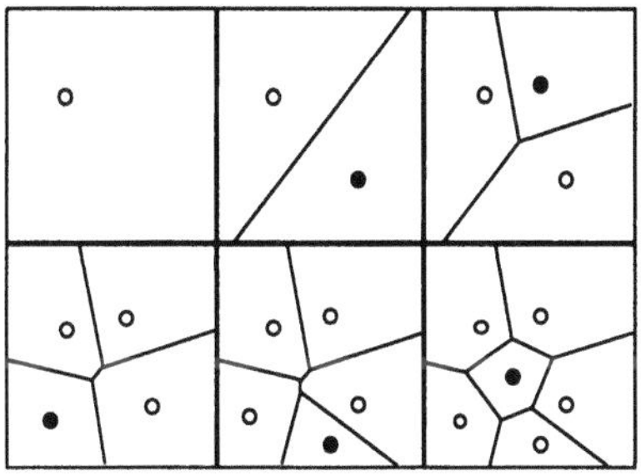

Fig. 2. Construction of the Voronoi diagram by adding successively seeds (local modification of the diagram). The black dot is the last seed to add.

These properties are directly issued from the locality induced by the Delaunay graph. We recall the definition of the neighborhood $N_S(p)$ of a seed p in S:

$$N_S(p) = \{q \in S,\, (p,q) \in E\},$$

where E consists of the edges of the Delaunay graph as previously defined.

In practice the mean of the cardinal of $N_S(s)$ is 6. As we will observe further this result is very important for the efficiency of the optimization algorithms.

Based on such representation of the image using a Delaunay graph we will focus on two directions: Mathematical Morphology (MM) and Markov random fields.

The originality of our work is to extend the Markov random fields on irregular graphs. It is the same idea used by Vincent who generalized the MM from regular lattices to irregular graphs (Vincent, 1990).

3. Some problems in graphs

3.1. Graphs and mathematical morphology

Morphological transformations have been recently studied whithin the framework of lattice theory (Serra, 1988). Morphological graphs constitute a particular kind of lattice and therefore are well suited for the general framework within which MM is defined. The neighborhood graph chosen for implementing the MM algorithms is the Delaunay triangulation. The edges of this graph are defined by all pair of points (p,q) in S whose Voronoi polygons are adjacent.

The classical transformations of MM (dilation, erosion, watershed transformation) can be extended to irregular graphs (Vincent, 1990) for image analysis. To avoid some theoretical problems we need to turn attention on the following problems.

Figure 3 illustrates a problem with dilation transform. Starting from the vertex p, the dilation of size one is obtained and generates a connected graph (black dots except p). If we consider the dilation of size two, the resulting vertices (white dots) do not form a connected component.

This first problem induces another one for the closure transform illustrated in Fig. 4. In regular lattice the closure tends to aggregate close connected components. As we can see in Fig. 4, this property is not always satisfied on irregular graphs.

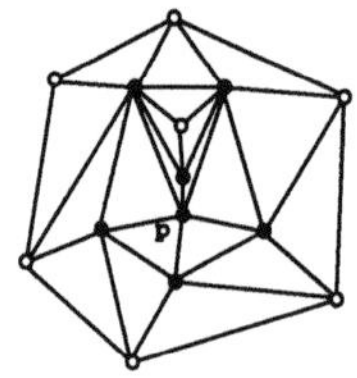

Fig. 3. Problem with the dilation from p. The ball B_1 of size one and centered on p is illustrated by the black dots. The ball B_2 of size two and centered on p is illustrated by the black and the white dots. We notice that a dot of B_2 is included in the convex hull of the dots of B_1.

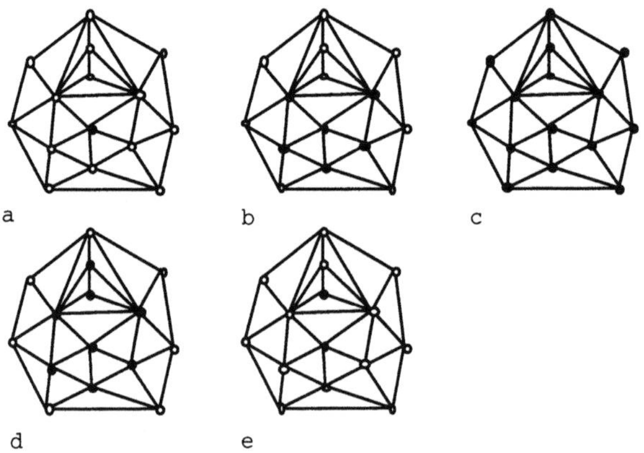

Fig. 4. Problem with the closure of size 2. (a) The black dot initializes the closure (one connected component). (b) dilation of size 1. (c) dilation of size 2. (d) Erosion of size 1. (e) Erosion of size 2 and result of the closure of size 2. The result presents two connected components.

3.2. Graphs and Optimization

To avoid the problems encountered with MM transformations on graphs, we direct our approach towards an optimized model based on local modifications of vertices of the graph. Such model will used the evaluation of an energy function and the aim is to produce a partition which minimizes this energy. Two approaches will be developed: the first one will be more restrictive since it preserves the graph topology and the second one will authorize the addition and removal of seeds.

For the first approach we must take into account the topological stability of the Delaunay graph. For each seed or vertex we define its topological order as the number of adjacent vertices. Figure 5 is an illustration of the area in which a seed p can move without changing its neighborhood $N_S(p)$.

4. Segmentation and Optimization

The aim is to find an optimal partition of the image as a set of Voronoi polygons satisfying the following energy criterion of Voronoi region: the sum of grey level standard deviations computed on Voronoi regions is minimal. To find a global minimum, we use the simulated annealing algorithm introduced by Metropolis in 1953, very well adapted to find global minimum of a complex non-linear and non-convex energy (Metropolis *et al.*, 1953).

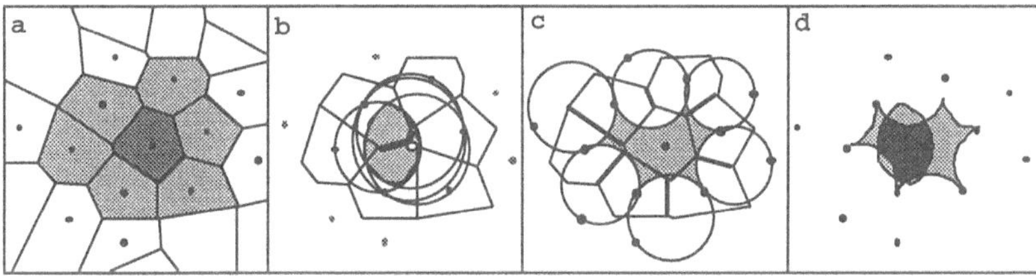

Fig. 5. Stability area of a seed in the Delaunay graph. (a) Voronoi diagram. (b) Delaunay circles built after removing a selected seed. (c) Delaunay circles built on neighbors of a selected seed. (d) The black surface describes the stability area of the selected seed. When a seed is moved in this area locally change its position, the Delaunay graph remains unchanged. The black surface shows the stability surface of a given seed.

4.1. Optimization preserving the Delaunay Stability

Moreover, we impose to preserve the Delaunay stability as illustrated in Fig. 6. Consequently, the number N of seeds corresponding to the vertices of the Delaunay graph is constant.

Let Ω be the space of all configurations of S in the plane: ($\Omega = \Lambda^S$), where Λ is the set of candidate positions of the seeds of S in the plane. For regular grids, Λ is the set of pixel positions. Let U be the energy to minimize defined as $U = \sum_{p\in S} \sigma^2(Vor_S(p))$. The simulated annealing algorithm can be described as follows:

Simulated Annealing Algorithm

1. Choosc a random configuration x in Ω.
2. Initialization of temperature: $T = T_0$ (high temperature).
3. For every seed s of S
   a) Change the value of x_s in $x_s^{'}$ where x_s and $x_s^{'}$ are both in Λ (elementary transformation).
   b) Compute the energy difference $\Delta U = U' - U$, where U' is the energy after the elementary transformation and U the energy before such transformation.
   c) If $\Delta U < 0$, accept the transition (the energy decreases).
   d) If $\Delta U \geq 0$, accept the transition with the probability equal to $\exp(-\frac{\Delta U}{T})$.
4. Decrease the temperature T.
5. Repeat 3-4 until convergence (the global minimum of U is found).

The elementary transformation (step 3.a) consists mainly in a random local displacement of the seed s from position x_s to position x_s'. Each displacement must preserve the topology of the Delaunay graph.

Geman *et al.* (1984) proved that this algorithm produces a Markov chain $X^{n,T}$ of invariante measure Π_T, where Π_T is the Gibbs measure associated with the energy $\frac{U(x)}{T}$ and with the neighborhood system $(N_S(p))_{p\in S}$:

$$\lim_{n\to\infty} P(X^{n,T} = x) = \Pi_T(x).$$

Then the simulated annealing algorithm converges using a simple property of the Gibbs measure. The Gibbs measure tends to the uniform probability of the global minima of the energy U.

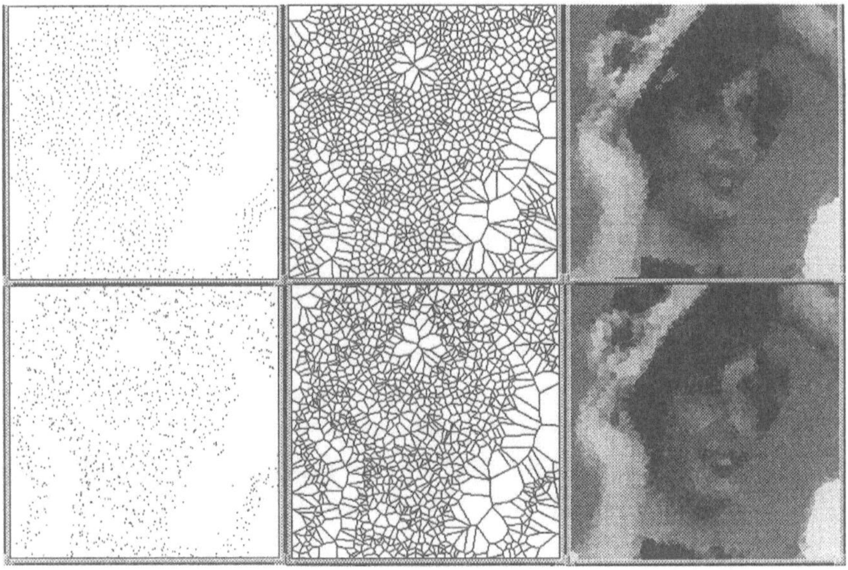

Fig. 6. Simulating annealing process. Upper line illustrates the result of the split and merge algorithm. The lower line illustrates the reorganization of the seeds after decreasing the energy U. The seeds have preserved their respective topological neighborhood.

Due to the locality of the Delaunay graph, the difference of energy in the simulated annealing optimization algorithm (step 3.b) can be written as follows if the elementary transformation (step 3.a) follows the topology of the Delaunay graph:

$$\Delta U = \sum_{x \in N_S(s)} \{\sigma(Vor_{S-\{s\}\cup\{s'\}}(x) - \sigma(Vor_S(x))\} \\ +\sigma(Vor_{S-\{s\}\cup\{s'\}}(s')) - \sigma(Vor_S(s)).$$

4.2. Optimization without the Delaunay Stability

The convergence state of the Markov chain generated by the simulated annealing algorithm does not require the stability of the Delaunay graph. In this case we have a variant of the previous algorithm.

The set S is decomposed into two subsets S_{ON} and S_{OFF} ($S = S_{ON} \cup S_{OFF}$), where the seeds of S_{ON} are present in the Voronoi diagram and the seeds of S_{OFF} do not contribute to the Voronoi diagram.

We introduce a polygon energy measurement as:

$$U_{S_{ON}}(p) = \sigma(Vor_{S_{ON}}(p)).$$

To take care of the global information, we define the total image energy as:

$$U_I = \frac{1}{N} \sum_{p \in S_{ON}} \left[\frac{A(Vor_{S_{ON}}(p))}{A_I} \left(U_{S_{ON}}(p) - \frac{\sum_{q \in S_{ON}} U_S(q)}{N_{ON}} \right) \right],$$

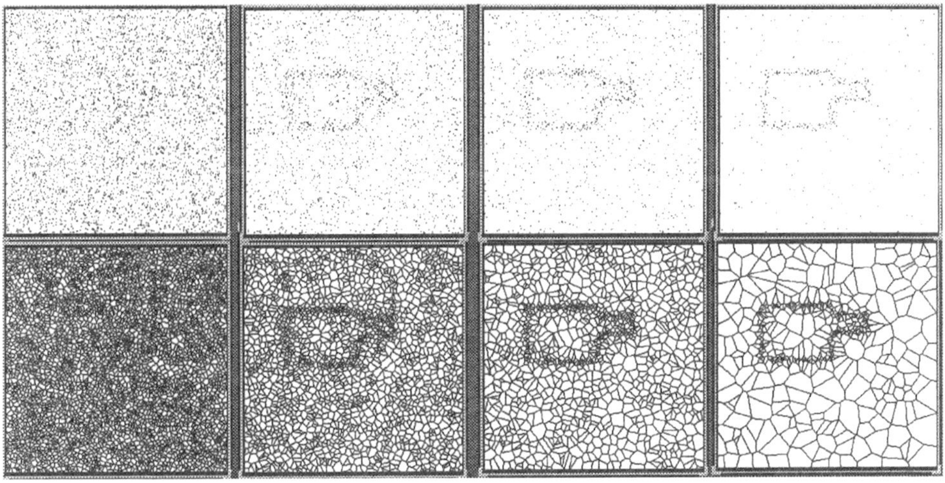

Fig. 7. Simulating annealing process. In upper line from left to right the number of seeds is successively: 5024, 2246, 1244, and 483. The cardinal of S is 10000. The lower line illustrates the corresponding Voronoi diagrams.

where N_{ON} is cardinal S_{ON}, $A(Vor_{S_{ON}}(p))$ is the area of the Voronoi polygon attached to the seed p, A_I is the image area.

The expression of U_I tends to maximize the area of low grey level variance regions and to minimize the area of high grey level variance regions.

For a seed p of S we define a binary state: p is ON ($x_p = ON$) if $p \in S_{ON}$ and p is OFF ($x_p = OFF$) if $p \in S_{OFF}$. We can now introduce the elementary transformation of a seed p in the simulated annealing algorithm: if $x_p = ON$ switch x_p in state OFF and if $x_p = OFF$ switch in state x_p in ON.

Then the algorithm developed to minimize U_I is the same as the previous one with this elementary transformation. The energy difference $\Delta U = U' - U$ is locally computed due to the property of the Delaunay graph.

A first result of our algorithm is given in Figs. 7 and 8. We see in these figures that the locations of the points seem to match with the object border (the object is an attractor of the seeds).

5. Conclusion

In conclusion we can notice that Markov Random Fields open to multiple perspectives for optimization problems in Voronoi diagrams. The results obtained are encouraging and future works will integrate new forms of energy.

Acknowledgements

We want to thank here Raphaël Marcelpoil for his enlightening discussions, useful comments and for the closure example (Fig. 4).

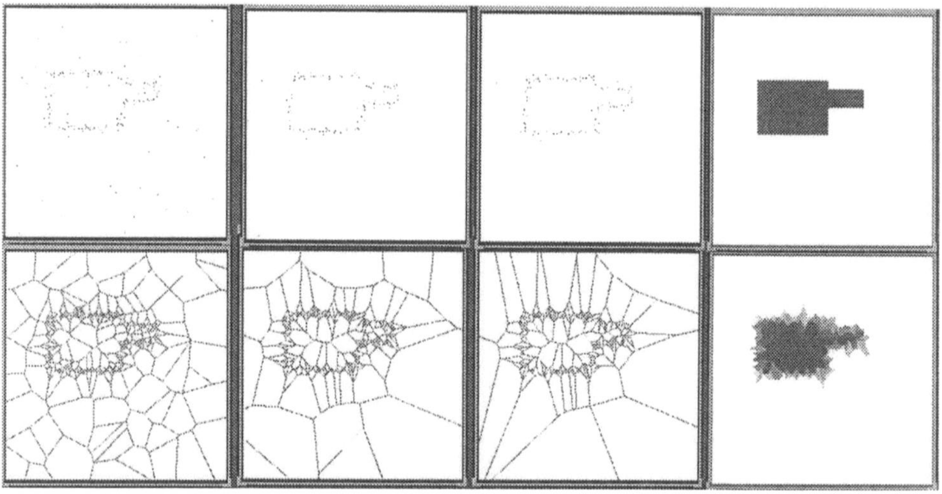

Fig. 8. Simulating annealing process and convergence. Upper line from left to right the number of seeds is successively: 361, 215, 145. The lower line illustrates the corresponding Voronoi diagrams. The last column presents the initial image and the grey-level image at the convergence step.

References

Ahuja, N., An, B. and Schachter, B.: 1992, 'Image representation using Voronoi tessellation', *Computer Vision Graphics and Image processing* Vol. 29, pp. 286–295

Bertin, E., Parazza, F. and Chassery J.-M.: 1993, 'Segmentation and measurement based on Voronoi diagram: Application to confocal microscopy', *Special issued of Computerized Medical Imaging and Graphics*, Vol. 17 no. **3**, pp. 175–182

Bertin, E.: 1994, 'Diagramme de Voronoï 2D et 3D : Applications en Analyse d'Images', PhD thesis, Joseph Fourier University, Grenoble, France.

Bowyer, A.: 1984, 'Computing Dirichlet tessellation', *The computer journal*, Vol. 24 no. **2**, pp. 162-166

Brandt, J.W., Algazi, V.R.: 1992, 'Continuous Skeleton Computation by Voronoi Diagram', *Computer Vision Graphics and Image processing* Vol. 55, pp. 329-338

Chassery, J.-M. and Melkemi M.: 1991, 'Diagramme de Voronoï appliqué à la segmentation d'images et à la détection d'événements en imagerie multi-source', *Traitement du signal*, Vol. 8 no **3**, pp. 155-164

Geman, S. and Geman, D.: 1984, 'Stochastic relaxation, Gibbs distribution, and the Bayesian restoration of images', *IEEE Transaction PAMI*, Vol. 6 no **6**, pp. 721-741

Marcelpoil, R. and Usson Y.: 1992, 'Methods for the study of cellular sociology: Voronoi diagrams and parametrization of the spatial relationships', *J. Theor Biol*, Vol. 154, pp. 359-369

Metropolis, N., Rosenbluth, A.W., Rosenbluth, M.N., Teller A.H. and Teller E.: 1953, 'Equation of the state calculations by fast computing machine', *J. Chem. Phys.*, Vol. 21, pp. 1087-1091

Okabe, A., Boots B. and Sugihara K.: 1992, 'Spatial Tessellations: Concept and Applications of the Voronoi Diagram', John Wiley and Sons, New York

Preparata J.P. and Shamos M.I.S.: 1988, 'Computational Geometry, an introduction', Springer Verlag, New York

Serra, J. (editor): 1988, 'Image analysis and mathematical morphology, volume 2: theoretical advances', *Academic Press, London*

Vincent L.: 1991 'Graphs and mathematical morphology', *Signal Processing*, Vol. 16 no **4** pp. 365-388

A STOCHASTIC TESSELLATION OF DIGITAL SPACE

THOMAS C.M. LEE
Department of Statistics, Macquarie University/
CSIRO Division of Mathematics and Statistics,
Locked Bag 17, North Ryde, 2113 Australia

and

RICHARD COWAN
Department of Statistics, University of Hong Kong,
Pokfulam Road, Hong Kong

Abstract. A tessellation which is capable of producing **rough** boundaries is proposed. Some properties of the proposed tessellation are also described.

Key words: tessellation, stochastic growth, roughness

1. Introduction

The work described below is motivated by complex images such as that in Fig. 1, which displays grains in rolled aluminium, viewed through polarized light. Statistical analysis of grain characteristics (eg. size, shape) first requires segmentation of the grains. In order to compare **quantitatively** the performance of different segmentation techniques, it is useful to develop and analyse models which mimic the important characteristics of real images, such as that in Fig. 1. In this paper, we describe a tessellation which attempts to mimic those **shape** characteristics. One observation about the grains is that they have **rough** boundaries. Therefore common tessellations such as the Voronoi, Delaunay and Poisson line tessellations (see [9]) are inappropriate for our purpose, as they have smooth boundaries.

It is known that the formation of those aluminium grains follows some sort of growth process. Therefore it is natural to build our tessellation using some "seeded region growing" mechanism, that is, we start with a number of seeds (or nuclei, or centres) and grow grains outward from the seeds. Eventually the grains meet each other and those points of contact define grain boundaries, which define a tessellation of the space. The Voronoi tessellation is one example of this: all seeds grow with uniform growth rate in all directions simultaneously. Smooth boundaries are obtained as a result of the uniform growth rate. In order to produce rough boundaries, the tessellation proposed in this paper employs a growth mechanism having a **stochastic growth rate**.

Various growth models with stochastic growth mechanisms have been proposed (eg. [5] [7], [8] and [11]). However, all these growth models are for single grains only, while ours are for multiple grains growing simultaneously. A brief comparison between the various models is given in a later section of this paper.

J.Serra and P. Soille (eds.), Mathematical Morphology and Its Applications to Image Processing, 217-224

Fig. 1. Green component of a colour image of aluminium grains

2. The Tessellation

2.1. General

Besides producing rough boundaries, another major characteristic of the proposed tessellation is that it is defined on a d-dimensional regular grid (eg. square, triangular or hexagonal) rather than the traditional $\mathbb{R}^d$, for the purpose of facilitating computer simulation. In this paper we restrict ourselves to the case of $d = 2$ and the grid is square with a 4-connected neighbour system. Extension to higher dimensions and other regular grids is straightforward.

Suppose we have a domain of interest — a "blank" image — to be tessellated. The tessellation building process is divided into two stages: **initial seed/pixel allocation** and **seed–growing/pixel–labelling** (from now on we use the word "pixel" rather than "seed"). The pixel–labelling stage can be further divided into two components: **pixel choosing** and **pixel assigning**. In this paper we use a digital version of a two dimensional homogeneous Poisson process to perform the initial pixel allocation. (We could certainly use other spatial point processes for this initialization, but we will only consider the Poisson case here.)

2.2. The Pixel–labelling Stage

Suppose n initial pixels are generated (and hence there are n grains in the final realization) and we group these n pixels into n sets: $G_1, G_2, \ldots, G_n$ (so initially each G_i has exactly one pixel). The pixel labelling mechanism labels one pixel at a time (according to the stochastic rule described below) and the whole process stops when all pixels have been labelled.

At any moment during the labelling process, the domain of interest (ie. the image to be tessellated) is partitioned into three sets L, C and N (defined below), and every pixel of the image belongs to exactly one of these three sets. L, C and N represent "**L**abelled", "**C**andidates for labelling" and "**N**ot candidates for labelling" respectively, and they are defined as:

$$\begin{aligned} L &= \bigcup_{i=1}^{n} G_i, \\ C &= \{x \notin L \mid nbr(x) \cap L \neq \emptyset\}, \\ N &= \{x \notin L \cup C\}, \end{aligned}$$

where $nbr(x)$ denotes the set of all 4-connected neighbours of the pixel x. Hence before the first labelling, L is the set of all initial pixels. With this setting, labelling a pixel is equivalent to **choosing** an $x \in C$ and **assigning** it to exactly one of the G_i's (of course after this pixel assignment we have to remove x from C and perform necessary updates on all related sets).

The stochastic labelling mechanism is as follows. First we further partition C into 4 sets C_1, C_2, C_3 and C_4, and define n_1, n_2, n_3 and n_4 as:

$$\begin{aligned} C_i &= \{x \in C \mid \text{ number of labelled neighbours of } x \text{ is } i\}, \\ n_i &= \text{ number of elements in } C_i \end{aligned}$$

for $i = 1, \ldots, 4$. Now assume that the time to labelling, t, for any pixel in C_i has an exponential distribution with parameter λ_i (denoted as $t \sim \exp(\lambda_i)$) for $i = 1, \ldots, 4$ (these λ_i's will be parameters of our tessellation) and that the times to labelling are mutually independent. Using the general result that, if $y_i \sim \exp(\mu_i)$, then $z = \min_i(y_i) \sim \exp(\sum_i \mu_i)$ and $P(z = y_i) = \mu_i / \sum_j \mu_j$ (where $P(E)$ means probability for event E), we have:

$$P(x \in C_i \text{ is the next pixel for labelling}) = \frac{\lambda_i}{\sum_{j=1}^{4} n_j \lambda_j}. \tag{1}$$

After having chosen the next pixel (x, say) for labelling from C_i's using (1), we have to assign/label this chosen pixel x to exactly one of the G_i's. If all labelled neighbours of x belong to the same G_i, then x will be assigned to this same G_i. If those labelled neighbours of x come from more than one G_i (in this case x is a boundary pixel), then we can assign x to G_i with probability proportional to the number of neighbours of x already assigned to this G_i. We call this boundary formation rule the "random rule". We could also have a "majority rule" — assign x to the set G_i which contains most of those labelled neighbours of x. See Fig. 2 for an explanation.

Repeat this pixel choosing and assigning mechanism until all pixels have been labelled (or equivalently, when C and N both become empty). See Fig. 3 for an example. This completes the algorithm but a further step of rescaling the vertical axis

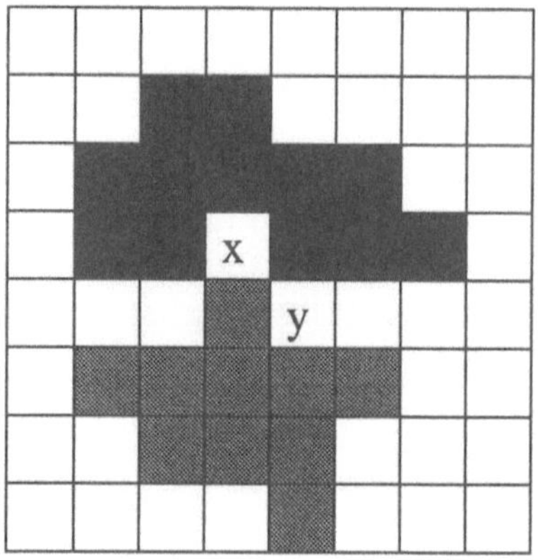

Fig. 2. White squares are unlabelled pixels. Using the random rule, pixels x and y will be labelled black with probabilities 3/4 and 1/3 respectively. Using the majority rule, x will be labelled black while y will be labelled grey.

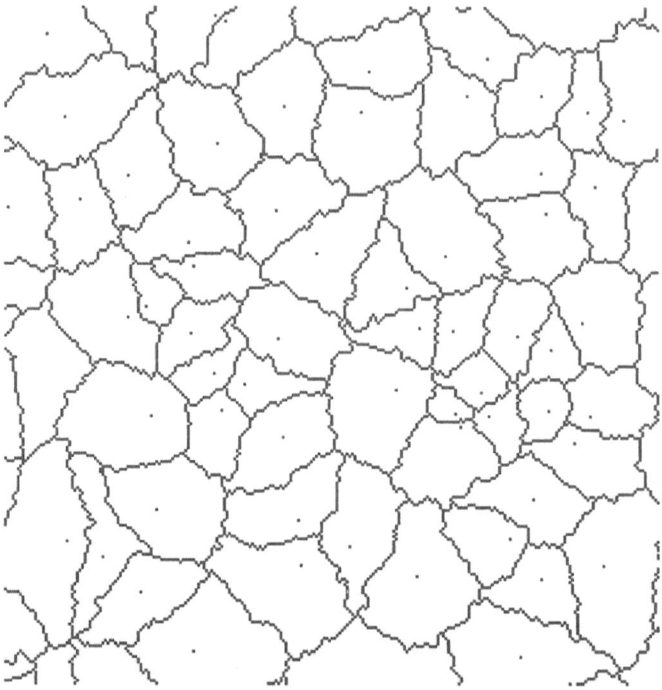

Fig. 3. Realization of the tessellation with Poisson intensity 0.0008, $r_1 = r_2 = 0$ (r_1, r_2 are defined in section 3) and the random rule for boundary formation. Dots inside grains are initial pixels/seeds generated by the Poisson process. Size of image: 256x256.

of such tessellations with respect to the horizontal axis helps to produce simulated images which appear to be similar to images of rolled aluminium grains.

3. Some Properties of the Tessellation

3.1. Comparison with some Growth Models

Eden proposed a model [7] in order to mimic the growth process of an organism which starts with a single cell (ie. there is only one initial pixel). Eden's growth process is the same as the growth process described here when all λ_i's are equal.

Williams and Bjerknes [11] studied the growth of a tumour and suggested a model for describing the phenomenon. As in Eden's model, only one initial pixel is considered. In their model, labelled pixels can be "delabelled" and the relative probability of labelling/delabelling is governed by a parameter κ. When $\kappa = \infty$ (ie. labelled pixels cannot be "delabelled"), the probability for a particular unlabelled pixel to be labelled next is proportional to the number of its labelled neighbours. This is the same as the growth process described here when the λ_i's are in the ratio 1, 2, 3 and 4.

Richardson [8] introduced a *Gp* model in which more than one unlabelled pixel can be labelled in the same time step. Again, only one initial pixel is considered. In this *Gp* model, each candidate for labelling (ie. unlabelled pixel having at least one labelled neighbour) will be labelled in the next time step with probability p. So if there are N candidates for labelling, we expect Np candidates will be labelled in the next time step.

Clearly, there is some overlap between our model and some of those above. However, all the above models consider a single initial pixel only, while ours uses multiple initial pixels.

3.2. Number of Independent Parameters

At first sight, there are six independent parameters for the proposed tessellation: the Poisson intensity μ, an indicator parameter I for choosing the random or the majority boundary formation rule, and the four λ_i's. However, there are in fact only four independent parameters which have an influence on the final crystallisation pattern: μ, I, $r_1 = \log(\lambda_2/\lambda_1)$ and $r_2 = \log(\lambda_3/\lambda_1)$. This follows, firstly because an $x \in C_4$ has a defined fate regardless of the value of λ_4, and so λ_4 is redundant, and secondly because the sum of all probabilities defined by (1) is one.

3.3. Boundary Roughness

It is clear that by changing r_1, r_2 and/or applying a different boundary formation rule (random or majority), we can change the boundary roughness, and hence it is desirable to have some quantitative measure of the boundary roughness. Fractal dimension is not suitable for the following reason. If we look at the boundaries at the microscopic level, all these boundaries just consist of horizontal and vertical straight lines. That is, they are "smooth" and always have fractal dimension one (eg. see [2]) no matter how rough to the human eyes it is. Therefore we propose the following roughness measure.

First, we measure the distance of the boundary of the grain from the centre of its initial pixel (or its centroid if the initial pixel is unknown) as a function of angle or arc-length. Call these distances the grain radii. It is usually convenient to choose "equally spaced" radii. Now suppose we have chosen n radii $l_1, \ldots, l_n$ and let $\bar{l}$ be

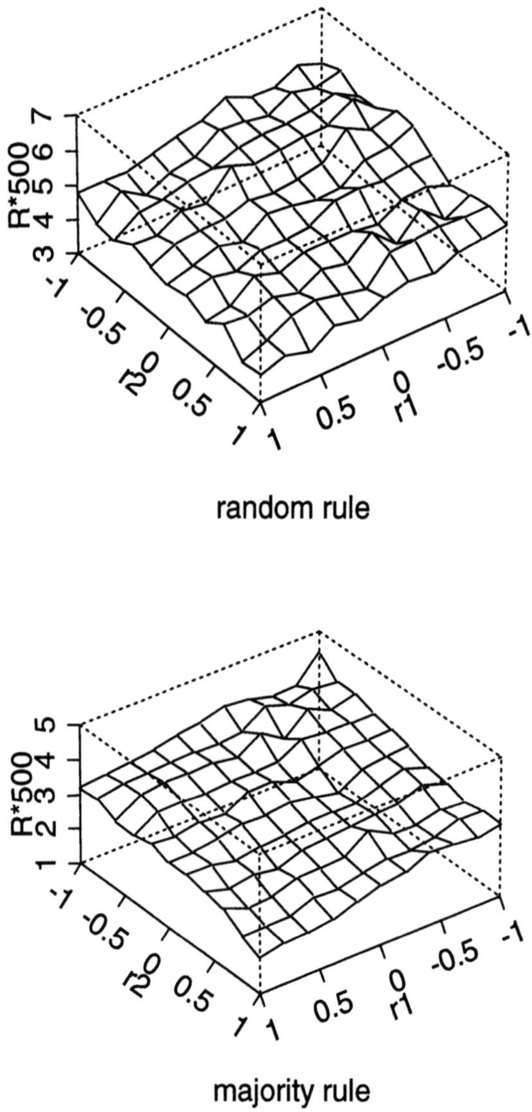

Fig. 4. Perspective plots demonstrating the effect of various r_1 and r_2 on R. Each data point is the average of fifty different simulations. It is clear that, for both boundary formation rules, the roughness measure R is a decreasing function of r_1 and r_2. Another observation is: the random rule always gives a larger R than the majority rule. (In order to speed up simulation times and minimize random errors, all simulations are done with the same nine regularly spaced initial pixels.)

their mean. Then we compute

$$R = \frac{\sum_i (l_{i+1} - l_i)^2}{\sum_i (l_i - \bar{l})^2}$$

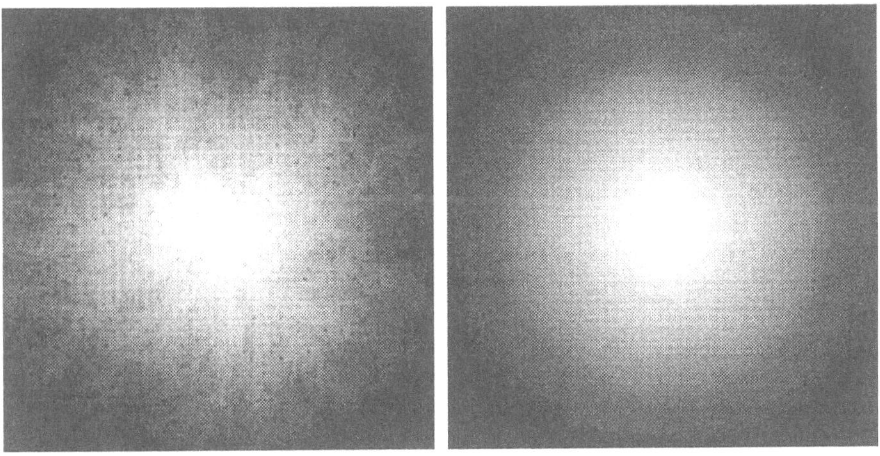

Fig. 5. These two images attempt to show the time of labelling for each pixel in the domain: the brighter the pixel is, the sooner it was labelled. Left: one realization of the presented growth process (with equal λ_i's) with one single initial pixel located in the centre of the image. Right: average of two hundred such realizations. From these images the isotropic property of the growth process is apparent. Size of each realization: 256x256.

as our roughness measure. Notice that R is a function of r_1, r_2 and the boundary formation rule indicator parameter I (we assume that the Poisson intensity μ is small enough not to have any effect on the boundary roughness).

Simulations show that R heavily depends on the choice of the boundary formation rule — the random rule **always** gives a larger value of R than the majority rule with the same r_1 and r_2. Also, smaller values of r_1 and r_2 tend to produce larger R with r_1 being more influential; see Fig. 4.

3.4. Is the Tessellation Isotropic?

Since we are using a 4-connected system, we only have two growth directions: horizontal and vertical, and hence the stochastic growth mechanism and the final tessellation pattern are not isotropic. Somewhat surprisingly, our simulations suggest that both the growth process and the tessellation are (for practical purposes) isotropic, provided that the Poisson intensity is not too large (of course this isotropic property of the tessellation pattern no longer holds if we apply the last vertical scaling step). The results of formal hypothesis testing (eg. testing differences between radii at different angles) support the claim that the tessellation is isotropic for practical purposes.

Fig. 5 shows a small scale simulation demonstrating the isotropic property of the growth process. Batchelor and Henry [3] have performed a more extensive simulation for the Eden model (2^{25} pixels involved), which also demonstrates isotropy. Various researchers have attempted to obtain the asymptotic shape of different growth processes (eg. [4] and [6]) as the grain size increases, but the results are so far limited. The strongest result is due to Bramson and Griffeath [4] who show that, a grain growing according to the Williams and Bjerknes model is eventually contained within an annulus with probability one.

Acknowledgements

The authors thank Mark Berman and Vic Solo for helpful discussions and comments.

References

1. Adams, R. and Bischof, L.: 1994, 'Seeded Region Growing', *IEEE Transactions on Pattern Analysis and Machine Intelligence*, (in press).
2. Barnsley, M.: 1988, *Fractals Everywhere*, Academic Press.
3. Batchelor, M. T. and Henry, B. I.: 1991, 'Limits to Eden growth in two and three dimensions', *Physics Letters A*, **157**, 229-236.
4. Bramson, M. and Griffeath, D.: 1981, 'On the Williams-Bjerknes tumour growth model I', *The Annals of Probability*, **9**, 173-185.
5. Cressie, N. A. C.: 1991, *Statistics for Spatial Data*, Wiley-Interscience.
6. Durrett, R. and Liggett, T. M.: 1981, 'The shape of the limit set in Richardson's growth model', *The Annals of Probability*, **9**, 186-193.
7. Eden, M.: 1961, 'A two dimensional growth process', *Proceedings of the Fourth Berkeley Symposium on Mathematical Statistics and Probability*, **IV**, J. Neyman, ed. University of California Press, Berkeley, CA, 223-239.
8. Richardson, D.: 1973, 'Random growth in a tessellation', *Mathematical Proceedings of the Cambridge Philosophical Society*, **74**, 515-528.
9. Stoyan, D., Kendall, W.S. and Mecke, J.: 1987, *Stochastic Geometry and its Applications*, Wiley: Chichester.
10. Szép, J., Cserti, J. and Kertész, J.: 1985, 'Monte Carlo approach to dendritic growth', *Journal of Physics A*, **18**, L413-L418.
11. Williams, T. and Bjerknes, R.: 1972, 'Stochastic model for abnormal clone spread through epithelial basal layer', *Nature*, **236**, 19-21.

LIQUID PHASE SINTERED MATERIALS MODELLING BY RANDOM CLOSED SETS

J.-L. QUENEC'H, J.-L. CHERMANT and M. COSTER
LERMAT, URA CNRS 1317, ISMRA
6 Bd Maréchal Juin, F-14050 Caen Cedex, France

and

D. JEULIN
Centre de Géostatistique, Ecole des Mines de Paris
35 rue Saint Honoré, F-77305 Fontainebleau, France

Abstract. Three different probabilistic models are used in order to describe the microstructure of WC-Co hard metals. While a two-phase mosaic model and a dead leaves model with Poisson polyhedra as primary grains seem not adapted, a Boolean model with Poisson polyhedra fits very well the WC phase. The two parameters of this model allow us to estimate the thermodynamics parameters of the coarsening of the WC phase during annealing. It is also possible to evaluate the Euler-Poincaré characteristic in $\mathbf{R}^3$, $N_V(X)$, which cannot be measured by another means. Mechanical parameters are also correlated with the parameters of the Boolean model.

Key words: probabilistic models, Boolean model, coarsening, WC-Co cermets.

1. Introduction

It is well known in material sciences that the size of the grains in a material is strongly connected with its physical and mechanical properties (German, 1985). In the case of materials elaborated by liquid phase sintering, which is a process commonly used in powder metallurgy in order to obtain dense materials from a mixture of packed powders, the size of the grains depends firstly on the size of the green powders and secondly on the temperature and the duration of the thermal treatment. The knowledge of the variations of the grain size during this treatment is therefore of great interest.

Classically, the stage of coarsening of the grains in liquid phase sintering is described by the LSW models (Lifshitz and Slyosov, 1961; Wagner, 1961). These authors predicted that the size of the grains follows a coarsening law $\bar{d}^n(t) - \bar{d}^n(0) = kt$, where $\bar{d}$ is the mean diameter of the grains, n is the kinetics exponent, k is the growth rate. They showed also that n may have only two values (2 or 3) depending on the kinetics rate limiting stage (reaction): diffusion across the matrix ($n = 3$), reactions of solution-reprecipitation at the interfaces of the first ($n = 2$) or the second ($n = 3$) order. Moreover, they demonstrated that the normalized distributions of the grain sizes were stationary and depended only on the limiting stage.

The typical way to study the coarsening of the grains during liquid phase sintering is then the following: the different grains appearing on the micrographs are segmented, often by hand or semi-automatically, their areas are measured and the

J.Serra and P. Soille (eds.), Mathematical Morphology and Its Applications to Image Processing, 225-232

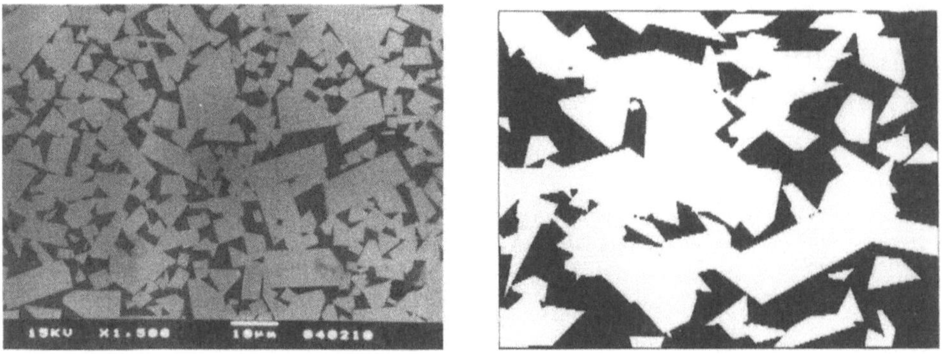

(a) (b)

Fig. 1. *(a)* Micrograph of WC-15 wt% Co sample sintered 30 hours at 1450 deg C. *(b)* Simulation of a two-phased Poisson mosaic in $\mathbf{R}^3$.

experimental distributions of the grain sizes are consequently obtained and compared to the theoretical ones.

In this study, we have chosen a fully different way to estimate the thermodynamics parameters of the sintering in the case of the WC-Co system. These cermets were modelled using mathematical models: the random closed sets or probabilistic models.

2. Experimental

The materials used which illustrate this original approach are the WC-Co hard metals. This method was also applied with more or less success to other materials: the TiC-Co and TiC-Ni cermets and the W-(Ni,Fe) heavy alloys (Quenec'h, 1994). The WC-Co were supplied by UGICARB (Grenoble) and were sintered in a graphite resistor furnace with a pressure of 10^{-4} Pa at 1450 deg C. In order to estimate the activation energy of the process, temperatures from 1350 deg C to 1600 deg C were used. Several composition (from 3 to 25 wt% of cobalt) were furnished. The alloys are so listed in the text by the letter A and the weight fraction of cobalt in the sample. Figure 1a presents a micrograph of A15 grade sintered at 1450 deg C for 7 hours. The samples were polished and observed in electron backscattering mode (Jeol JSM T 330A). The obtained micrographs were afterwards analyzed using an image processor (NS-1500, Microcontrole) which uses an hexagonal digitization grid.

3. The probabilistic models

The probabilistic models were introduced by Matheron (1967; 1975) and afterwards developed in many disciplines. The reader interested in the fundamental theory, which will not be improved in this paper, can refer to Matheron (1967; 1975), Serra (1982) or Jeulin (1991). Examples in many fields of application can be found in Stoyan *et al.* (1987) or Jeulin (1991).

Probabilistic models are random closed sets which allow the description of random structures. As WC-Co cermets are two-phased (Fig. 1a), the models used in this study were chosen in the range of multiphase models (Serra, 1982; Jeulin, 1979). The WC grains are polyhedral and consequently Poisson polyhedra are used to model this phase. The random closed sets (RACS) are characterized by a functional called the Choquet's capacity (Matheron, 1975; Serra, 1982). This functional defines a RACS exactly like a distribution law defines a random variable. It represents the probability Pr that a compact K intersects the random set X: $T(K) = Pr(K \cap X \neq \emptyset) = 1 - Pr(K \subseteq X^c)$.

According to the basic morphological operations processed on metallographical images, this Choquet's capacity may be estimated for a compact K and a RACS X in $\mathbf{R}^2$ by $T(K) = 1 - A_A[\varepsilon^K(X^c)]$, where A_A represents the surface fraction of the transformed set and ε^K the erosion operation. The experimental Choquet's capacities are consequently relatively easy to estimate and moreover, their analytical expressions are known as a function of the parameters of the model for few compacts in the case of the studied models (Jeulin, 1991).

Three different models were afterwards tested for WC-Co materials: a dead leaves model, a Boolean scheme with Poissonian primary grains and a two-phased Poisson mosaic. The properties of these models are well known and we will only describe shortly their way of building. The great advantage of these models is that they have good stereological properties: a given model in $\mathbf{R}^3$ induces the same kind of model in a sub-space ($\mathbf{R}^2$ or $\mathbf{R}^1$). This property allows us to estimate the parameters of the model in $\mathbf{R}^3$ from measurements in cross sections.

3.1. The two-phase Poisson mosaic

This model is built from a Poisson mosaic obtained from a tessellation of the $\mathbf{R}^3$ space by random planes: let $D(\omega)$ be a straight line with orientation ω and $\lambda(\omega)d\omega$ be the density of a Poisson point process performed on the line $D(\omega)$. In each point, the plane orthogonal to $D(\omega)$ is implanted. The union of these planes, for $0 \leq \omega \leq \Pi$, encloses a network of Poisson polyhedra. Then, each polyhedron is randomly and independently allocated to one phase or another, according to the wanted volume fraction. In the case of isotropic mosaic, λ is independent of ω. Figure 1b presents a simulation of a two-phased Poisson mosaic. The two parameters of this model are p, the volume fraction of phase X which is obtained from the classical stereological parameters ($p = A_A(X)$), and λ, the parameter of the Poisson polyhedra.

3.2. The dead leaves model

The second model used is the homogeneous dead leaves tessellation model, introduced by Matheron (1968) and developed by Jeulin (1979, 1991). This two-phased tessellation is built as follows: for both phases, the primary grains, which are Poisson polyhedra obtained from two Poisson mosaics of parameter λ_1 and λ_2, are implanted randomly with constant density Θ_1 and Θ_2. The grains appeared between t and $t+dt$ may hide a portion of the former grains. A random tessellation of space is obtained as the time goes to infinity. The three parameters of this model are consequently λ_1, λ_2 and Θ, the ratio of Θ_1 and Θ_2. Figure 2a presents a simulation of a dead leaves model in $\mathbf{R}^2$.

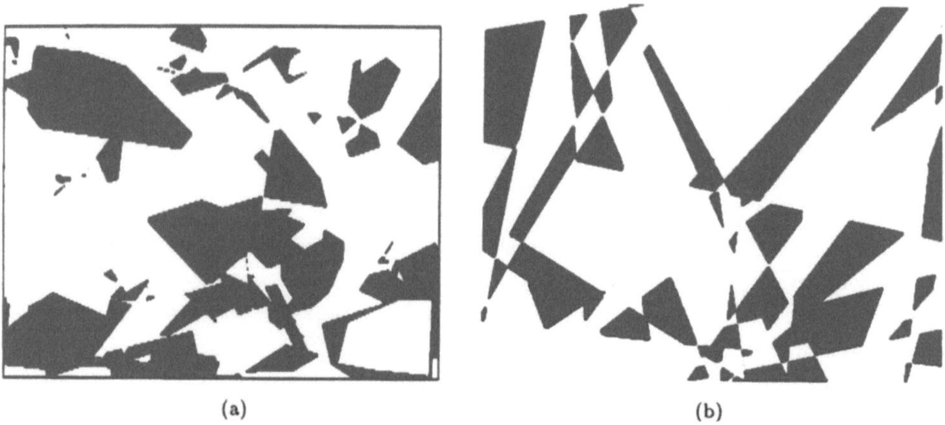

Fig. 2. *(a)* Simulation of a dead leaves model with Poissonian primary grains in $\mathbf{R}^2$. *(b)* Simulation of a Boolean model with polygonal grains in $\mathbf{R}^2$.

3.3. The Boolean model

The Boolean model is a very well known model. In order to build it, a Poisson point process of intensity Θ is generated in the space. In each germ, a primary grain is afterwards implanted and the model results of the union of these primary grains (Matheron, 1967; 1975; Delfiner, 1971; Serra, 1982; Jeulin, 1979). In the case of WC-Co samples, Poisson polyhedra of parameter λ were chosen as primary grains. The two parameters of the model are then λ and Θ. Figure 2b shows a simulation of a Boolean scheme in $\mathbf{R}^2$ with Poisson polygons.

4. Results

4.1. The dead leaves model

For this model, only one compact was used: the bipoint h, which allows us to estimate a functional $\Phi(h)$, which is experimentally obtained from the variogram $\gamma(h)$:

$$\Phi(h) = \frac{\gamma(h)}{p(1-p)} \tag{1}$$

$\Phi(h)$ may be theoretically estimated from the mean geometric covariograms $r_1(h)$ and $r_2(h)$ of both phases and using the following relation

$$\Phi(h) = \frac{2 - r_1(h) - r_2(h)}{2 - pr_1(h) - (1-p)r_2(h)}. \tag{2}$$

Using the fact that the analytical expression of the mean covariogram for Poisson polyhedra is given by: $r_i(h) = exp(-\Pi\lambda_i h)$ and that $\lim_{h\to 0}\Phi(h) = \Pi(\lambda_1 + \lambda_2)$, the experimental $\Phi(h)$ functional, obtained by relation (1), is compared with the theoretical ones, which are evaluated by relation (2) and varying (λ_1, λ_2), knowing the sum $(\lambda_1 + \lambda_2)$. This sum was estimated for A15 samples sintered at 1450 deg C. Figure 3 shows the comparison between the experimental $\Phi(h)$ functional and

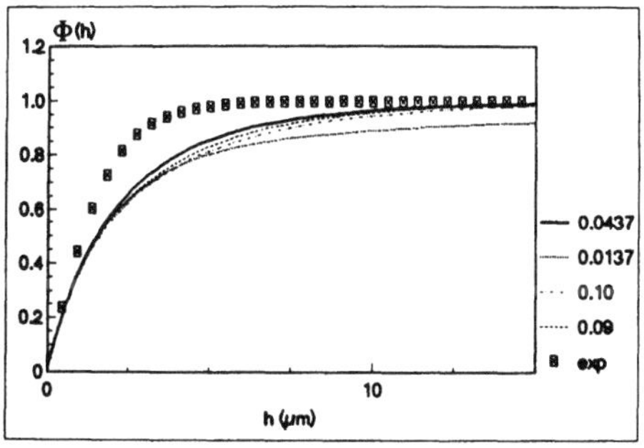

Fig. 3. Comparison between the experimental and several theoretical $\Phi(h)$ functionals for different values of λ_1 in the case of A15 sample annealed 100 hours at 1450 deg C.

TABLE I
Mean values of λ estimated on WC phase, λWC, and on Co phase, λ_{Co}, with their coefficients of correlation, CV_{WC} and CV_{Co}.

	1hr	2hrs30	3hrs30	7hrs	14hrs	30hrs	100hrs
$\lambda_{WC}(\mu m^{-1})$	0.59	0.60	0.60	0.52	0.39	0.26	0.21
$\lambda_{Co}(\mu m^{-1})$	0.56	0.56	0.53	0.46	0.31	0.22	0.17
$CV_{WC}(\%)$	19	13	19	19	12	10	09
$CV_{Co}(\%)$	25	18	26	24	30	24	27

different theoretical curves obtained for the sample annealed 100 hours ($\lambda_1 + \lambda_2 = 0.1637$), which is characteristic of the results obtained for the whole batch.

The printed theoretical curves are the ones which presented the best fit with the experimental points. It is consequently clear that the dead leaves model is not adapted at all in order to describe the microstructure of WC-Co cermets. Furthermore, realizations of this model would present inclusions of one phase into another which is not observed in the microstructure.

4.2. The mosaic model

The parameter λ of the model is evaluated using three different compacts: the straight segment ℓ, the bipoint h and the triplet of points $T(h_1, h_2)$. Moreover, as the mosaic model is symmetric from its way of construction, the value of λ estimated from both phases must be the same. The comparison between the different values of λ is consequently the major test for this model. The mean values for both phases of each sample are presented in Table I with their coefficients of variation, CV, which represent the variation between the four values obtained by the different compacts.

It can be noticed that the values of λ fit approximately for both phases, but the discrepancy between the coefficients of variation is too important to be negligible. In order to conclude more surely, the comparison between the experimental number of connectivity in $\mathbf{R}^2$, $N_A(X)_{exp}$, measured on metallographic sections, and the theoretical number of connectivity for an hexagonal grid, $N_A(X)_{mos}$, obtained from

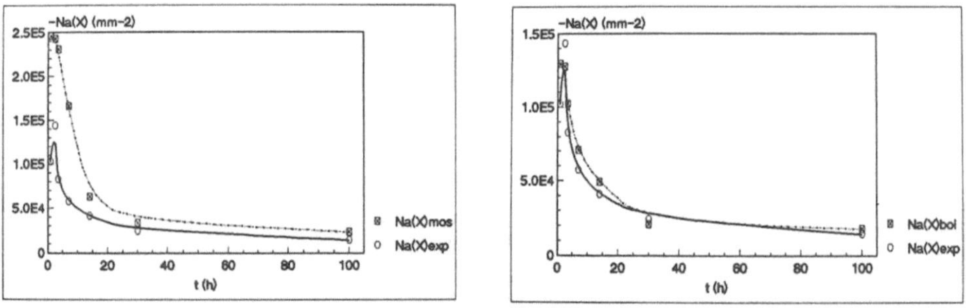

(a) (b)

Fig. 4. Comparison between the experimental numbers of connectivity, $N_A(X)_{exp}$, and the theoretical numbers of connectivity for the mosaic model, $N_A(X)_{mos}$, *(a)*, and the Boolean scheme, $N_A(X)_{bol}$, *(b)*, in the case of A15 samples sintered at 1450 deg C.

the equation $N_A(X)_{mos} = \frac{\sqrt{3}}{2}\Pi^2\lambda^2 p(1-p)(2p-1)$ was tested.

The differences between the two curves, displayed on Fig. 4a, allow us to discard this second model. Moreover, the systematic alignments of the "grains boundaries" in the simulations of the mosaic model are inconsistent with the observations of the microstructure of WC-Co samples. For all these reasons, the two-phased Poisson mosaic was discarded to model the structure of WC-Co cermets.

4.3. Modelling by a Boolean model

In order to test this model, we have first to check that the experimental $T(K)$ functionals are consistent with their theoretical exponential expressions (Serra, 1982). This condition was verified for the four compacts used in this work: ℓ, h, $T(h_1, h_2)$ and $H(r)$, the hexagon of size r. It was then assumed that the WC phase could be modelled by a Boolean scheme with Poisson primary grains (Quenec'h, 1994). The theoretical connectivity numbers in $\mathbf{R}^2$ were also calculated using the relation $N_A(X) = \frac{3q\Theta}{2\Pi\lambda}\left(1 - \frac{12\sqrt{3}\Theta}{\Pi^5\lambda^3}\right)$, and compared with the experimental ones (Fig. 4b). The very good correlation confirms that this model is well adapted.

The variation of the parameters λ and Θ was then used in order to estimate the different thermodynamic parameters of the system. It was indeed shown that these parameters were varying with power laws such as the mean diameter in the LSW models (Quenec'h et al, 1992). Figure 5 shows that the best value for the kinetics exponent is $n = 3$, which is consistent with the results of the literature (Exner and Fischmeister, 1966; Coster, 1974). The slope of the curve gives an estimation of the growth rate in the system, but the values obtained for this growth rate are much lower than those in the previous studies (approximately $10^{-19} m^3 s^{-1}$ compared to $10^{-22} m^3 s^{-1}$). This may be perhaps explained by the fact that the Boolean model gives a description of the whole WC phase whereas the other workers took only into account the growth of the mean particle. An estimation of the activation energy of the system was also obtained from an Arrhenius plot using λ or Θ (Fig. 5b). The value of 300 kJ/mol agrees well with the literature (350 ± 100 kJ/mol).

We can consequently conclude that this mathematical model is able to give the

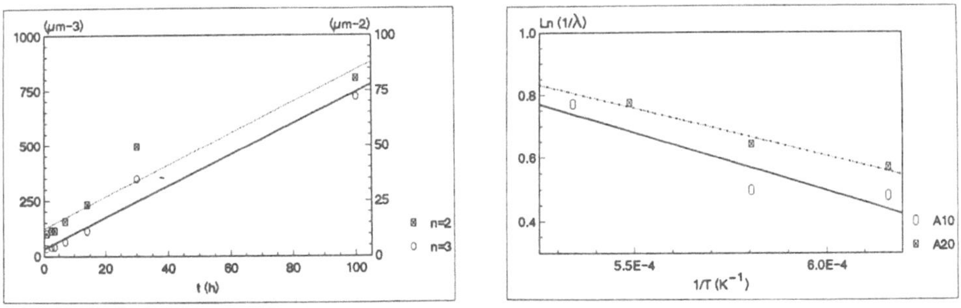

(a) (b)

Fig. 5. *(a)* Variation of λ^{-n} with the sintering time, t, for $n = 2$ and $n = 3$. *(b)* Variation of $ln(1/\lambda)$ with $1/T$.

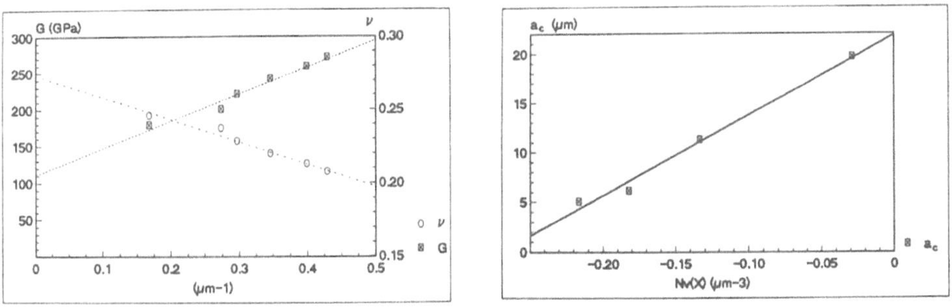

(a) (b)

Fig. 6. *(a)* Variation of the shear modulus, G, and the coefficient of Poisson ν, versus the parameter λ of the Boolean model. *(b)* Variation of the critical size defect, a_c, with the estimated number of connectivity in $\mathbf{R}^3$, $N_V(X)$.

same informations than the classical models only with two parameters. Another great advantage of this model is that the number of connectivity in $\mathbf{R}^3$, $N_V(X)$, may be estimated (Jeulin, 1979): $N_V(X) = q\Theta\left(1 - \frac{18\Theta}{\Pi^4\lambda^3} + \frac{36\Theta^2}{\Pi^8\lambda^6}\right)$.

The values of the estimated $N_V(X)$ are negative (Quenec'h, 1994), which means that the WC particles are very interconnected. Hence, these estimations confirm the presence, at the observation scale used, of a continuous skeleton of WC grains in these cermets, which was already assumed by another way (Osterstock, 1980).

The mechanical properties of several WC-Co alloys with different volume fraction of cobalt were measured. A good correlation is found between the parameters of the Boolean model and the mechanical parameters: E, the elastic modulus, G, the shear modulus and ν, the coefficient of Poisson (Fig. 6).

The results of Chermant and Osterstock (1977) were also used. They have evaluated the critical size defect, a_c, for the same alloys than those used in this study. This parameter represents the maximum size defect from which the fracture becomes catastrophic. These authors showed that the curve presenting the variations of a_c with the volume fraction of cobalt exhibited a marked minimum. With the knowledge of $N_V(X)$, it is now possible to explain the presence of this minimum: Fig. 6b, which presents the variations of a_c with $N_V(X)$, shows clearly the existence of a linear dependence between these two parameters. The size of the critical defect seems therefore strongly correlated with the connectivity between the WC grains.

5. Conclusion

The probabilistic models were used to model the structure of WC- Co cermets. It was shown that a Boolean model with Poisson primary grains was adapted to describe the WC phase. The parameters of this mathematical model allow us to obtain values of kinetics parameters which agree with the literature. This modelling leads also to the evaluation of $N_V(X)$. The variations of the mechanical properties were after that correlated with the parameters of the Boolean model.

References

Chermant J.-L. and Osterstock F. (1977), Fracture toughness and fracture of WC-Co composites. *J. Mat. Sci.*, 11, 1939-1951.

Coster M. (1974), Applications des méthodes quantitatives et stéréologiques à l'étude de la croissance et des caractéristiques mécaniques d'échantillons polyphasés: cas des matériaux cabure de tungstène-cobalt. Thèse de Doctorat ès Sciences, Université de Caen.

Delfiner P. (1971), Etude morphologique des milieux poreux et automatisation des mesures en plaques minces. Thèse de Docteur-Ingénieur, Université de Nancy.

Exner H.E. and Fischmeister H. (1966), Gefügeausbildung von gesinterten Wolframkarbid-Kobalt Härtelegierungen. *Arch. Eisenhüttenwesen*, 37, 417-426.

German R.M. (1985), *Liquid Phase Sintering.* Plenum Press, New York.

Jeulin D. (1979), Morphologie mathématique et propriétés physiques des agglomérés de minerais de fer et du coke métallurgique. Thèse de Docteur-Ingénieur, Ecole des Mines de Paris.

Jeulin D. (1991), Modèles morphologiques de structures aléatoires et de changement d'échelle. Thèse de Doctorat ès Sciences Physiques, Université de Caen.

Lifshitz I.M. and Slyosov V.V. (1961), The kinetics of precipitation from supersaturated solutions. *J. Phys. Chem. Solids*, 19, 35-50.

Matheron G. (1967) *Eléments pour une Théorie des Milieux Poreux.* Masson, Paris.

Matheron G. (1968), Schéma booléen séquentiel de partition aléatoire. Rapport Technique de l'Ecole des Mines de Paris, N-83-CMM.

Matheron G. (1975), *Random Sets and Integral Geometry.* J. Wiley and Sons, New York.

Osterstock F. (1980), Comportement mécaniques d'alliages biphasés: contribution à l'étude de la rupture fragile et de la déformation plastique des composites WC-Co. Thèse de Doctorat ès Sciences Physiques, Université de Caen.

Quenec'h J.-L. (1994), Modèles probabilistes et frittage en phase liquide. Thèse de l'Université de Caen.

Quenec'h J.-L., Coster M., Chermant J.-L. and Jeulin D. (1992), Study of the liquid phase sintering process by probabilistic models: application to WC-Co cermets. *J. Microsc.*, 168, 3-14.

Serra J. (1982), *Image Analysis and Mathematical Morphology.* Academic Press, London.

Stoyan D., Kendall W.S. and Mecke J. (1987), *Stochastic Geometry and its Applications.* J. Wiley and Sons, Chichester.

Wagner C. (1961), Theory of precipitate change by redissolution. *Z. Electrochem.* 65, 581-591.

MONTE CARLO ESTIMATION OF MORPHOLOGICAL GRANULOMETRIC DISCRETE SIZE DISTRIBUTIONS

K. SIVAKUMAR and J. GOUTSIAS*
Department of Electrical and Computer Engineering
Image Analysis and Communications Laboratory
The Johns Hopkins University
Baltimore, MD 21218, U. S. A.

Abstract. Morphological granulometries are frequently used as descriptors of granularity, or texture, within a binary image. In this paper, we study the problem of estimating the (discrete) size distribution and size density of a random binary image by means of empirical, as well as, Monte Carlo estimators. Theoretical and experimental results demonstrate superiority of the Monte Carlo estimation approach, and suitability of mathematical morphology in studying important properties of a particular binary random image model, widely known as a Markov random field model.

Key words: Granulometries, Markov random fields, Monte Carlo estimation, Size distribution.

1. Introduction

The notion of granulometry has been first conceived by Matheron [1], in order to axiomatize the physical meaning of size distribution, which describes the granularity, or texture, within a binary image. Size distributions provide us with a wealth of information about image structure, and have been extensively used in a number of image analysis tasks, such as shape and texture analysis [2], multiscale shape representation [3], morphological shape filtering and restoration [4]-[6], analysis, segmentation, and classification of textures [7]-[9], and as a goodness-of-fit tool for testing whether an observed image has been generated by a given random field model [10]. From all these applications, it has become clear that is necessary to calculate the size distribution of images modeled by means of binary random fields. As noted in [1], except in very limited cases, it is extremely difficult to express the granulometric size distribution in terms of the distribution functional, or the capacity functional, of a *random closed set*. In order to effectively employ size distributions in realistic problems, it is imperative to be able to estimate these quantities for general stochastic image models.

In this paper, we shall assume that the image X is a realization of a *discrete random set* (DRS) $\mathbf{X}$ [11]. We shall employ a Monte Carlo method, in order to estimate the (discrete) size distribution and the associated size density. We would like to mention here the related work of Sand and Dougherty [12], who have derived asymptotic expressions for the moments of the size distribution. Their work, however, is based on an image model which is quite restrictive in practice. Bettoli and Dougherty [13], have derived explicit expressions for moments of the size distribu-

* This work has been supported by the Office of Naval Research, Mathematical, Computer, and Information Sciences Division, under ONR Grant N00014-90-1345.

J.Serra and P. Soille (eds.), Mathematical Morphology and Its Applications to Image Processing, 233-240

tion. However, they have assumed a deterministic image corrupted by random pixel noise, and they have only considered linear granulometries.

2. Granulometric Size Distributions

A granulometry on $\mathcal{P} = \mathcal{P}(\mathcal{Z}^d)$ is a parameterized family $\{\alpha_n\}_{n=0,1,\cdots}$ of mappings, from $\mathcal{P}$ into itself, such that:

1. α_0 is the identity mapping on $\mathcal{P}$; i.e., $\alpha_0(X) = X$, $X \subseteq \mathcal{Z}^d$,
2. α_n is increasing; i.e., $X \subseteq Y \subseteq \mathcal{Z}^d \Rightarrow \alpha_n(X) \subseteq \alpha_n(Y)$, $n = 1, 2, \cdots$,
3. α_n is anti-extensive; i.e., $\alpha_n(X) \subseteq X$, $n = 1, 2, \cdots$, $X \subseteq \mathcal{Z}^d$,
4. $\alpha_n \alpha_m = \alpha_m \alpha_n = \alpha_{\max(n,m)}$, $n, m = 1, 2, \cdots$.

Given a granulometry $\{\alpha_n\}_{n=0,1,\cdots}$ on $\mathcal{P}$, the dual parametrized family $\{\beta_n\}_{n=1,2,\cdots}$ of mappings on $\mathcal{P}$, where $\beta_n(X) = (\alpha_n(X^c))^c$, $n = 1, 2, \cdots$, $X \in \mathcal{P}$, is known as the *anti-granulometry* on $\mathcal{P}$ associated with $\{\alpha_n\}_{n=0,1,\cdots}$. In practice, the most useful granulometries and anti-granulometries are the ones given by $\alpha_0(X) = X$, $\alpha_n(X) = X \circ nB$, $n = 1, 2, \cdots$, and $\beta_n(X) = X \bullet n\check{B}$, $n = 1, 2, \cdots$, respectively, where B is a finite subset of $\mathcal{Z}^d$, nB is defined recursively by $0B = \{\mathbf{0}\}$ and $nB = (n-1)B \oplus B$, for $n = 1, 2, \cdots$, and $\check{B} = \{-b \mid b \in B\}$ is the reflection of B about the origin $\mathbf{0}$ in $\mathcal{Z}^d$. In the following, we shall exclusively deal with these mappings, which are known as the *morphological granulometry* and *morphological anti-granulometry*, respectively.

Let $\mathbf{X}(\omega)$, $\omega \in \Omega$, be a DRS from $(\Omega, \Sigma(\Omega), \mu[.])$ into $(\mathcal{P}, \Sigma(\mathcal{P}))$, where $\Sigma(\mathcal{P})$ is the σ-field generated by the *relative hit-or-miss topology* on $\mathcal{P}$ [1]. It is easy to show that $\alpha_n(\mathbf{X}(\omega))$, $\omega \in \Omega$, and $\beta_n(\mathbf{X}(\omega))$, $\omega \in \Omega$, are also DRS's, for every $n = 1, 2, \cdots$. For every $\omega \in \Omega$, let $\Lambda_X(x;\omega)$ be a function from $\mathcal{Z}^d$ into $\bar{\mathcal{Z}}$, given by

$$\Lambda_X(x;\omega) = \begin{cases} \sup\{n \geq 0 \mid x \in \alpha_n(\mathbf{X}(\omega))\}, & \text{for } x \in \mathbf{X}(\omega) \\ -\inf\{n \geq 1 \mid x \in \beta_n(\mathbf{X}(\omega))\}, & \text{for } x \in \mathbf{X}^c(\omega) \end{cases}.$$

The function

$$S_X(n;x) = \mu[\{\omega \in \Omega \mid \Lambda_X(x;\omega) \geq n\}] = \begin{cases} P[x \in \alpha_n(\mathbf{X}(\omega))], & \text{for } n \geq 0 \\ P[x \in \beta_{-n}(\mathbf{X}(\omega))], & \text{for } n \leq -1 \end{cases},$$

for every $x \in \mathcal{Z}^d$, where $P[.]$ is the probability distribution of $\mathbf{X}$ (i.e., $P[\mathcal{A}] = \mu[\{\omega \in \Omega \mid \mathbf{X}(\omega) \in \mathcal{A}\}]$, for every $\mathcal{A} \in \Sigma(\mathcal{P})$), is called the *size distribution* of the DRS $\mathbf{X}$ (with respect to the granulometry $\{\alpha_n\}_{n=0,1,\cdots}$), whereas, the function

$$s_X(n;x) = S_X(n;x) - S_X(n+1;x),\ n \in \bar{\mathcal{Z}},\ x \in \mathcal{Z}^d, \tag{1}$$

is called the *size density* (or *pattern spectrum* [3]) of the DRS $\mathbf{X}$. Observe that, for every $x \in \mathcal{Z}^d$, $S_X(n_1;x) \leq S_X(n_2;x)$, for every $n_1 \geq n_2$, (i.e., $S_X(n;x)$ is a decreasing function of n), $\lim_{n\to-\infty} S_X(n;x) = 1$, and $\lim_{n\to+\infty} S_X(n;x) = 0$, whereas, $s_X(n;x) \geq 0$, for every $n \in \bar{\mathcal{Z}}$, $\sum_{n=-\infty}^{+\infty} s_X(n;x) = 1$, and $S_X(n;x) = \sum_{m=n}^{+\infty} s_X(m;x)$, for every $n \in \bar{\mathcal{Z}}$.

The dependence of $S_X(n;x)$ and $s_X(n;x)$ on $x \in \mathcal{Z}^d$ may be bothersome. To ameliorate this problem, we may consider a "spatial average" of these quantities over a bounded observation window W. We now define the spatial averages $S_{X \cap W}(n)$

and $s_{X \cap W}(n)$, over W, by

$$S_{X\cap W}(n) = \frac{1}{|W|} \sum_{x \in W} S_X(n;x) \quad \text{and} \quad s_{X\cap W}(n) = \frac{1}{|W|} \sum_{x\in W} s_X(n;x),$$

where $|W|$ is the cardinality of W, which is assumed to be non-zero. It is not difficult to show that

$$S_{X\cap W}(n) = \begin{cases} \frac{1}{|W|} E[|\alpha_n(\mathbf{X}) \cap W|], & \text{for } n \geq 0 \\ \frac{1}{|W|} E[|\beta_{-n}(\mathbf{X}) \cap W|], & \text{for } n \leq -1 \end{cases}, \tag{2}$$

where $E[.]$ denotes expectation. Furthermore, $s_{X\cap W}(n) = S_{X\cap W}(n) - S_{X\cap W}(n+1)$, for every $n \in \bar{\mathcal{Z}}$. When $\mathbf{X}$ is a stationary DRS, it can be easily shown that

$$S_X(n) \triangleq S_X(n;\mathbf{0}) = S_X(n;x) = S_{X\cap W}(n) = \begin{cases} P[\mathbf{0} \in \alpha_n(\mathbf{X})], & \text{for } n \geq 0 \\ P[\mathbf{0} \in \beta_{-n}(\mathbf{X})], & \text{for } n \leq -1 \end{cases}, \tag{3}$$

for every $x \in \mathcal{Z}^d$, $n \in \bar{\mathcal{Z}}$, and every bounded window $W \subset \mathcal{Z}^d$.

By using a discrete version of the analysis in [14], it can be shown that,

$$\hat{S}_X(n;W_m) = \begin{cases} |((\mathbf{X}\cap W_m)\circ nB) \cap W'_m(n)|/|W'_m(n)|, & \text{for } n \geq 0 \\ |((\mathbf{X}\cap W_m)\bullet(-n)\check{B}) \cap W'_m(-n)|/|W'_m(-n)|, & \text{for } n \leq -1 \end{cases}, \tag{4}$$

is an unbiased (for every $m \geq 1$) *empirical estimator* of the size distribution $S_X(n)$, provided that $\mathbf{X}$ is a stationary DRS. Furthermore, (4) is a consistent (as $m \to +\infty$) estimator of $S_X(n)$, provided that there exists a function $c_n(x,y) : \mathcal{Z}^d \times \mathcal{Z}^d \to \mathcal{R}$, such that

$$P[x \in \psi_n(\mathbf{X}); y \in \psi_n(\mathbf{X})] \leq c_n(x,y) + \eta^2(n), \ \forall x,y \in \mathcal{Z}^d, \tag{5}$$

and

$$\lim_{m\to+\infty} \frac{1}{|W'_m(n)|^2} \sum\sum_{x,y\in W'_m(n)} c_n(x,y) = 0, \tag{6}$$

where $\psi_n(X) = X \circ nB$, for $n \geq 0$, and $\psi_n(X) = X\bullet(-n)\check{B}$, for $n \leq -1$. In (4)-(6), $W_1 \subset W_2 \subset \cdots \subset W_m \subset \cdots \subset \mathcal{Z}^d$ is an increasing sequence of bounded windows, and $W'_m(n) = W_m \ominus (nB \oplus n\check{B})$. Additionally, the empirical estimator

$$\hat{s}_X(n;W_m) = \hat{S}_X(n;W_m) - \hat{S}_X(n+1;W_m), \tag{7}$$

is an unbiased (for every $m \geq 1$) and consistent (as $m \to +\infty$) estimator of the size density $s_X(n)$, provided that conditions (5) and (6) are satisfied, at both sizes n and $n+1$. These conditions are difficult to verify in practice (however, see [14] for some examples for which these conditions are easily verified). Furthermore, the previous results indicate that the estimators (4) and (7) will be reliable only when data are observed through large enough windows (i.e., large enough m). Since, in practice, the observation window is usually fixed, estimators (4) and (7) will not be reliable for large "sizes" n.

3. Monte Carlo Estimators

Suppose now that $\mathbf{X}$ is a stationary DRS, such that it is possible to draw independent samples from its probability distribution, inside a window W; i.e., we can draw samples $X^{(1)} \cap W, X^{(2)} \cap W, \cdots, X^{(K)} \cap W$, where $X^{(k)}$, $k = 1, 2, \cdots, K$, are K independent and identically distributed realizations of $\mathbf{X}$. A *Monte Carlo estimator* of the size distribution $S_X(n)$ is now given by (see (2) and (3))

$$\hat{S}_K^{(1)}(n) = \begin{cases} \frac{1}{K}\sum_{k=1}^{K} \frac{|((\mathbf{X}^{(k)} \cap W) \circ nB) \cap W'(n)|}{|W'(n)|}, & \text{for } n \geq 0 \\ \frac{1}{K}\sum_{k=1}^{K} \frac{|((\mathbf{X}^{(k)} \cap W) \bullet (-n)\check{B}) \cap W'(-n)|}{|W'(-n)|}, & \text{for } n \leq -1 \end{cases}, \tag{8}$$

where $W'(n) \subseteq W \ominus (nB \oplus n\check{B})$. It can be easily shown that

$$E[\hat{S}_K^{(1)}(n)] = S_X(n),$$

and

$$\text{Var}[\hat{S}_K^{(1)}(n)] = \begin{cases} \frac{1}{K|W'(n)|^2}\text{Var}[|(\mathbf{X} \circ nB) \cap W'(n)|], & \text{for } n \geq 0 \\ \frac{1}{K|W'(-n)|^2}\text{Var}[|(\mathbf{X} \bullet (-n)\check{B}) \cap W'(-n)|], & \text{for } n \leq -1 \end{cases}.$$

$\hat{S}_K^{(1)}(n)$ is an unbiased (for every $K \geq 1$) and consistent (as $K \to +\infty$) estimator of the size distribution $S_X(n)$. It is now clear that the mean-squared-error (MSE), associated with this estimator, is directly controlled by the underlying number of Monte Carlo iterations K, regardless of the size of the observation window W. In fact, the MSE decreases to zero, as the number of Monte Carlo iterations increases.

An alternative estimator $\hat{S}_K^{(2)}(n)$ can be derived by observing that, for $n \geq 0$ (see (3))

$$\begin{aligned} S_X(n) &= P[(\mathbf{X} \ominus nB) \oplus nB \supseteq \{0\}] = P[\mathbf{X} \ominus nB \supseteq \{x\}, \text{ for some } x \in n\check{B}] \\ &= E[\bigvee_{x \in n\check{B}} (\bigwedge_{y \in nB \oplus \{x\}} \mathbf{x}_y)], \end{aligned}$$

where $\mathbf{x}_y$ is a Boolean random variable, such that $\mathbf{x}_y = 1$, if $y \in \mathbf{X}$, and 0, otherwise, and $\bigvee$ and $\bigwedge$ denote the Boolean OR and AND operators, respectively. A similar expression can be derived for the case when $n \leq -1$. This leads to the following Monte Carlo estimator:

$$\hat{S}_K^{(2)}(n) = \begin{cases} \frac{1}{K}\sum_{k=1}^{K}(\bigvee_{x \in n\check{B}}(\bigwedge_{y \in nB \oplus \{x\}} \mathbf{x}_y^{(k)})), & \text{for } n \geq 0 \\ \frac{1}{K}\sum_{k=1}^{K}(\bigwedge_{x \in (-n)\check{B}}(\bigvee_{y \in (-n)B \oplus \{x\}} \mathbf{x}_y^{(k)})), & \text{for } n \leq -1 \end{cases}. \tag{9}$$

It can be easily shown that

$$E[\hat{S}_K^{(2)}(n)] = S_X(n), \quad \text{and} \quad \text{Var}[\hat{S}_K^{(2)}(n)] = \frac{\eta(n)(1 - \eta(n))}{K} \leq \frac{1}{4K} < +\infty, \tag{10}$$

where $\eta(n) = P[\mathbf{0} \in \mathbf{X} \circ nB]$. $\hat{S}_K^{(2)}(n)$ is an unbiased (for every $K \geq 1$) and consistent (as $K \to +\infty$) estimator of the size distribution $S_X(n)$. When $|W'(n)| = 1$ in (8),

$\hat{S}_K^{(1)}(n)$ and $\hat{S}_K^{(2)}(n)$ are identical. When $|W'(n)| > 1$, $\hat{S}_K^{(1)}(n)$ is different than $\hat{S}_K^{(2)}(n)$. Furthermore, $\hat{S}_K^{(1)}(n)$ may enjoy a smaller variance than $\hat{S}_K^{(2)}(n)$, although no closed-form expression is available for $\text{Var}[\hat{S}_K^{(1)}(n)]$ to verify this argument. Due to the computationally attractive properties of $\hat{S}_K^{(2)}(n)$, this estimator is exclusively used, instead of estimator $\hat{S}_K^{(1)}(n)$. Estimator $\hat{S}_K^{(2)}(n)$ provides us with a Monte Carlo estimator $\hat{s}_K^{(2)}(n) = \hat{S}_K^{(2)}(n) - \hat{S}_K^{(2)}(n+1)$, of the size density, which is unbiased (for every $K \geq 1$) and consistent (as $K \to +\infty$). Finally, notice that $\text{Var}[\hat{S}_K^{(2)}(n)]$ is bounded by $1/4K$, and, therefore, MSE $= O(1/K)$, in this case.

In many instances, it is not possible to draw independent samples from the probability distribution of $\mathbf{X}$. However, a Monte Carlo algorithm, known as *Monte Carlo Markov chain sampling* (MCMCS), may be effectively used, in order to obtain a sequence $X^{(k)}$, $k = 1, 2, \cdots, K$, of statistically dependent samples of $\mathbf{X}$ [15]. In MCMCS, an ergodic Markov chain $\{\mathbf{X}_1, \mathbf{X}_2, \cdots, \mathbf{X}_{n_b+(K-1)l+1}\}$, of $n_b + (K-1)l + 1$ samples, is generated, whose equilibrium probability distribution is that of $\mathbf{X}$. The first n_b samples (known as the "burn-in") are discarded, in order to guarantee that the chain has approximately reached equilibrium, whereas, the remaining samples are subsampled at every l^{th}-step, in order to reduce correlation between consecutive samples. In this case, $\mathbf{X}^{(k)} = \mathbf{X}_{n_b+(k-1)l+1}$, for $k = 1, 2, \cdots, K$, will be DRS's which are approximately independent, and whose probability distribution is approximately that of $\mathbf{X}$. It can be shown that (compare with (10))

$$|E[\hat{S}_K^{(2)}(n) - S_X(n)]| \leq \frac{1}{K}\frac{\delta_{n_b}}{1-\rho_l} S_X(n) \leq \frac{1}{K}\frac{\delta_{n_b}}{1-\rho_l},$$

where $\rho_l = \lambda_{\max}^l$ and $\delta_{n_b} = \lambda_{\max}^{n_b}/\pi_{\min}$, with $\lambda_{\max} < 1$ being the second largest absolute eigenvalue of the transition probability matrix of the underlying Markov chain, and $\pi_{\min} = \min_X\{\pi(X)\} > 0$, where $\pi(X)$ is the probability mass function of $\mathbf{X}$. Furthermore, the MSE, associated with $\hat{S}_K^{(2)}(n)$, satisfies (compare with (10))

$$\begin{aligned}
E[(\hat{S}_K^{(2)}(n) - S_X(n))^2] &\leq \frac{1}{K}[S_X(n)(1 - S_X(n)) + \frac{2\rho_l}{1-\rho_l}\frac{1}{\pi_{\min}} S_X^2(n)] + \\
&\quad \frac{1}{K^2}\frac{\delta_{n_b}}{1-\rho_l}[S_X(n)(1 - S_X(n)) + \frac{2\rho_l}{1-\rho_l}(1 + \frac{1}{\pi_{\min}}) S_X^2(n)] \\
&\leq \frac{1}{K}\left[\frac{1}{4} + \frac{2\rho_l}{1-\rho_l}\frac{1}{\pi_{\min}}\right] + \frac{1}{K^2}\frac{\delta_{n_b}}{1-\rho_l}\left[\frac{1}{4} + \frac{2\rho_l}{1-\rho_l}(1 + \frac{1}{\pi_{\min}})\right].
\end{aligned}$$

Clearly, $\hat{S}_K^{(2)}(n)$ is an asymptotically unbiased and consistent estimator of $S_X(n)$, as $K \to +\infty$, regardless of the values of n_b, l, $\lambda_{\max}$, and $\pi_{\min}$.

4. Markov Random Fields, Phase Transitions, and Size Densities

In order to study the performance of the Monte Carlo estimator (9), we shall consider $\mathbf{X}$ as being a homogenous *Markov random field* (MRF), with probability mass function given by

$$\pi(X) = P[\mathbf{X} = X] = \frac{\exp(-U(X)/T)}{Z}, \tag{11}$$

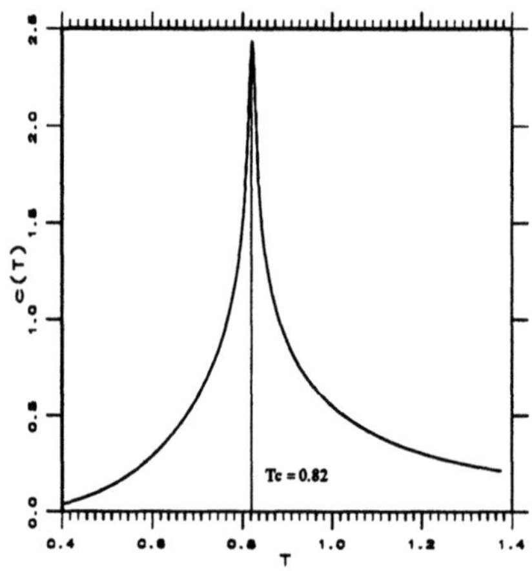

Fig. 1. The specific heat of the MRF considered in Fig. 2, as a function of temperature. Clearly, $T_c = 0.82$.

where $U(.)$ is the *energy function*, $T > 0$ is known as the *temperature*, and $Z = \sum_X \exp(-U(X)/T)$ is a normalization constant, referred to as the *partition function*. The *specific heat* of the MRF is defined by $c(T) = \text{Var}[U(\mathbf{X})]/|W|T^2$, where W is an observation window. It is well known that a MRF may experience *phase transition*, which is due to the fact that the specific heat becomes infinite at a *critical temperature* $T = T_c$, as $|W| \to +\infty$. At high temperatures (i.e., $T > T_c$), only short range pixel interactions are possible and, therefore, only small size structures are expected (i.e., the MRF is said to be at a *fine phase*). At critical temperature, "structures of a vast range of sizes" coexist. At low temperatures (i.e., $T < T_c$), there exist long range pixel interactions and, therefore, only large size structures are expected (i.e., the MRF is said to be at a *coarse phase*) [16]. It is our idea to study this behaviour, by using the morphological notion of size density.

We shall limit our attention here to the case when $U(X) = \sum_i \sum_j u(X_{ij}, X_{i-1,j}, X_{i,j-1})$, with $u(x, y, z) = b_1(2x-1)(2y-1) + b_2(2x-1)(2z-1)$. We have considered a MRF, with $b_1 = 0.25$ and $b_2 = 0.5$. This corresponds to an *Ising model*, for which the critical temperature can be computed analytically, and exact asymptotic expressions are available for the specific heat. Figure 1 shows a plot of the specific heat $c(T)$. The critical temperature for this model is clearly $T_c = 0.82$. The first row of Figure 2 shows typical realizations of the MRF, at three different temperatures: $T = 1.0, 0.8$, and 0.6. The Monte Carlo estimates of the size density (w.r.t. to a rhombus structuring element) is shown in the second row, whereas, the third row depicts the corresponding empirical estimates. Observe that the Monte Carlo size density estimates are symmetric, as expected, since this model is self-dual (i.e., $\pi(X) = \pi(X^c)$). It is now clear how the size density characterizes the granular structure of a MRF, at different temperatures. Above the critical temperature (e.g., at $T = 1.0$), most non-negligible values of the size density are assigned at small sizes, which verifies the presence of a fine phase. Below the critical temperature (e.g., at $T = 0.6$), the size density spreads out to larger sizes, whereas, it is negligible at small sizes, which verifies the presence of a coarse phase. Close to the critical temperature (e.g., at $T = 0.8$), the size density takes non-negligible values at a wide range of

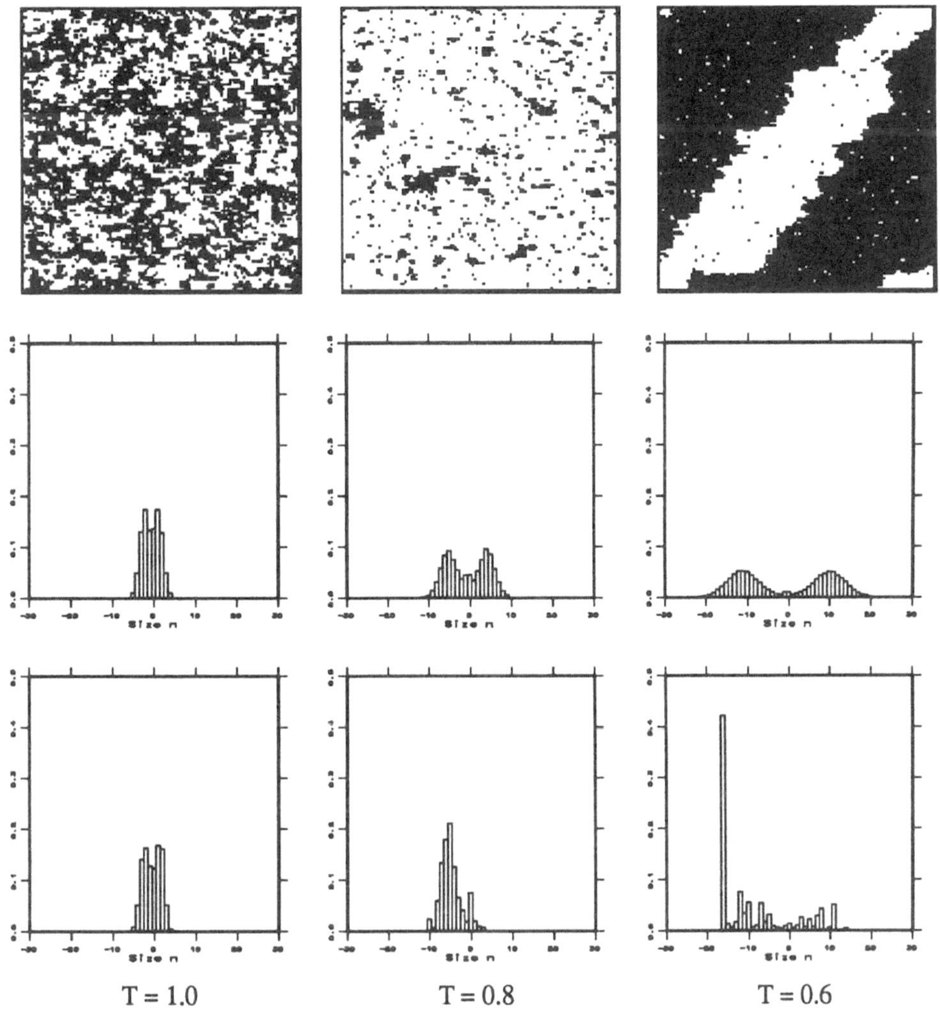

Fig. 2. (First Row): MRF realizations. (Second Row): Monte Carlo estimates of the discrete size density. (Third Row): Empirical estimates of the discrete size density. The critical temperature is $T_c = 0.82$ (see Fig. 1).

sizes, which verifies the presence of phase transition (i.e., the coexistence of both fine and coarse phases). The empirical estimator (4) works reasonably well at high temperatures. However, at low temperatures the resulting estimates are wrong. Notice that, at low temperatures, most of the non-negligible, empirically estimated size density values are assigned at negatives sizes (e.g., see the case of $T = 0.8$ or $T = 0.6$ in Fig. 2). This is definitely wrong (since the size density is expected to be symmetric), and is partially due to the fact that, although there exist two equiprobable realizations X and X^c with substantially different granularities, the empirical estimator (4) is blindly applied to only one of these realizations. On the other hand, conditions (5) and (6) may not be satisfied here, in which case the empirical estimator (4) may not be consistent.

5. Conclusion

We have proposed a Monte Carlo estimator for the size distribution, and, therefore, for the size density, of a random binary image. This estimator can be used, either with independent samples, or with dependent samples generated by a MCMCS algorithm. It is asymptotically unbiased and consistent and the MSE can be directly controlled by the total number of Monte Carlo iterations. Simulation experiments show that the performance of this estimator is significantly better than of the empirical estimator. The phenomenon of phase transition, experienced by a MRF, can be easily described by means of morphological size densities.

References

1. G. Matheron, *Random Sets and Integral Geometry*. New York: Wiley, 1975.
2. J. Serra, *Image Analysis and Mathematical Morphology*. London: Academic Press, 1982.
3. P. Maragos, "Pattern spectrum and multiscale shape representation," *IEEE Transactions on Pattern Analysis and Machine Intelligence*, vol. 11, pp. 701-716, 1989.
4. D. Schonfeld, and J. Goutsias, "Optimal morphological pattern restoration from noisy binary images," *IEEE Transactions on Pattern Analysis and Machine Intelligence*, vol. 13, pp. 14-29, 1991.
5. R. M. Haralick, "Model-based morphology: Simple and complex shapes," In *Visual Form: Analysis and Recognition*, C. Arcelli, L. P. Cordella, and G. Sanniti di Baja, Eds., pp. 275-285. New York: Plenum Press, 1992.
6. E. R. Dougherty, R. M. Haralick, Y. Chen, C. Agerskov, U. Jacobi, and P. H. Sloth, "Estimation of optimal morphological τ-opening parameters based on independent observation of signal and noise pattern spectra," *Signal Processing*, vol. 29, pp. 265-281, 1992.
7. E. R. Dougherty, and J. B. Pelz, "Morphological granulometric analysis of electrophotographic images–Size distribution statistics for process control," *Optical Engineering*, vol. 30, pp. 438-445, 1991.
8. E. R. Dougherty, J. B. Pelz, F. Sand, and A. Lent, "Morphological image segmentation by local granulometric size distributions," *Journal of Electronic Imaging*, vol. 1, pp. 46-60, 1992.
9. E. R. Dougherty, J. T. Newell, and J. B. Pelz, "Morphological texture-based maximum-likelihood pixel classification based on local granulometric moments," *Pattern Recognition*, vol. 25, pp. 1181-1198, 1992.
10. S. Archambault, and M. Moore, "Statistiques morphologiques pour l'ajustement d'images," *International Statistical Review*, vol. 61, pp. 283-297, 1993.
11. J. Goutsias, "Morphological analysis of discrete random shapes," *Journal of Mathematical Imaging and Vision*, vol. 2, pp. 193-215, 1992.
12. F. Sand, and E. R. Dougherty, "Asymptotic normality of the morphological pattern-spectrum moments and orthogonal granulometric generators," *Journal of Visual Communication and Image Representation*, vol. 3, pp. 203-214, 1992.
13. B. Bettoli, and E. R. Dougherty, "Linear granulometric moments of noisy binary images," *Journal of Mathematical Imaging and Vision*, vol. 3, pp. 299-319, 1993.
14. M. Moore, and S. Archambault, "On the asymptotic behavior of some statistics based on morphological operations." In *Spatial Statistics and Imaging*, A. Possolo, Ed., vol. 20, pp. 258-274. Hayward, California: Institute of Mathematical Statistics, Lecture Notes–Monograph Series, 1991.
15. J. Besag, and P. J. Green, "Spatial statistics and Bayesian computation," *Journal of the Royal Statistical Society, Series B*, vol. 55, pp. 25-37, 1993.
16. K. G. Wilson, "Problems in physics with many scales of length," *Scientific American*, vol. 24, pp. 158-177, 1979.

ON THE IMPLEMENTATION OF MORPHOLOGICAL OPERATIONS

MARC VAN DROOGENBROECK
Belgacom, New Developments
121, Boulevard E. Jacqmain, B-1210 Brussels, Belgium
Fax: (+32) 2 202 84 52

Abstract.
This work presents different novel approaches to the implementation of morphological operations, like opening and close-open filter. In the restricted case of binary mathematical morphology, we propose a propagation algorithm well-suited for opening. Another algorithm, based on a "sliding window", is described for the implementation of grey-level openings. Finally we present some theoretical results that simplify the computation of complex operations.

Key words: Fast algorithm, Filter, Histogram, Opening

1. Introduction

Over the years, mathematical morphology has become very attractive. The gain of popularity is due to the recent development of powerful tools, like the watershed, but also to the discovery of fast algorithms that make morphology competitive in comparison with linear operations.

The fast implementation of morphological operations is an important task for both hardware and software. Unfortunately, the requirements of these two are often in conflict. In this paper, we propose a way of optimizing the implementation of morphological operations. The leading idea is that *knowledge about previous operations can be used to decrease the complexity of further morphological stages*, a property which could for instance significantly decrease the computation time of alternate sequential filters. In fact, it has been thought for many years that an opening is always computed as an erosion followed by a dilation. This is not true as will appear from the algorithms described in sections 3 and 4.1.

2. Reminder

We briefly recall the definitions and notations used in this paper. Let f be a function defined on $\mathbf{R}^2$ and $B \subseteq \mathbf{R}^2$ a planar structuring element. The erosion $f \ominus B$ (resp. dilation $f \oplus B$) of a function f by B transforms f into another function defined as:

$$f \ominus B(x) = \bigwedge_{b \in B} f_{-b}(x) = \bigwedge_{b \in B} f(x+b)$$

$$f \oplus B(x) = \bigvee_{b \in B} f_b(x) = \bigvee_{b \in B} f(x-b)$$

J.Serra and P. Soille (eds.), Mathematical Morphology and Its Applications to Image Processing, 241-248

for every $x \in \mathbf{R}^2$.

The opening $f \circ B$ and closing $f \bullet B$ result from cascading erosion and dilation operations:

$$f \circ B = (f \ominus B) \oplus B$$
$$f \bullet B = (f \oplus B) \ominus B$$

By definition, the opening of a set X with respect to a structuring element B, denoted $X \circ B$, is the union of the translates of B included in X. It can also be obtained from the above definition by replacing the infimum and the supremum respectively with the intersection and the union.

3. Propagation algorithm for binary opening

As could be assumed from the definition, the computation of the opening is proportional to the surface area. In practice, testing the correspondence for each position would be too slow and several methods were proposed to overcome this difficulty:

- *Linear decomposition.* A large structuring element is decomposed into a succession of dilations of smaller sets. Suppose for example that $C = B \oplus B$ then $X \circ C = (((X \ominus B) \ominus B) \oplus B) \oplus B$;
- *Logarithmic decomposition.* Originated by PECHT [5], this method enhances the linear decomposition by removing some redundant computations ;
- SCHMITT [6] and VINCENT [9] proposed methods which analyze the border of both X and B.

Other techniques were also suggested in the literature [1, 8]. All these methods perform an opening as an erosion followed by a dilation. The algorithm described hereafter is based on the propagation of the structuring element inside of X and will not proceed by intermediate erosions and dilations.

3.1. ALGORITHM DESCRIPTION

The proposed algorithm is adaptive in the sense that it relies locally on the set X: an early step detects the border elements of X where B could be anchored and propagates the structuring element inside the set in order to minimize the number of tests for each displacement.

In mathematical terms, the idea is the following. Let B_p, B_q denote the translation of B by p, q, and $\setminus$ the set subtraction. Suppose $B_p \subseteq X$. If $B_q \setminus B_p \subseteq X$ then $B_q \subseteq X \circ B$. The algorithm proceeds in two steps: (1) detection of B_p-like candidates and (2) check if $B_q \setminus B_p \subseteq X$ for several positions q close to p. Ideally we could expect the number of tests to be small: 1 per element added to $X \circ B$. This lower limit will be reached if X is homothetic to B.

Step 1: detection of an anchored homothetic version of B. It is obvious that $X \circ B$ touches X at several border points. These points, called *anchor points*, characterize the opening to some extent. The first step of the algorithm is the detection of anchor points and associated homothetic sets of B. Figure 1 represents X, B and possible anchor points of X respectively. It is not necessary to detect all homothetic sets of B anchored at a point because of a propagation step. For the same reason, further anchor points will only be detected during the image scan, after the previous propagations.

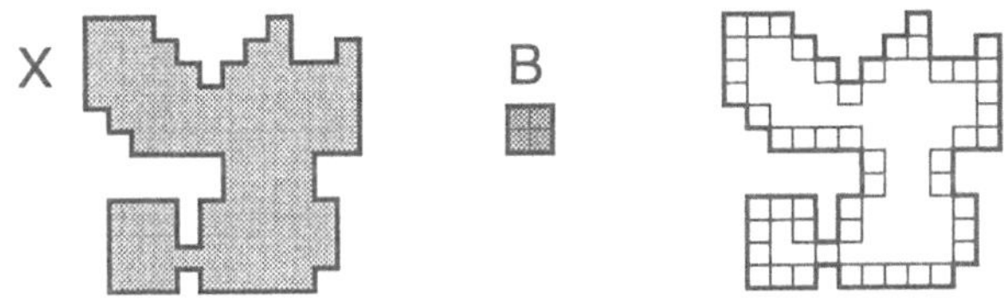

Fig. 1. A set X, the structuring element B and the possible anchor points of X.

Step 2: propagation of B inside X. The propagation process is complex. Eight propagation directions are defined for our purpose which is an opening with a square in 8-connectivity ; the principle is similar for 4 or 6-connectivity openings. The algorithm checks possible propagations in these directions and starts with the larger propagation front. Throughout the propagation in a given direction, new fronts may appear in perpendicular or forward-diagonal directions. They are pushed on a stack until the initial propagation ends. Then each popped front will initiate a new propagation process. When the stack is empty, the algorithm searches for another anchor point.

Example. The first steps of the algorithm are decomposed in Fig. 2. During a horizontal image scan, the algorithm finds the upper left corner of X which is an anchor point and initializes a propagation process. Each propagation direction is checked and the larger front propagates first. In this example, a diagonal propagation is initiated. After propagation step 3, the algorithm detects that the diagonal propagation is no longer possible and changes the direction. But as soon as the front width allows it, the front direction is changed to a diagonal (step 6).

It is easy to adapt the algorithm to the opening of each region of a label image. For this kind of operation, a label propagates only in the corresponding region. All regions will be treated in a single scan in contrast with other methods which would require dealing with each region in turn after binarization.

3.2. Numerical results

The two curves of Fig. 3 compare the linear decomposition with the propagation algorithm for the computation of a binary opening by a square. The given results were obtained on a NeXT 68040 station with `gcc` and `gprof`. The original image was "photograph" of 256 × 256 pixels, threshold at 128. Note that in the propagation method, the time is independent of the square size. Moreover, also at the origin, the propagation algorithm performs better.

4. Grey-level operations

4.1. Grey-level opening

The key idea of improving the efficiency of an erosion algorithm is that it is useless to recompute a minimum on the set of points representing the structuring element

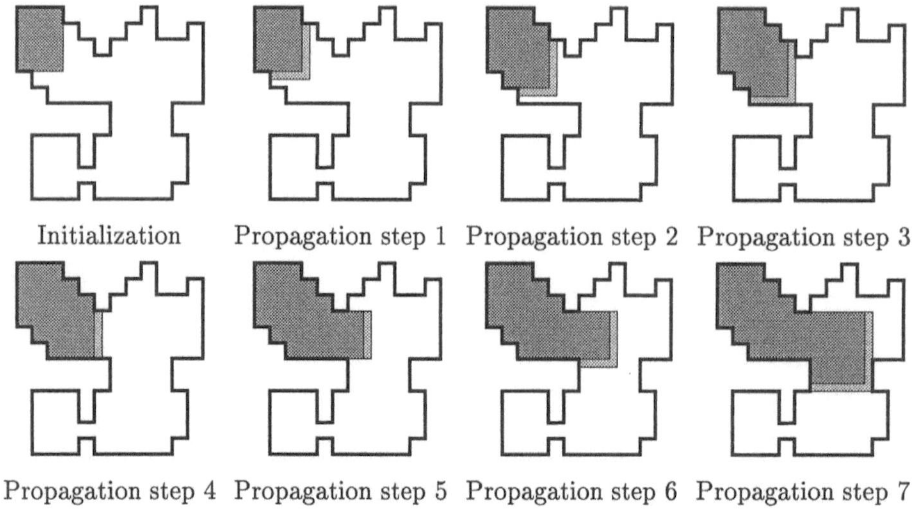

Fig. 2. First steps of a binary opening by propagation. For better understanding, the propagation fronts indicated in light grey are a half pixel wide.

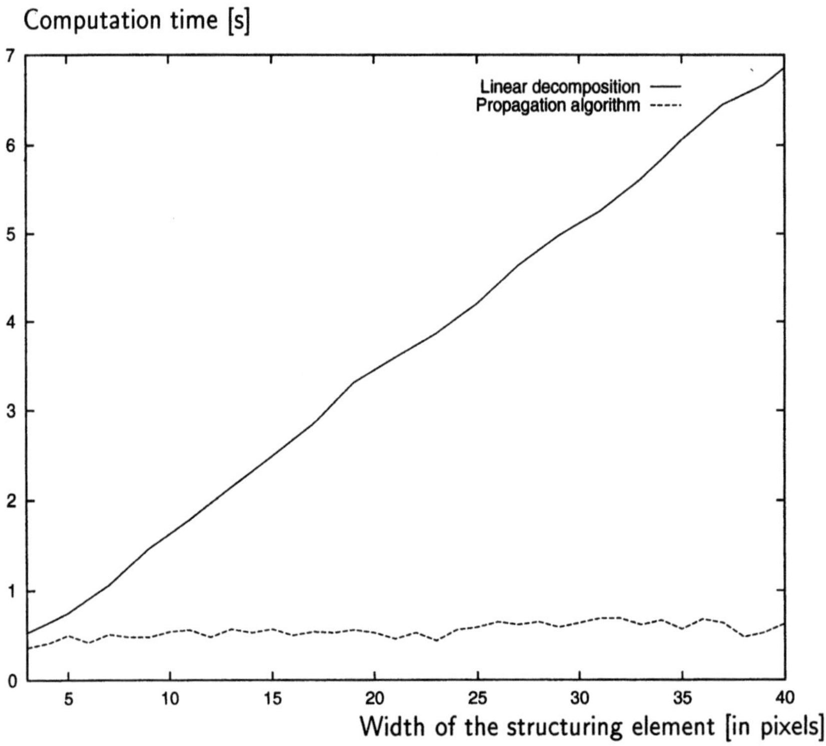

Fig. 3. Computation times of a linear decomposition opening algorithm compared with the proposed propagation algorithm applied on a simple binary image.

for two neighbouring points. This has led HUANG *et al.* [4] to use a sliding window combined with a histogram analysis to compute rank-order filters. For each window position, a pixel of the output image receives the local minimum value. However, if the minimum is compared to each output pixel contained in the window, it is possible to compute an *opening in a single pass.* The general algorithm is the following:

1. All the pixels that enter a window for the first time receive the minimum value.
2. The other pixels receive the maximum between the previously retained value and the local minimum.

This algorithm takes a simplified form when B is a segment because it is easy to track the local minimum values. In that case, the complete step 2 is only needed when the local minimum has increased after the window translation. Otherwise the algorithm attributes the minimum value to the new pixel covered by the window. Fig. 4 illustrates the principle. Other structuring elements lead to similar simplifications.

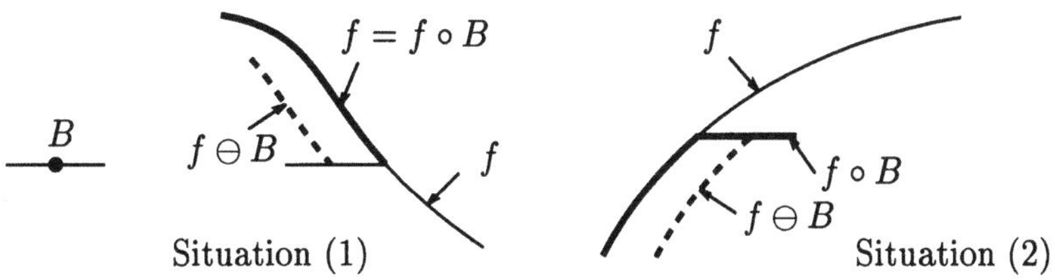

Fig. 4. Two different situations occur during the computation of the opening of f with a linear segment B as the one represented on the left (the origin is located in the middle). Suppose we scan the function from left to right. The negative slope of situation (1) corresponds to a decreasing sliding minimum as is confirmed by the erosion curve $f \ominus B$. It is easy to see that only the opening value of the utmost right point has to be modified after a translation. On the contrary, all values of $f \circ B$ covered by B need to be reallocated in situation (2).

4.2. THEORETICAL RESULTS

In this section, we provide some theoretical results and utilize them to speed up the computation of close-open filters.

An initial theorem establishes a connection between structuring elements involved in grey-level erosions and dilations.

Theorem 1

$$(f \ominus A) \oplus B \leq (f \oplus C) \ominus D \tag{1}$$

if and only if

$$A \oplus C \supseteq B \oplus D.$$

Proof.
The proof is made of two parts:

(1) $\underline{\forall f,\ (f \ominus A) \oplus B \leq (f \oplus C) \ominus D \ \Rightarrow\ B \oplus D \subseteq A \oplus C}$:

Write o for the origin. $A = o \oplus A \subseteq A$ is equivalent to $o \subseteq A \ominus A$ because $(\ominus, \oplus)$ is an adjunction [3]. If we replace f by A in Eq.1, the relation becomes

$B = o \oplus B \subseteq (A \ominus A) \oplus B \subseteq (A \oplus C) \ominus D$. By the adjunction again, it results in $B \oplus D \subseteq A \oplus C$.

(2) $\forall f,\ (f \ominus A) \oplus B \leq (f \oplus C) \ominus D \Leftarrow B \oplus D \subseteq A \oplus C$:
$B \oplus D \subseteq A \oplus C$ implies $(f \ominus A) \oplus B \oplus D \leq (f \ominus A) \oplus A \oplus C$. Moreover, $(f \ominus A) \oplus A \oplus C = (f \circ A) \oplus C \leq f \oplus C$. This means that $(f \ominus A) \oplus B \oplus D \leq f \oplus C$, or $(f \ominus A) \oplus B \leq (f \oplus C) \ominus D$ by the adjunction.

As the proof uses the algebraic framework introduced by HEIJMANS and RONSE [3], the demonstration scheme is also valid for grey-level erosions and dilations, i.e. with non-flat structuring elements. ∎

It is interesting to note that there exists a relationship between structuring elements that induces $(f \ominus A) \oplus B \leq (f \oplus C) \ominus D$. We concentrate below on the combination of openings and closings.

Theorem 2 *If $A \oplus C \supseteq B \oplus C$ and $A \subseteq B$ (which implies that $A \oplus C = B \oplus C$) then*

$$[(f \circ C) \oplus A] \ominus B = (f \circ C) \bullet B.$$

Proof.
If $A \subseteq B$ then $(f \circ C) \oplus A \leq (f \circ C) \oplus B$, and $[(f \circ C) \oplus A] \ominus B \leq (f \circ C) \bullet B$ as erosion is increasing.
On the other hand, $A \oplus C \supseteq B \oplus C \Leftrightarrow C \oplus A \supseteq C \oplus B$, so that we have $(f \oplus A) \ominus B \geq f \circ C$ following relation (1). As this inequality holds for any function f, we may use it for $f \circ C$: $[(f \circ C) \oplus A] \ominus B \geq (f \circ C) \circ C = f \circ C$. It is known that closing is an increasing operation: $([(f \circ C) \oplus A] \ominus B) \bullet B \geq (f \circ C) \bullet B$. Moreover, for any function g, $(g \ominus B) \bullet B = g \ominus B$ [2]. In conclusion, $[(f \circ C) \oplus A] \ominus B \geq (f \circ C) \bullet B$. ∎

The previous theorem only makes sense if $A \oplus C \supseteq B \oplus C$ and $A \subseteq B$ are realistic. In fact, the induced condition $A \oplus C = B \oplus C$ is not a severe one. Suppose for instance $B = C$. Then the condition becomes $A \oplus B = B \oplus B$, called the *reduction condition*. Fig. 5 shows different sets that satisfy the reduction condition.

In both cases, A is a subset of the border of B. But it is by no means necessary to take all the border points since some of them are redundant. Yet, if A is the border of B, the reduction condition is always satisfied as confirmed by next theorem (the proof can be found in [7]).

Theorem 3 *Let ∂B be the border of the compact set $B \subseteq \boldsymbol{R}^2$. Then*

$$B \oplus B = B \oplus \partial B$$

If $B = C$, $A \subseteq B$ and $A \oplus C \supseteq B \oplus C$, then $[(f \circ B) \oplus A] \ominus B = (f \circ B) \bullet B$. In other words a dilation by B is replaced by a less expensive dilation by A. Because in alternate sequential filters (a typical case where filtering operators follow one another) the number of involved operations is very high, theorem 2 will prove very useful.

The conditions $A \oplus C \supseteq B \oplus C$ and $A \subseteq B$ do not imply that C is included in B or contains B. Fig. 6 confirms this remark in $\mathbf{Z}^2$.

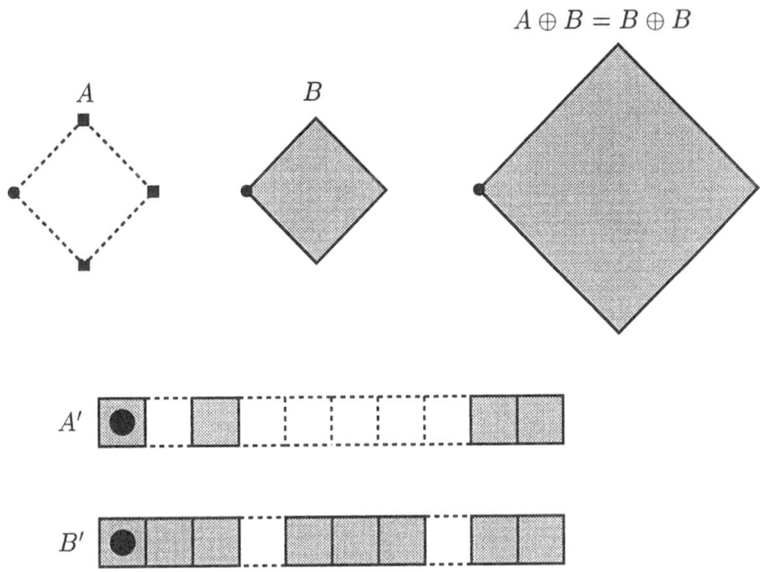

Fig. 5. Two pairs of sets ($A, B \subseteq \mathbf{R}^2$ and $A', B' \subseteq \mathbf{Z}^2$) that satisfy the reduction condition. Each black disk indicates the origin of the corresponding structuring element.

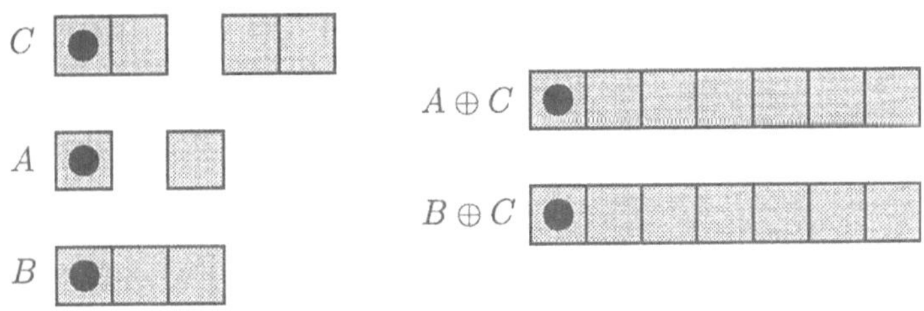

Fig. 6. B and C do not need to be included in each other, even if $A \oplus C \supseteq B \oplus C$ and $A \subseteq B$.

4.3. Numerical results

We have implemented different morphological operations with a horizontal segment. The algorithms are based on a sliding window of which the minimum is the relevant information. All the steps have been integrated so that *only one image scan* is required. The aim of this description is to compare erosion, opening and close-open computation times.

Figure 7 presents the computation times on a large image (1440×1280). The lower curve corresponds to the erosion algorithm. The second curve represents the time needed for an opening implemented as indicated in section 4.1. With other algorithms, it is twice that of the erosion curve because an opening is an erosion followed by a dilation. Everything happens here as if the dilation was performed during the same scan process as the erosion. The last curve is the close-open filter. Usually this curve is four times the lower one, but due to the combination of the new opening algorithm and theorem 2, it is only about 1.4 higher.

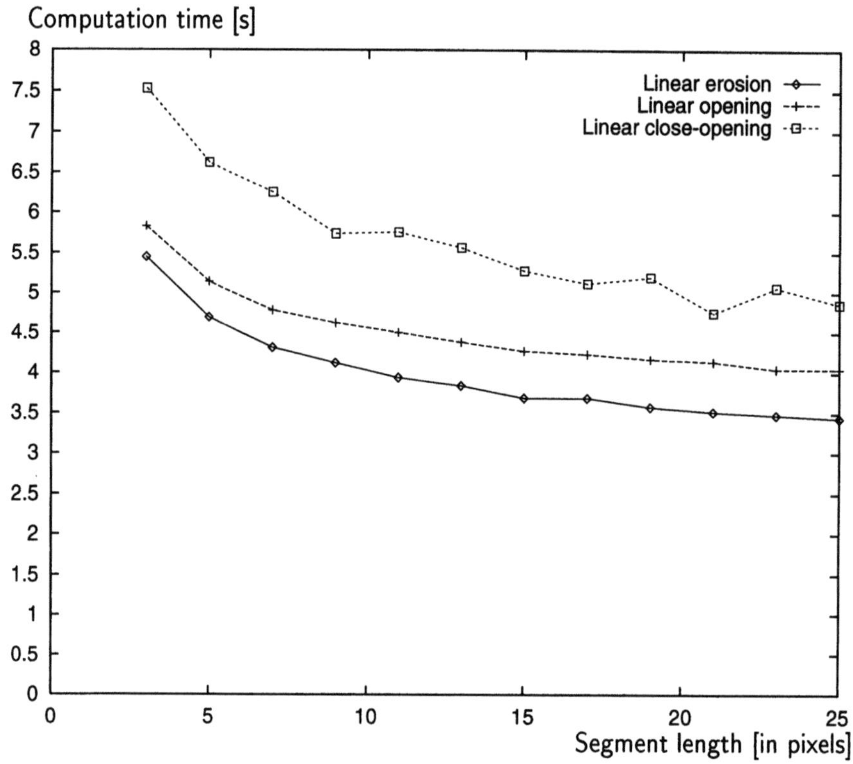

Fig. 7. Computation times of different morphological operations on a large image.

References

1. E. Breen and P. Soille. Generalization of van Herk recursive erosion/dilation algorithm to lines at arbitrary angles. In *Digital Image Computing: Techniques and Applications*, pages 549–555, Sydney, December 1993.
2. R. Haralick, S. Sternberg and X. Zhuang. Image analysis using mathematical morphology. *IEEE Transactions on Pattern Analysis and Machine Intelligence*, 9(4):532–550, July 1987.
3. H. Heijmans and C. Ronse. The algebraic basis of mathematical morphology; I. Dilations and erosions. *Computer Vision, Graphics, and Image Processing*, 50:245–295, 1990.
4. T. Huang, G. Yang, and G. Tang. A fast two-dimensional median filtering algorithm. *IEEE Transactions on Acoustics, Speech and Signal Processing*, 27(1):13–18, February 1979.
5. J. Pecht. Speeding up successive Minkowski operations. *Pattern Recognition Letters*, 3(2):113–117, 1985.
6. M. Schmitt. *Des algorithmes morphologiques à l'intelligence artificielle.* PhD thesis, École nationale supérieure des mines de Paris, February 1989.
7. M. Van Droogenbroeck. *Traitement d'images numériques au moyen d'algorithmes utilisant la morphologie mathématique et la notion d'objet : application au codage.* PhD thesis, Université catholique de Louvain, May 1994.
8. M. van Herk. A fast algorithm for local minimum and maximum filters on rectangular and octogonal kernels. *Pattern Recognition Letters*, 13(7):517–521, July 1992.
9. L. Vincent. Morphological transformations of binary images with arbitrary structuring elements. *Signal Processing*, 22(1):3–23, January 1991.

AN EVALUATION OF PRIORITY QUEUES FOR MATHEMATICAL MORPHOLOGY

EDMOND J. BREEN AND DAVID H. MONRO
CSIRO, Division of Mathematics and Statistics, Institute of Information Science and Engineering, Locked Bag 17, Nth Ryde N.S.W. 2113 Australia.

Abstract. This report will be of interest to those who program mathematical morphology routines, since it concentrates on data structures for their efficient implementation. With respect to basic priority queue operations, we provide an empirical evaluation, using execution time, of an implicit heap, splay–tree, SplayQ, AVL–tree, Fibonacci–heap and hierarchical queue. It is shown that the hierarchical queue implementation performs fastest. However, it is an unrealistic implementation for images that contain data items with a key value greater than 12 significant bits or for floating point values. Therefore, we introduce the SplayQ, a hybrid data structure, to overcome this limitation, and with respect to speed of performance, it is the SplayQ that is the fastest from the other data structures considered.

Key words: Data Structures, Priority queues, Mathematical morphology

1. Introduction

Mathematical morphology (MM) routines usually involve a sequence of steps (Serra, 1982). While the implementation of these steps can be carried out using a variety of techniques, the generality and simplicity of recursive queue based abstract data types (ADT) has been shown to be extremely efficient (Vincent, 1991*b*).

The queue ADT has been used for variety of MM transforms (Vincent, 1991*b*; Vincent, 1991*a*; Vincent, 1992; Vincent, 1989). It is a first in, first out list (FIFO). The two principle operations are enqueue (add an item to the rear of the list) and dequeue (extract the item from the front of the list). In image analysis the items stored in the queue are often pixel addresses or vertices and in practice, the size of the queue can be controlled via dynamic array techniques (Breen, Joss & Williams, 1992), circular arrays and linked lists. In the general case, we wish to order the items according to some specified key value, i.e. we want a priority queue, as for watershed segmentation (Soille & Vincent, 1990; Vincent & Soille, 1991), closings and openings by area (Vincent, 1993), and seeded region growing (Adams & Bischof, 1994). Here, the pixels priorities are either obtained from their grey-scale values (Soille & Vincent, 1990; Vincent & Soille, 1991; Vincent, 1993) or the absolute difference between grey-scale values (Adams & Bischof, 1994). In (Soille & Vincent, 1990; Vincent & Soille, 1991), an effective priority queue was achieved by first placing all pixel addresses associated with a given grey-scale value into a separate array. Thus, for each grey-scale within the image there was an associated array of pixels. This separated pixel priorities from pixel addresses and allowed breadth–first propagation (or flooding) to be efficiently carried out sequentially at each pixel level with the use of a single queue. An hierarchical queue (Meyer, 1991), is another approach for constructing a

J.Serra and P. Soille (eds.), Mathematical Morphology and Its Applications to Image Processing, 249-256

TABLE I
Summary of Abstract Data Types

Implementation	Enqueue	Dequeue	Source Code	Stable
Hqueue	$O(1)$	$O(1)^1$	In house	Yes
SplayQ	$O(\log d)^{1,3}$	$O(\log d)^{1,3}$	In house	Yes
Splay–tree	$O(\log n)^1$	$O(\log n)^1$	C version[4] of Pascal code used in (Jones, 1986)	Yes
AVL–tree	$O(\log n)^2$	$O(\log n)^2$	from the XRN newsreader	No[5]
Heap	$O(\log n)^2$	$O(\log n)$	In house	No[5]
Fibonacci–Heap	$O(1)^1$	$O(\log n)^1$	C translation of Modula - 2 code given in (Kingston, 1990)	No[5]

[1]amortized bound. [2]worst case bound. [3] d is the number of distinct priorities in the queue.
[4] comp.sources.unix, volume 14, translated by Dave Brower.
[5] Stability can be achieved at a cost of one integer per item

priority queue. Here, an array of queues is maintained, one for each priority. The problem with these methods, is that they are somewhat limited to the range of priorities and to discrete values. This is not a problem for 8-bit grey-scale images, but it is for 16-bit, 32-bit data and floating point values.

To overcome this range problem an implicit heap (Williams, 1964) or heap ADT, was introduced in (Vincent, 1993). However, a heap is inherently unstable, in the sense that items with the same priority are not handled in FIFO order. In (Jones, 1986), it was shown that the splay–tree (Sleator & Tarjan, 1985), a self–adjusting binary search tree, when optimized for dequeuing and enqueuing, outperformed the heap with respect to priority queue operations. However, a comparison between different self–adjusting ADTs to the classic height–balanced AVL–tree (Knuth, 1973), showed that the AVL–tree generally outperformed splay–trees and other self–adjusting ADTs (Bell & Gupta, 1993). From theoretical considerations, the most efficient implementation of a priority queue should be the Fibonacci–heap (Fredman & Tarjan, 1987), since all standard priority queue operations (insert, find min and merge) other than the deletemin operation are performed in $O(1)^1$ time; with deletemin performed in $O(\log n)^1$ time. Hence, we decided to do an empirical evaluation, using execution time and with respect to standard priority queue operations, of the optimized splay–tree, SplayQ, heaps, AVL–trees, Fibonacci–heaps and hierarchical queues.

2. Data Structures

2.1. Hierarchical Queue

The hierarchical queue is a structure consisting of a fixed length array of queues (see Fig. 1).

[1] amortized bound

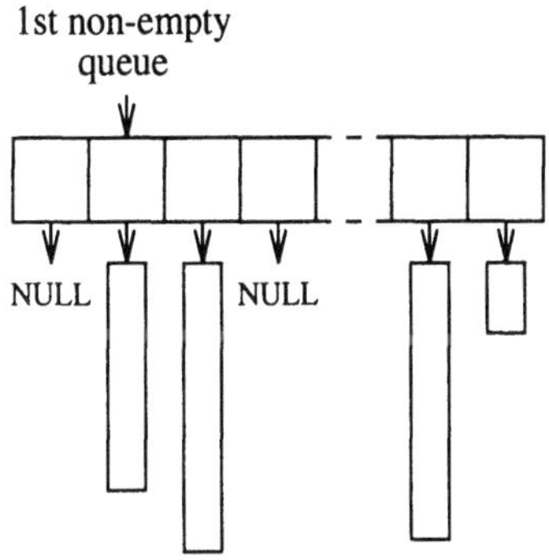

Fig. 1. Implementation of a hierarchical queue.

Insertion of an item is achieved by using the key as an index into the array and placing the data item in the queue at that index, i.e.,

$$item \rightarrow queue[key.value].$$

Deleting the minimum item involves finding the lowest index in the array with a non-empty queue attached (which is normally stored in the data structure and updated every delete and insert), and removing the first item in the queue. Finding an arbitrary item is achieved by indexing into the array with the key, and then scanning through the entire queue looking for the required item.

2.2. Heap

A heap consists of an array representation of a complete left justified heap ordered binary tree. We can represent a complete binary tree with an array by placing the root node in the first position in the array, the children of the root node in the second and third positions and so on (see Fig. 2). Thus the children of the node at index i are at indices $2i$ and $2i + 1$. Using the array representation, the heap invariant for a tree of n nodes can be stated as:

1. $k_i \leq k_{2i}, \forall i : 1 \leq i \leq \lfloor n/2 \rfloor$
2. $k_i \leq k_{2i+1}, \forall i : 1 \leq i \leq \lfloor \frac{(n-1)}{2} \rfloor$

This has the following consequences:

(a) Keys from the root to a leaf will be monotonically increasing.

(b) The root node has the smallest key.

(c) Keys at a given level are in no defined order.

Insertion is achieved by adding the node to the end of the array, and then shuffling it up the tree until the heap invariant holds. Deleting the minimum item involves removing the item at the front of the array, taking the item at the back of the array and moving it to the front, and then shuffling it down the tree until the invariant holds. Deleting an arbitrary item requires searching the tree for all nodes with the requested key and checking each node to see if it is the right one. This is slow because of (c) above. Once we have found the right node we remove it and replace it with the node in the last occupied position in the array, then shuffle this node in the appropriate direction until the heap invariant is satisfied.

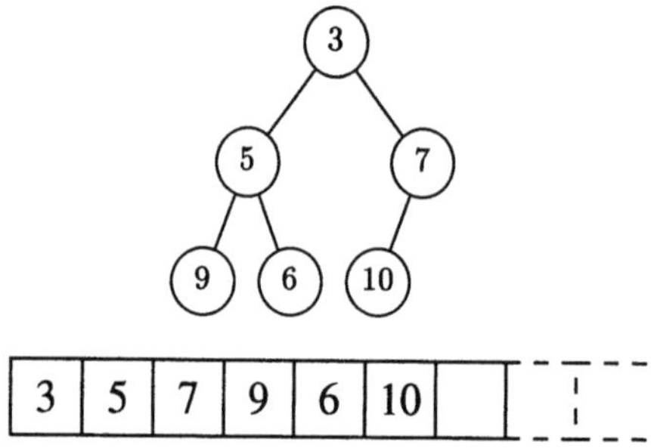

Fig. 2. A heap ordered complete left justified binary tree and its array equivalent.

2.3. AVL TREE

An AVL tree is defined as a balanced binary search tree where, for every node in the tree, the heights of its two subtrees differ by at most one. The balance of the tree is maintained by left and right rotations (Knuth, 1973).

Insertion into a tree is a reasonably complex procedure. We shall assume without loss of generality that we are inserting a node into the left subtree of our tree.

Let l and r denote the left and right subtrees, and H denotes tree height. Assume that the new node is inserted into l, increasing H_l by 1. There are three cases to be considered:

1. If $H_l = H_r$, increase H_l by 1, and the balance criterion is not violated.
2. If $H_l = H_r - 1$, increase H_l by 1, and the balance criterion is not violated.
3. If $H_l = H_r + 1$, increase H_l by one and rebalance the tree as H_l is now 2 greater than H_r, violating the balance criterion.

There are basically two possible cases, shown in Fig. 3. In both cases, either the node X_l or X_r has been added, making the left subtree too long. The other two possible cases are the symmetric variants of the two given above. To delete a node, the tree is first searched to find it, and it is replaced with the rightmost node in its left subtree, or its right child if it has no left subtree. The tree is then rebalanced if necessary. To delete the minimum the same procedure is followed, but the node deleted is always the leftmost node in the entire tree.

2.4. SPLAY TREE AND SPLAYQ

The splay tree is an example of a different sort of modified binary tree. The splay tree employs a heuristic to improve its performance. All operations on the splay tree are based on calls to an operation called splay, which handles three cases and which are described in detail by (Sleator & Tarjan, 1985). Insertion is achieved as follows: first split the tree into two portions. To do this, find the node in the tree with the nearest key value to that of the node to be inserted. Splay this node to the root, and split off one of its subtrees as a new tree. Then attach the new node as the root with the two portions of the tree as its children. Deleting the minimum item involves splaying the minimum item to the root (which is always the extreme leftmost item in a binary search tree, and is thus quick to find), removing it, and joining its subtrees together with one of its children being the new root. Deleting an arbitrary item follows the same procedure, except that the required node will have to be searched for in the tree, since we do not know in advance where it is. Fig. 4

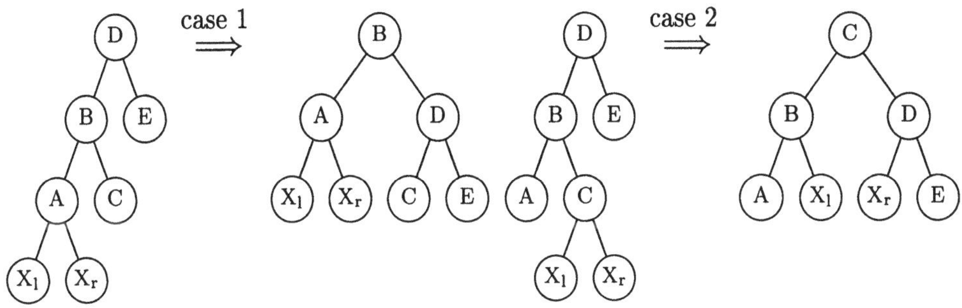

Fig. 3. Rebalancing operations on AVL trees.

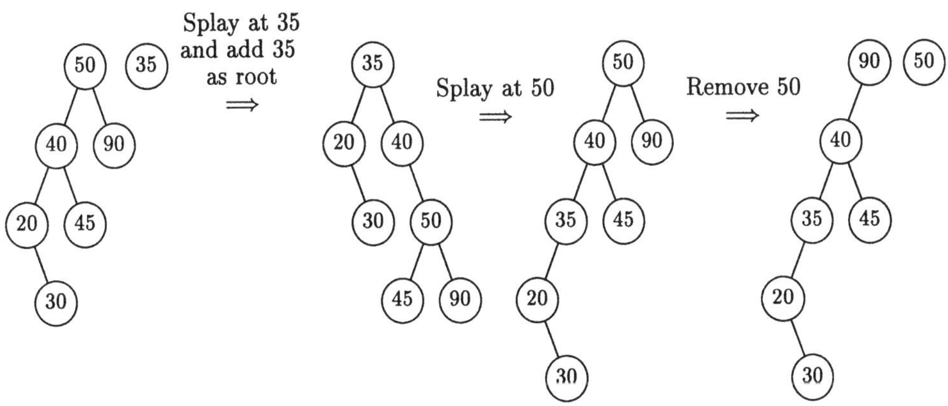

Fig. 4. Example operations on a splay tree.

shows example operations on a splay tree.

The SplayQ is a hybrid data structure consisting of a splay tree of FIFO queues organized in a similar manner to the hierarchical queue. To insert an item, first check if a queue exists in the splay tree with that priority. If one does not exist, add a new queue to the splay tree. Then insert the item into the appropriate queue. Deletion is performed in a similar manner, removing queues from the tree as they become empty. Arbitrary deletion requires scanning the entire queue attached to the node of the tree with the desired priority.

2.5. Fibonacci Heap

The Fibonacci heap is asymptotically the most efficient of the various priority queue implementations, having $O(1)$ insert and $O(\log n)$ deletemin operations, see Table I. It consists of a forest of heap ordered trees, represented by a series of doubly linked lists. The insert, deletemin and delete operations for the Fibonacci heap are somewhat complicated, and unfortunately the Fibonacci heap does not perform at all well as a priority queue in practice, so we shall not describe these operations here, see (Fredman & Tarjan, 1987; Kingston, 1990).

3. Methodology

Table I provides a summary of the ADTs considered here. To compare the ADTs, a large number of tests were run on each. All priority queue implementations require insert and deletemin operations, so these operations were tested. Implementation of the seeded region growing algorithm presented in (Adams & Bischof, 1994) requires the facility to alter an item's priority once it has been inserted into a priority queue, therefore all ADTs (except the Fibonacci–heap) were tested for their efficiency of locating and deleting arbitrary items. The key values used were random integers in the range [0,99], with a uniform distribution. Each test consisted of the following steps, with n representing the number of items:

1. Do n random insertions into the data structure.
2. Do n random arbitrary finds on the data structure.
3. Do n iterations of the hold model: delete the minimum value, then insert another random item. This is performed on a queue with n items already inserted.
4. Do n deletemins.
5. Do n random insertions.
6. Do n random arbitrary deletes.

The heap and Fibonacci–heap were only tested with n ranging from 3000 to 300000, due to CPU time constraints. The Fibonacci–heap was not tested for arbitrary finds and arbitrary deletes for the same reason, once it became clear that it was not competitive on the basis of its performance on the other tests.A second series of tests were run, consisting of simply inserting n items and the doing n deletemins, using data sorted in non-decreasing order, i.e. monotonically increasing. This was used to simulate how data would be encountered during watershed segmentation.All tests were run on a Sun SparcStation 10 running Solaris 2.3, using the GNU C compiler with optimizations enabled.

4. Results

The results for the first series of tests appear in Fig. 5. From these graphs, it is clear that the hierarchical queue is the quickest data structure for all operations, but it is only viable for data with a fixed narrow range of key values. It is closely followed by the SplayQ. For the remaining ADTs, the order of performance is: splay–tree, AVL–tree, heap, Fibonacci–heap. For insertions, Fig. 5(a), the AVL–tree is by far the worst, but the range of differences between the ADTs is small. As seen from Fig. 5(b) and (c) the Fibonacci–heap is not suitable for priority queue implementations in image analysis. From Fig. 5(d), the AVL–tree is seen to be marginally quicker for arbitrary finds than the splay–tree. This is probably due to the fact that a splay–tree can be quite skewed on occasion, while the AVL–tree is always fairly well balanced. However, once we start modifying the tree, as seen in Fig. 5(e), the advantage is substantially reduced. Also note in Fig. 5(d) and Fig. 5(e) that the hierarchical queue and SplayQ enjoy a very large advantage over the other implementations for smaller values of n. This is a consequence of the use of separate queues for each priority, as it cuts down the number of items encountered while scanning the structure for all items with a given priority.

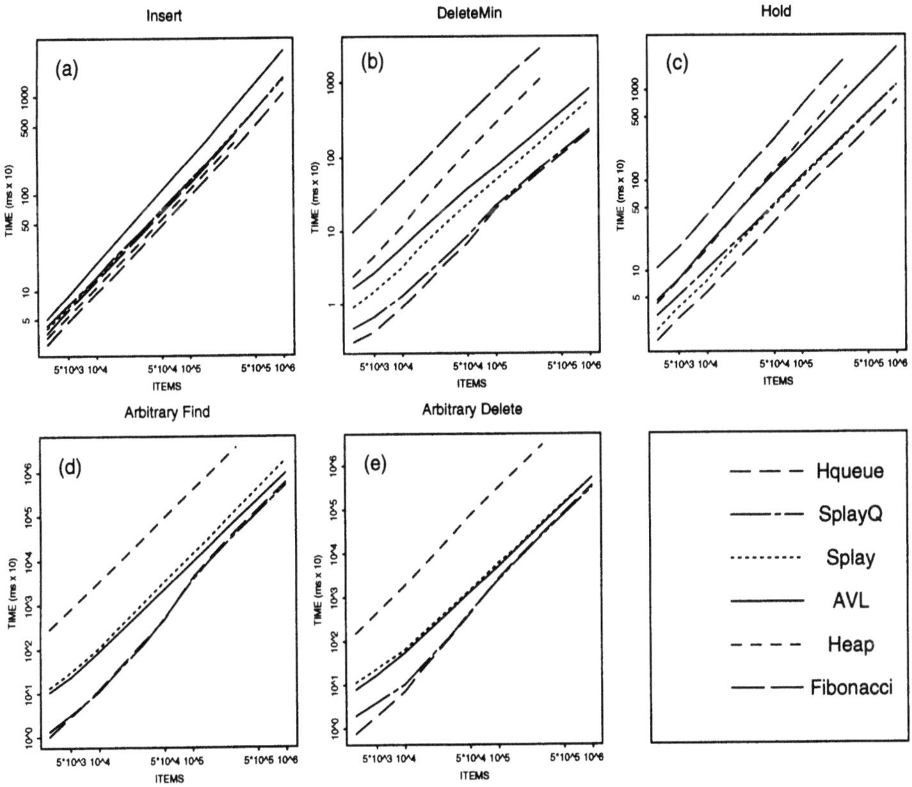

Fig. 5. Results for the first set of tests, using uniform random numbers.

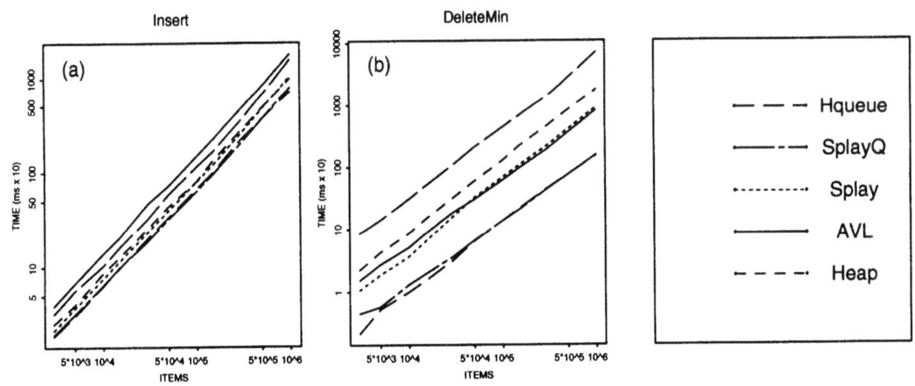

Fig. 6. Results for the second set of tests, using monotonically increasing numbers.

The results for the second series of tests are shown in Fig. 6. While the results are similar to those shown in Fig. 5(a) and (b), it appears that for a monotonically increasing data set the performance of the Fibonacci–heap for insertions, Fig. 6(a), has degraded slightly, while the performance of the AVL–tree has improved with respect to deletions, Fig. 6(b).

5. Conclusion

Here we have considered a variety of ADTs as priority queues for MM. Although the hierarchical queue (Meyer, 1991) was the fastest on all tests performed, it has limited usage. The other ADTs considered do not have the same restrictions. From these ADTs it was shown that the SplayQ performed best. The SplayQ, as well as being the fastest, is inherently stable, see §2, and has a low memory overhead. This then suggests that the SplayQ is the implementation most suited for MM routines.

References

Adams, R. & Bischof, L. (1994), 'Seeded region growing', *IEEE Transactions on Pattern Analysis and Machine Intelligence.*

Bell, J. & Gupta, G. (1993), 'An evaluation of self-adjusting binary search tree techniques', *Software Practice and Experience* **23**, 369–382.

Breen, E., Joss, G. & Williams, K. (1992), 'Dynamic arrays for fast, efficient, data manipulation during image analysis: a new software tool for exploratory data analysis', *Computer Methods and Programs in Biomedicine* **37**, 85–92.

Fredman, M. L. & Tarjan, R. E. (1987), 'Fibonacci heaps and their uses in improved network optimization algorithms', *J. Assoc. Comp. Mach.* **34**, 596–615.

Jones, D. W. (1986), 'An empirical comparison of priority–queue and event–set implementations', *Communications of the ACM* **29**, 300–311.

Kingston, J. H. (1990), *Algorithms and data structures: design, correctness, analysis*, International Computer Science, Addison-Wesley, Sydney.

Knuth, D. (1973), *The art of computer programming. Volume 3 : Sorting and searching*, Addison-Wesley.

Meyer, F. (1991), Algorithmes ordonnés de ligne de partage des eaux, Technical Report N-06/90/MM, Ecole des Mines de Paris, Centre de Morphologie Mathématique.

Serra, J. (1982), *Image Analysis and Mathematical Morphology*, Academic Press.

Sleator, D. D. & Tarjan, R. E. (1985), 'Self–adjusting binary search trees', *J. Assoc. Comp. Mach.* **32**, 652–686.

Soille, P. & Vincent, L. (1990), Determining watersheds in digital pictures via flooding simulations, *in* 'Visual Communications and Image Processing'90', Lausanne, pp. 240–250.

Vincent, L. (1989), 'Graphs and mathematical morphology', *Signal Processing* **16**, 365–388.

Vincent, L. (1991*a*), Efficient computation of various types of skeletons, *in* 'Medical Imaging V'.

Vincent, L. (1991*b*), New trends in morphological algorithms, *in* 'Nonlinear Image Processing II', pp. 158–170.

Vincent, L. (1992), Morphological grayscale reconstruction: definition, efficient algorithm and applications in image analysis, *in* 'Proc. IEEE Computer Vision and Pattern Recognition'92', Champaign IL, pp. 633–635.

Vincent, L. (1993), Grayscale area openings and closings, their efficient implementation and applications, *in* J. Serra & P. Salembier, eds, 'Mathematical Morphology and its applications to signal processing', UPC Publications, pp. 22–27.

Vincent, L. & Soille, P. (1991), 'Watersheds in digital spaces: an efficient algorithm based on immersion simulations', *IEEE Transactions on Pattern Analysis and Machine Intelligence* **13**(6), 583–598.

Williams, J. W. J. (1964), 'Algorithm 232: Heapsort', *Communications of the ACM* **7**, 347–348.

ONE PIXEL THICK SKELETONS

MICHEL SCHMITT
Thomson-CSF, L.C.R.
Domaine de Corbeville, F-91404 Orsay-Cedex, France

Abstract.
When computing digital skeletons, one is often interested in obtaining digital lines of a thickness of one pixel. Then, the connectivity of these lines is unambiguous and the notions of end points or triple points are defined by examining only a neighborhood of size one of each pixel. This paper presents how to adapt the queue algorithms in order to directly obtain skeletons of thickness one by computing only their end points.

Key words: Skeleton, Digital Metric, Osculating Circle.

1. Introduction

The skeleton transformation [1, 5] has been designed in order to reduce a shape to a set of lines describing the structure of this shape: one line corresponding to one protrusion, multiple points to the conjunction of several parts of the object. In the continuous plane, the standard definition for skeletons is the locus of the centers of the maximal disks included in the shape. Under adequate conditions, this skeleton has nice properties and is a finite graph, as intuitively expected [6, 2]. For a comprehensive study of skeletons, see [8] and the included references. When dealing with lattices, this approach does not work anymore (the skeleton transformation is not digitizable) and other notions have to be developed: the maximal balls do not produce connected lines. If we want to describe the digital skeleton of a shape as a finite graph, this skeleton must verify the two following properties:

1. it must be homotope to the shape, *i.e.* preserve the connectivity and the holes of the shape,
2. its thickness must be of one pixel on its arcs.

These two properties ensure an unambiguous description of the digital skeleton with end points, multiple points and points on its arcs, by only examining a neighborhood of size one of each pixel. This paper presents how to adapt standard algorithms in order to directly obtain skeletons of thickness one by computing only their end points.

The paper is organized as follows:

- We first present the existing algorithms and show that they do not efficiently provide the desired requirements.
- Then, we go to the continuous plane equipped with the distance induced by hexagons and show how the skeleton should be defined in this case.
- Finally, the properties obtained in the continuous plane are used to design an enhancement of queue algorithms.

J.Serra and P. Soille (eds.), Mathematical Morphology and Its Applications to Image Processing, 257-264

TABLE I

Computing time for the different algorithms for the skeleton (Sun Sparc 2 workstation, Compilation option `cc -O`, image size 256 × 256).

Algorithm	Thickness: 2 pixels	Thickness: 1 pixel
Homotopic thinning	—	36.40 s
Meyer's algorithm	0.50 s	1.80 s
Anchor skeletons with centers of maximal hexagons	1.10 s	1.80 s
Anchor skeletons with centers of osculating hexagons	—	0.75 s

2. Existing Algorithms

From now on, we assume to be on the hexagonal lattice $\mathcal{H}$. The existing algorithms are mainly designed to ensure the homotopy of the result. So the one pixel thickness is obtained after an homotopic thinning [10], which can take a long computation time on sequential machines. Let us examine the three main families of skeleton algorithms. A more detailed description can be found in [9]. Computation times are summarized in table I.

2.1. Homotopic Thinnings

The homotopic thinnings were historically the first ones to appear. A description can be found in [10]. Their main drawback is their long computation time: they examine each pixel of the image about $6 \times R$ times, where R is the size of the maximal inscribed hexagon. So they are usually used to thin objects, which have a thickness less than 3 pixels. Their advantage is that the result is homotopic to the original object and has a one pixel thickness.

2.2. Meyer's Algorithms

The idea of these algorithms is to find some points which necessarily belong to the skeleton, called crest points and then to connect them by following the upstream of the crest points on the distance function [4]. Meyer's algorithm sweeps 5 times the image (two for the crest point calculus and three for the connection). The main problem is that the result has generally a thickness of two pixels (see fig. 6). Thus, an homotopic thinning has to be used afterwards. The originality of Meyer's algorithm is that it is based on a mathematical characterization.

2.3. Anchor Skeletons

The main difference with Meyer's algorithm is that the connection of the points, named here anchor points, is always one pixel thin [11, 12]. The points which are connected are usually the local maxima of the distance function, *i.e.* the centers of the maximal inscribed hexagons. Unfortunately, these anchor points build parts of thickness two pixels (see fig. 7.a). The use of the crest points of Meyer's algorithm

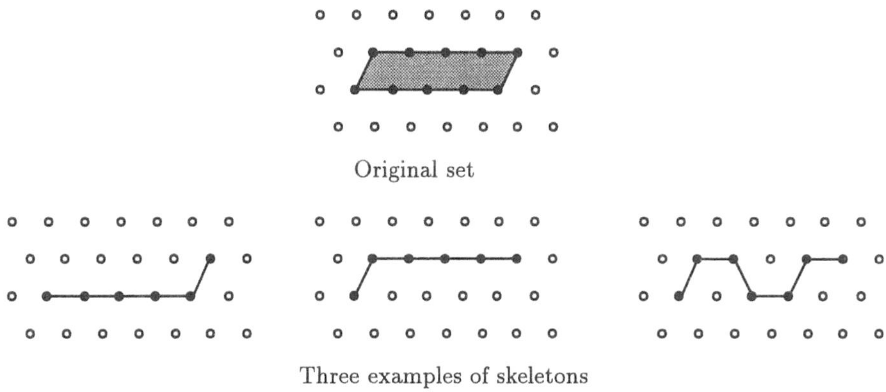

Fig. 1. A set of thickness two cannot be reduced to a skeleton of thickness one without making some arbitrary choices.

as anchor points is even worse, because it gives much more anchor points, here also, of thickness two.

It has to be pointed out that homotopic thinnings and anchor skeletons are not rotation invariant, *i.e.* do not commute with rotations of 60°. On the other hand, Meyer's algorithm is rotation invariant and corresponds to the smallest set one can define as skeleton without making arbitrary choices. Note that a skeleton of thickness one always assumes an arbitrary choice (see fig. 1).

3. Continuous Hexagonal Skeletons

In order to avoid the problem of choice of pixels, we work now in the continuous plane. To be compatible with the distances on the lattice, we equip the continuous plane R^2 with the distance induced by the hexagon. This approach has already proved its usefulness for the design of algorithms dedicated to the propagation function [7].

Let X be the shape under study. We suppose that X is a polygon whose edges have directions in the set $(0°, 60°, 120°, 180°, 240°, 300°)$. Such polygons will be called hexagonal polygons in the sequel. This is not a real restriction, because we can always associate such a polygon to a set of pixels on the hexagonal lattice.

3.1. Maximal Hexagons

We denote by ∂X the boundary of X. Following the Euclidean definition with circles, we first study the maximal hexagons included in X. The hexagons of size r centered at x is denoted by $H(x, r)$. When centered at the origin O, we omit it and write $H(O, r) = H(r)$.

Proposition 3.1 *An hexagon H is maximal in X if and only if $H \cap \partial X$ is not included in two successive edges of H.*

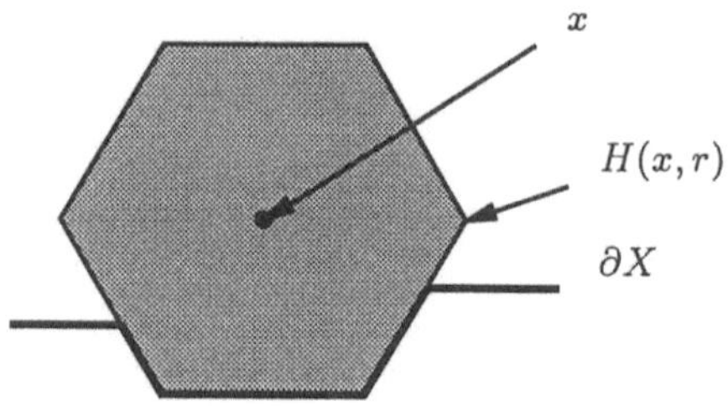

Fig. 2. Local configuration of an end point in $Sk_H(X)$.

Another characterization of the centers of these maximal hexagons is given by Lantuéjoul's formula, usually stated for the Euclidean distance [3]:

$$\bigcup_{r\geq 0} \bigcap_{\varepsilon>0} (X \ominus H(r)) \setminus (X \ominus H(r))_{H(\varepsilon)}. \tag{1}$$

As we supposed that X is an hexagonal polygon, so is $X \ominus H(r)$. The centers of the maximal hexagons are located at:
- the convex vertices of $X \ominus H(r)$ of angle 60°,
- the thin parts of $X \ominus H(r)$.

Unfortunately, these centers do not build a connected set of pixels (see fig. 4). In order to connect them, let us state the property of connectivity we want for the hexagonal skeleton, we denote by $Sk_H(X)$:

Property 3.2 *Let $H(x,r)$ be a maximal hexagon in X. We want that the number of connected components of $X \setminus H(x,r)$ is equal to that of $Sk_H(X) \setminus \{x\}$.*

So, the end points of such a skeleton are the centers of the hexagons which do not cut X in many pieces. Using proposition 3.1 we can state the following characterization which is at the basis of our algorithm:

Proposition 3.3 *An end point of $Sk_H(X)$ is the center x of an hexagon $H(x,r)$, included in X, such that its intersection with the boundary of X is a connected set, composed of a complete edge of $H(x,r)$ and parts of the two adjacent edges (see fig. 2). Such hexagons are also called* osculating hexagons.

Let us add a few words about the diagram composed of the maximal hexagons:

Proposition 3.4 *The set of centers of maximal hexagons is composed of isolated points or line segments at $k \times 30°$, $k \in \mathbb{N}$.*

3.2. Connexion of Maximal Hexagons

The simplest way to connected the disconnected parts of the diagram of the maximal hexagons is to do a kind of "climbing" along the steepest slope on the hexagonal distance function. More precisely:

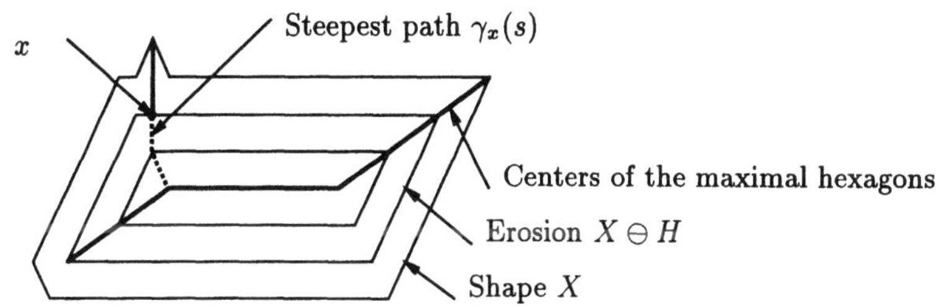

Fig. 3. Construction of the hexagonel skeleton $Sk_H(X)$. Solid lines: diagram of centers of maximal hexagons (proposition 3.4) – dashed lines: connexion procedure by steepest slope following.

Definition 3.5 *Let x be a point which is not a local maximum of the hexagonal distance function d_X^H on X. Then, there exists a unique path $\gamma_x(s)$ linking x to a local maximum of d_X^H such that:*

$$\gamma_x(s) \;=\; \text{argmax}\;\{d_X^H(y) \mid y \in B(x,s)\} \qquad (2)$$

It can be shown that the union of the centers of the maximal hexagons and their associated arcs γ_x build a graph which has the desired properties:

- it is connected,
- its end-points are those characterized in proposition 3.3,
- it verifies property 3.2. Fig. 3 gives an illustration of this construction.

So we put:

$$Sk_H(X) \;=\; \{\gamma_x(s) \mid x \text{ center of maximal hexagon }\}. \qquad (3)$$

Remark 3.6 *Note however that the set $\{\gamma_x(s) \mid x$ center of osculating hexagon $\}$ is included, but usually not equal to $Sk_H(X)$ and may be disconnected.*

4. Digital Framework

How can we use the previous results on the hexagonal lattice $\mathcal{H}$? We suppose now that X is a set of pixels on the hexagonal lattice. Let us first state some properties:

Proposition 4.1 *The end points of the hexagonal skeleton Sk_H (see proposition 3.3) are always on the lattice and are obtained by the local shape of the boundary depicted in fig. 5.*

Proposition 4.2 *The centers of the maximal hexagons are located on the half-lattice associated to the hexagonal lattice $\mathcal{H}$ (see fig. 4).*

Proposition 4.3 *The rule depicted by Meyer ([4], pp. 279–280) for connecting the crest points in his algorithm is the digital analog of the steepest slope arc $\gamma_x(s)$.*

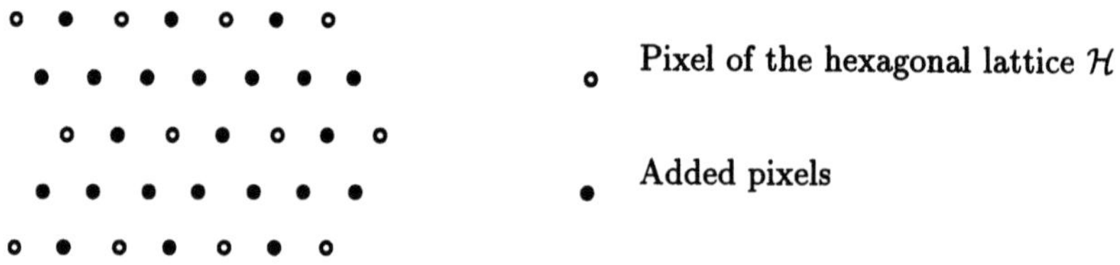

Fig. 4. The half-lattice is obtained by inserting new pixels in the middle of existing pixels. The total number of pixels is multiplied by 4.

However, this rule, applied to the centers of the osculating hexagons does not give a digital approximation of the hexagonal skeleton (see remark 3.6). The way to connect the end points we propose is to use Vincent's connexion algorithm ([12], pp. 278).

Algorithm for one pixel thin skeleton

1. Follow the boundary of the object
2. Test for the configurations depicted in fig. 5
3. For each of these configurations
   - Check if the whole hexagon based on the boundary configuration is totally included in the object
   - Mark the center of the included hexagons
4. Connect the marked pixels using Vincent's thinning algorithm

Finally, note that if object X is supposed to be simply connected (without holes), it is sufficient to check whether the boundary of the hexagon is included in X or not in step 3 of the algorithm.

References

1. H. Blum and R.N. Nagel. Shape description using weighted symmetric axis features. *Pattern Recognition*, 10:167–180, 1973.
2. L. Calabi and J.A. Riley. The skeletons of stable plane sets. Technical Report AF 19 (628-5711), Parke Math. Lab. Inc., One River Road, Carlisle, Massachusetts, December 1967.
3. Ch. Lantuéjoul. La squelettisation et son application aux mesures topologiques des mosaïques polycristallines. Thèse École des Mines de Paris, 1978.
4. F. Meyer. Skeletons in digital spaces. In J. Serra, editor, *Image Analysis and Mathematical Morphology, Volume 2: Theoretical Advances*. Academic Press, London, 1988.
5. W.K. Pratt. *Digital Image Processing*. John Wiley and Sons, New York, 1978.
6. J. Riley. Plane Graphs and their Skeletons. Technical Report 60429, Park Math. Lab. Inc., One River Road, Carlisle, Massachusetts, 1965.
7. M. Schmitt. Geodesic arcs in non-euclidean metrics: Application to the propagation function. *Revue d'Intelligence Artificielle*, 3 (2):43–76, 1989.

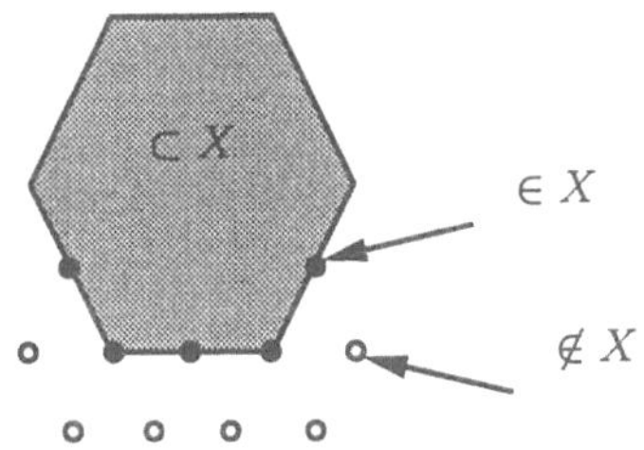

Fig. 5. Digital definition of an osculating hexagon at a maximum of curvature.

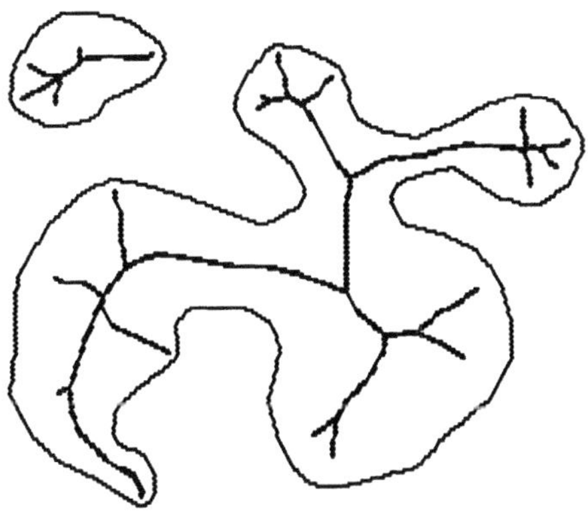

Fig. 6. Meyer's algorithm: the skeleton may be of thickness two.

8. M. Schmitt and J. Mattioli. *Morphologie Mathématique.* Logique - Mathématiques - Informatique. Masson, Décembre 1993.
9. M. Schmitt and L. Vincent. *Morphological image analysis: a practical and algorithmic handbook.* Cambridge University Press, To appear in 1994.
10. J. Serra. *Image Analysis and Mathematical Morphology.* Academic Press, London, 1982.
11. L. Vincent. *Algorithmes Morphologiques à Base de Files d'Attente et de Lacets : Extension aux Graphes.* Thèse, École des Mines, Paris, France, May 1990.
12. L. Vincent. Morphological Algorithms. In E.R. Dougherty, editor, *Mathematical Morphology in Image Processing*, Optical engineering, pages 255–288. Marcel Dekker, inc., New York - Basel - Hong Kong, 1993.

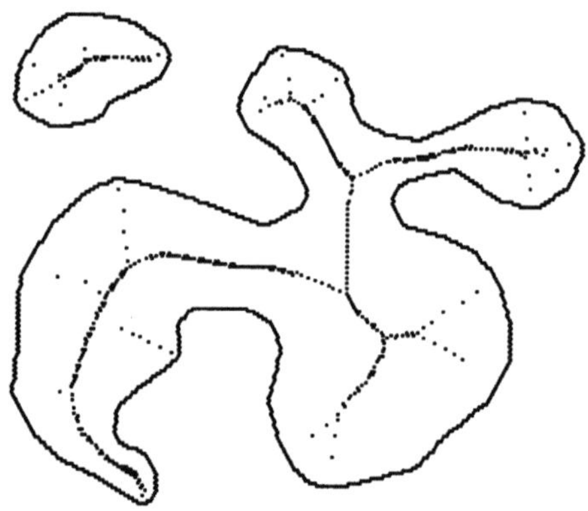

(a) – Lantuéjouls's formula (usually of thickness two)

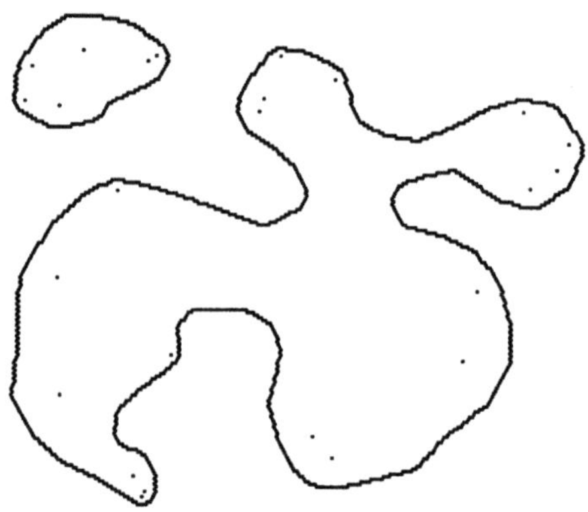

(b) – Centers of osculating hexagons at maxima of curvature

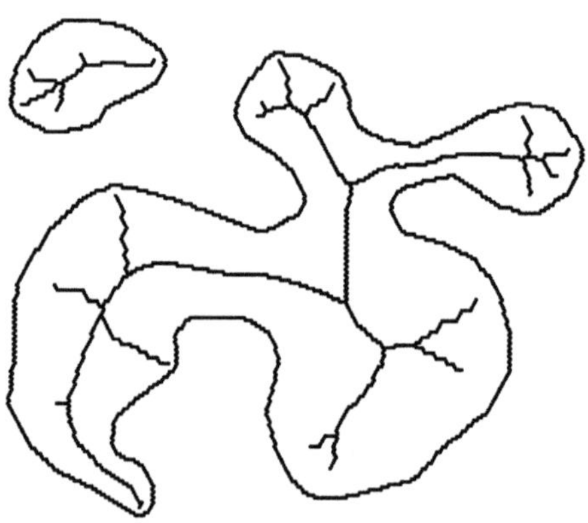

(c) – Result

Fig. 7. Illustration of our algorithm: Lantuéjoul's formula, centers of osculating hexagons at maxima of curvature and one pixel thin connection.

FAST GRAYSCALE GRANULOMETRY ALGORITHMS

LUC VINCENT
Xerox Imaging Systems
9 Centennial Drive, Peabody, MA 01960, USA

Abstract.
Granulometries constitute an extremely useful set of morphological operators, applicable to a variety of image analysis tasks. Traditional granulometry algorithms involve sequences of openings or closings of increasing size, and are therefore very slow on non-dedicated hardware. Efficient techniques have been proposed to compute granulometries in binary images, based on the concept of *opening functions.* In the present paper, a class of algorithms for computing granulometries in grayscale images is introduced. The most advanced among them are based on the new concept of *opening tree.* These algorithms are several orders of magnitude faster than traditional techniques, thereby opening up a range of new applications for grayscale granulometries.

Key words: Algorithms, Mathematical Morphology, Grayscale Granulometries, Pattern Spectrum, Opening Tree

1. Introduction, State of the Art

In a variety of image analysis problems, one is interested in extracting the *size distribution* of the "objects" or "structures" present in an image. In 1967, Matheron formally characterized meaningful size distributions by introducing the concept of *granulometry* [9, 10]:

Definition 1 *A granulometry is a family of openings $\Phi = (\phi_\lambda)_{\lambda \geq 0}$ satisfying:*

$$\forall \lambda \geq 0, \mu \geq 0, \quad \lambda \geq \mu \Longrightarrow \phi_\lambda \leq \phi_\mu. \tag{1}$$

Performing the granulometric analysis of an image I with Φ consists in mapping each size λ to a measure of the opened image $\phi_\lambda(I)$. Similarly, anti-granulometries, or granulometries *by closings,* can be defined as families of increasing closings. For more details on granulometries, see [10].

In the discrete case, a granulometry is a decreasing family of openings $\Phi = (\phi_n)_{n \geq 0}$, indexed on an integer parameter n. Denote by $m(I)$ the measure of a discrete image I: $m(I)$ is the area of I in the binary case[1] (number of "on" pixels) and the volume of I in the grayscale case (sum of pixel values). The granulometric analysis of I with Φ results in a granulometric curve:

Definition 2 *The granulometric curve or* pattern spectrum [8] *of an image, I, with respect to granulometry $\Phi = (\phi_n)_{n \geq 0}$ is the mapping $PS_\Phi(I)$ given by:*

$$\forall n > 0, \quad PS_\Phi(I)(n) = m(\phi_n(I)) - m(\phi_{n-1}(I)). \tag{2}$$

[1] In the binary case, it may be useful for some granulometries to define $m(I)$ as the number of connected components in I [2].

J. Serra and P. Soille (eds.), Mathematical Morphology and Its Applications to Image Processing, 265-272

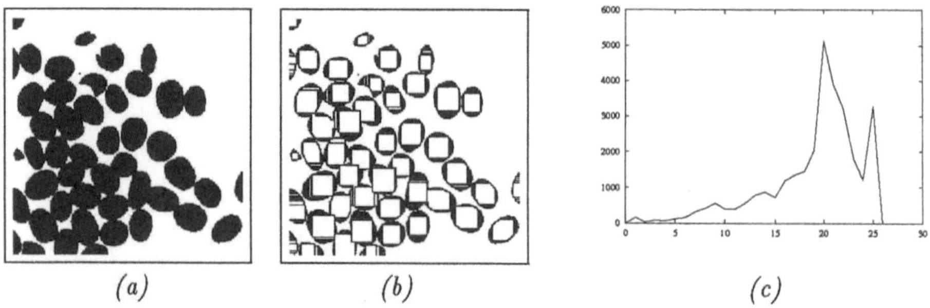

Fig. 1. (a) original binary image of coffee beans, (b) level lines of "square" opening function, (c) pattern spectrum obtained as histogram of the opening function.

In practice, the most useful granulometries are based on openings (or closings) with the homothetics of a simple convex structuring element B. Typically, B is a line segment, a square, or a hexagon. In such cases, we talk about "linear granulometries, "square granulometries", or "hexagonal granulometries" respectively. Granulometries based on maxima of openings with line segments at different orientations are also commonly used.

Until recently, determining a granulometric curve involved computing a sequence of openings of increasing size, which is very time consuming no matter how efficient the opening algorithm. Even when $\phi_n(I)$ (n-th opening in the series) can be computed in constant time (for a fixed image size), determining the pattern spectrum using openings of size 1 through n is still an $O(n)$ algorithm. For most applications, this is prohibitively costly, unless specialized hardware is used for computing the successive openings.

Over the past few years, a number of algorithms have been proposed for fast granulometries in binary images (see [6, 14, 5] and more recently [12]). These algorithms typically involve as an intermediate step the extraction of the "opening" function of the binary image studied [12]: this function maps each pixel with the size of the first opening that removes it from the image. It can be computed efficiently for all classic structuring element shapes, and the histogram of the resulting grayscale image provides the desired pattern spectrum. An example is shown in Fig. 1.

This paper treats the case of grayscale granulometries, which has not been previously addressed in literature. In section 2, a fast linear grayscale granulometry algorithm is first described (this algorithm was already briefly mentioned in [12]). Then, in section 3, the concept of *opening trees* is introduced as a way to compactly encode all the successive linear openings of a grayscale image. This concept is at the basis of another set of new algorithms for the fast computation of granulometries with maxima of linear openings, as well as approximations of square granulometric curves. Timing results prove that the introduced algorithms are several orders of magnitude faster than traditional techniques.

2. Linear Granulometries

In this section, the case of granulometries using openings with line segments is considered[2]. For simplicily, let us assume that the line segments used as structuring elements are horizontal (the algorithm easily extends to any orientation). The opening ϕ_n in the series is the opening with structuring element L_n:

$$L_n = \underbrace{\bullet \; \bullet \; \bullet \cdots \bullet \; \bullet}_{n+1 \text{ pixels}} \qquad (3)$$

Let us analyze the effect of an opening by L_n, $n \geq 0$ on a grayscale image I. Denote by $N_l(p)$ and $N_r(p)$ respectively the left and the right neighbors of a pixel p.

Definition 3 *A horizontal line segment S, of length $l(S)$, is a set of pixels $\{p_0, p_1, \ldots, p_{n-1}\}$ such that for $0 < i < n$, $p_i = N_r(p_{i-1})$.*

Definition 4 *A* horizontal maximum *M of length $l(M) = n$ in grayscale image I is a horizontal line segment $\{p_0, p_1, \ldots, p_{n-1}\}$ such that:*

$$\forall i, 0 < i < n, \quad I(p_i) = I(p_1) \quad \textit{and} \quad I(N_l(p_0)) < I(p_0), \;\; I(N_r(p_{n-1})) < I(p_0). \quad (4)$$

This notion is the 1-D equivalent of the classic *regional maximum* concept [7]. The study of how such maxima are altered through horizontal openings is at the basis of the algorithm introduced in this section. Denote by $I \circ B$ the opening of image I by a structuring element B. The following proposition holds:

Proposition 5 *Let $M = \{p_0, p_1, \ldots, p_{n-1}\}$ be a horizontal maximum of I.*

$$\forall k < n, \forall p \in M, \quad (I \circ L_k)(p) = I(p), \quad (5)$$
$$\textit{for } k = n, \forall p \in M, \quad (I \circ L_n)(p) = \max\{I(N_l(p_0)), I(N_r(p_{n-1}))\} < I(p). \quad (6)$$

That is, any opening of I by a line segment L_k such that $k < n$ leaves this maximum unchanged, whereas for any $k \geq n$, all the pixels of M have a lower value in $I \circ L_k$ than in I. Furthermore, we can *quantify* the effect of an opening of size n on the pixels of this maximum: the value of each pixel $p \in M$ is decreased from $I(p)$ to $\max\{I(N_l(p_0)), I(N_r(p_{n-1}))\}$. In granulometric terms, the contribution of maximum M to the n-th bin of the horizontal pattern spectrum $\mathrm{PS}_h(I)$ is:

$$n \times [I(p) - \max\{I(N_l(p_0)), I(N_r(p_{n-1}))\}]. \quad (7)$$

This is illustrated by Fig. 2.

Additionally, the local effect of a horizontal opening of size n on M is that a new "plateau" of pixels is created at altitude $\max\{I(N_l(p_0)), I(N_r(p_{n-1}))\}$. This plateau P contains M, and may be itself a maximum of $I \circ L_n$. If it is, we say that P is part of the *maximal region* $R(M)$ surrounding maximum M, and we can now compute the contribution of P to the $l(P)$-th bin of the pattern spectrum, etc. Following this principle, the proposed granulometry algorithm works as follows on each image line:

[2] The algorithm described in this section applies to 1-D signals as well.

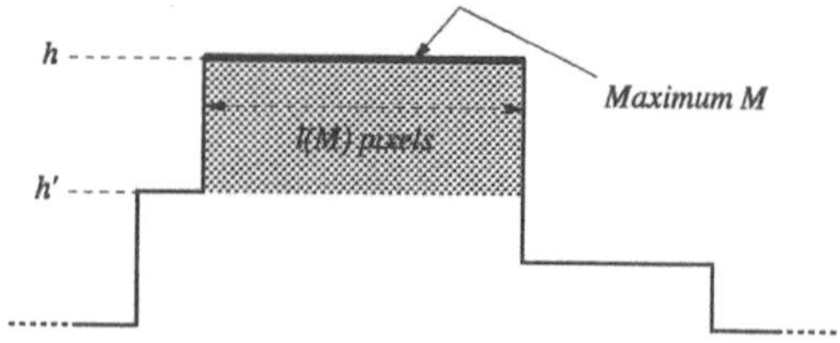

Fig. 2. Horizontal cross section of I with a maximum M. The shaded area, of volume $(h-h')\times l(M)$ shows the local contribution of this maximum to the $l(M)$-th bin of the horizontal pattern spectrum.

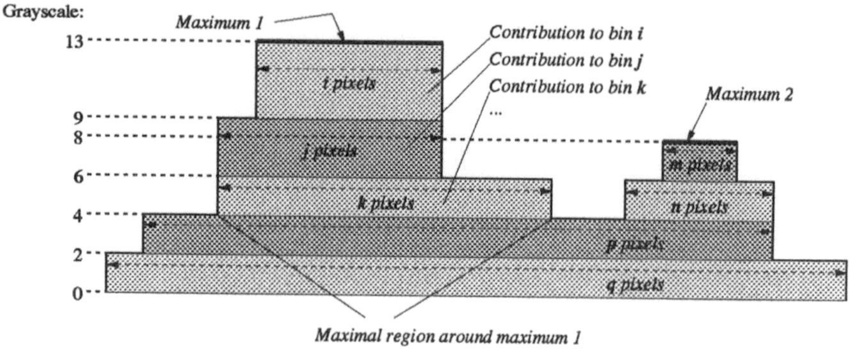

Fig. 3. Illustration of horizontal grayscale granulometry algorithm for a line with two maxima. In this case, maxima were scanned from left to right. Processing maximum 1 results in bins i, j, and k of the pattern spectrum being incremented. While processing maximum 2, bins m and n are first incremented, then the algorithm skips over the already processed maximal region, and bins p and q are incremented. The maximal region around maximum 2 is the entire line.

Algorithm: horizontal granulometry of an image line

- `for each maximum` M `of this line (in any order) do:`
  - `Adds contribution of this maximum to` $l(M)$`-th bin of pattern spectrum;`
  - `Let` P `be the plateau of pixels formed by opening of size` $l(M)$ `of` M`; if` P `is itself a maximum of` $I \circ L_{l(M)}$`, computes its contribution to bin` $l(P)$ `of pattern spectrum;`
  - `Iterate previous step until the new plateau formed is no longer a maximum;`
  - ```Mark'' the maximal region around`` M `as already processed;`

Note that this algorithm is inherently recursive: once a maximal region R has been processed, all of its pixels are regarded as having the gray-level they were given by the last opening considered for R. In practice though, there is no need to physically modify the values of all the pixels in R: keeping track of the first and last pixels of R is sufficient, allowing the algorithm to efficiently skip over already processed maximal regions (see Fig. 3). Thanks to this trick, the algorithm only considers each image pixel *twice* in the worst case.

This algorithm was compared to the traditional opening-based technique. For the latter, a fast opening algorithm was used, whose speed is proportional to the number of pixels in the image and (almost) independent of the length of the line segment used as structuring element. As illustrated by table I, the new algorithm described in this section is *three orders of magnitude faster.*

3. Granulometries with Maxima of Linear Openings

In order to deal with more complicated cases, we now introduce a technique that can be seen as a generalization of the concept of opening functions for the grayscale case. When performing openings of increasing size of a binary image, each "on" pixel p is turned "off" for an opening size given by the value of the opening function at pixel p. In other words, the opening function encodes for each pixel the successive values it takes for increasing opening sizes (namely, a series of of 1's followed by a series of 0's). Similarly, in the grayscale case, as the size of the opening increases, the value of each pixel decreases monotonically. If each pixel was assigned the list of values it takes for every opening size, then the corresponding grayscale granulometry could be extracted straightforwardly.

Unfortunately, even if it were possible to compute such lists of values quickly, assigning one to each image pixel would require far too much memory. A more compact representation needs to be designed, that takes into account the intrinsic "redundancy" of opened images, characterized by their large plateaus of pixels. If we again consider the linear case, an elegant solution can be proposed to both the problem of computing these lists of values, and the problem of storing them compactly:

Let M be a horizontal maximum of image I, with altitude (grayscale) h. We pointed out in the previous section that a horizontal opening of size $l(M)$ of M takes all of its pixels down to a new value h'. Beyond this, the following proposition can easily be proved:

Proposition 6 *Let $n > 0$, I a grayscale image such that $I = I \circ L_{n-1}$. Then, for every pixel p in I:*

$$(I \circ L_n)(p) < I(p) \Longleftrightarrow \exists M \text{ horiz maximum such that } l(M) = n \text{ and } p \in M. \quad (8)$$

Therefore, at opening n in the sequence, the only pixels affected are those which belong to maxima of length n. Furthermore, all the pixels belonging to the same maximum M, $l(M) = n$, will be affected in the same way for any opening of size greater than or equal to n. The list of decreasing values we wish to associate with each pixel in M can therefore "converge" into one single list for size n. For larger opening sizes, this list may itself be merged with other lists, etc.

Based on this principle, the algorithm introduced here represents each image line as a tree T, which we call its *opening tree.* The leaves of T are the image pixels, and the nodes are made of pairs (h, n), where h is a grayscale value and n is an opening size. Every pixel that can be reached by going upwards in the tree starting from node (h, n) is such that its value for the opening of size n is h. Conversely, starting from a pixel p, successive pairs (h_1, n_1), (h_2, v_2),..., (h_1, v_i),..., are reached by going down towards the root of the tree. By convention, for this pixel, $(h_0, n_0) = (I(p), 0)$. These pairs satisfy:

$$\forall i > 0, \quad h_i > h_{i+1} \text{ and } n_i < n_{i+1}. \quad (9)$$

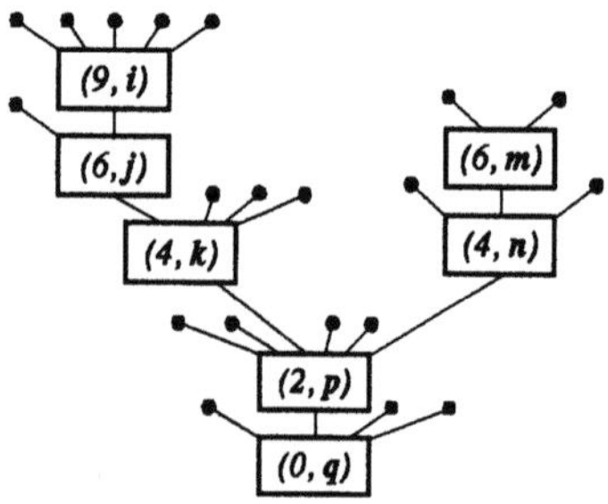

Fig. 4. Opening tree representation of the image line of Fig. 3. The leaves of this tree (•) correspond to the image pixels.

For $n \geq 0$, the value of the opening of size n of I at pixel p is given by:

$$(I \circ L_n)(p) = h_j, \quad \text{where } j \text{ is such that } n_j \leq n < n_{j+1}. \tag{10}$$

Opening trees can be computed using an algorithm very similar to the one described in the previous section. An example of opening tree is shown in Fig. 4.

Opening trees provide a hierarchical description that can be used to compactly represent *all* the horizontal openings of a grayscale image. In this respect, this notion is a grayscale equivalent of the opening function mentioned earlier (see Fig. 1). One can prove that, in the worst case, the opening tree has one node per image pixel. In practice though, only between 0.3 and 0.9 nodes per pixel are needed depending on the complexity of the image processed.

Any horizontal opening of I can be straightforwardly derived from its opening tree. In addition, the horizontal pattern spectrum of I, $\text{PS}_h(I)$, can be computed from T as follows:

Algorithm: horizontal granulometry of I from its opening tree

- initialize each bin of pattern spectrum $\text{PS}_h(I)$ to 0;
- for each pixel p of I do:
  - $v \leftarrow I(p)$; $(h, n) \leftarrow$ node pointed at by p;
  - while (h, n) exists, do:
    $\text{PS}_h(I)(n) \leftarrow \text{PS}_h(I)(n) + (v - h)$;
    $v \leftarrow h$; $(h, n) \leftarrow$ next node down in tree;

This algorithm is obviously less efficient for horizontal granulometries than the one introduced in the previous section. However, it easily generalizes to the computation of granulometries using maxima of linear openings in several orientations. For example, to determine the granulometric curve corresponding to maxima of horizontal and vertical openings, one first extracts the horizontal opening tree T_1 and the vertical opening tree T_2. Then, for each pixel p, the technique consists in descending the corresponding branches of T_1 and T_2 simultaneously as follows:

Algorithm: granulometry of I from opening trees T_1 and T_2

- initialize each bin of pattern spectrum $\text{PS}(I)$ to 0;
- for each pixel p of I do:
  - $v \leftarrow I(p)$;

```
– (h1, n1) ← node of T1 pointed at by p;
– (h2, n2) ← node of T2 pointed at by p;
– while (h1, n1) and (h2, n2) exist, do:
      size ← max(n1, n2);
      while n1 ≤ size and (h1, n1) exists do:
          (h1, n1) ← next node down in T1;
      while n2 ≤ size and (h2, n2) exists do:
          (h2, n2) ← next node down in T2;
      PS(I)(size) ← PS(I)(size) + (v − max(h1, h2));
      v ← max(h1, h2);
```

The same technique extends to any number of opening trees. The whole granulometry algorithm (extraction of trees followed by computation of the pattern spectrum from these trees) is once again orders of magnitude faster than traditional techniques, as illustrated by table I. In this table, a granulometry by maxima of linear openings at 4 orientations was computed. In terms of memory, the computation of this particular granulometry requires, in the worst case, 1 pointer (4 bytes) and 1 node (8 bytes) per pixel, for each orientation. This comes to a total of 48 bytes/pixel, i.e., a worst case scenario of 12 Megabytes for a 512×512 image. This is a reasonable tradeoff given the speed of the algorithm, and is not a strain on modern systems.

TABLE I

Execution time of traditional opening-based techniques and of introduced algorithms for the computation of a horizontal grayscale granulometry (left) and a granulometry by maxima of linear openings in 4 orientations (right). A complex 512×512 image was used for this comparison, done on a Sun Sparc Station 10. Granulometries were computed for opening sizes 1 to 512.

horizontal			in 4 orientations		
traditional	new	improvement factor	traditional	new	improvement factor
204s	0.206s	990	824s	2.78s	296

The algorithm given above can be easily adjusted to the computation of *pseudo-granulometries* by *minima* of linear openings (for more details, see [13]). Although minima of openings are not themselves openings [10], minima of openings with line segments of increasing length constitute a decreasing family of image operators. The resulting pseudo-granulometric curves often characterize the same image features as square granulometries[3]. They have been very successful as one of the feature sets used to characterize plankton in towed video microscopy images [3].

4. Conclusion

In the present paper, a novel class of algorithms was introduced for efficiently computing granulometries in grayscale images. These algorithms turn out to be several orders of magnitude faster than any previously available technique. One of their key underlying concepts is that of *opening tree:* such structures are shown to provide a compact representation for the successive openings of a grayscale image by

[3] The author wishes to thank Gaile Gordon for this useful insight.

line segments of increasing size. They are at the heart of the algorithm proposed for grayscale granulometries with maxima of linear openings. In addition, opening trees provide a way to extract pseudo-granulometries by minima of openings with line segments at different orientations, which can be used to approximate square granulometries. These algorithms can even be extended to the fast computation of granulometries by area openings and closings [11], as described in [13]. However, the efficient computation of *exact* grayscale granulometries with square openings remains an open problem (no pun intended).

Over the past few years, grayscale granulometries have proved to be useful in a variety of image analysis tasks, including texture classification [1] and picture segmentation [4]. However, these applications have often been handicapped by slow processing speeds. The efficiency of the algorithms introduced in the present paper not only makes it now possible to use granulometries on a routine basis, they also open new areas of application for these tools. For example, in [12], it was briefly shown how linear granulometries can be used to directly extract *global* estimates of object size in grayscale images without the need for any segmentation or binarization. Extracting such information is sometimes a goal in itself, but it can also be essential to calibrate the parameters of subsequent image analysis algorithms to be applied, thereby greatly enhancing their robustness. Undoubtedly, the family of algorithms introduced in this paper will contribute to popularize the use of granulometries for a growing number of image and signal analysis problems.

References

1. Y. Chen and E. Dougherty. Texture classification by gray-scale morphological granulometries. In *SPIE Vol. 1818, Visual Communications and Image Processing*, Boston MA, Nov. 1992.
2. M. Coster and J.-L. Chermant. *Précis d'Analyse d'Images*. CNRS Ed., Paris, 1985.
3. C. S. Davis, S. M. Gallager, and A. R. Solow. Microaggregations of oceanic plankton observed by towed video microscopy. *Science*, 257:230–232, Jan. 1992.
4. E. Dougherty, J. Pelz, F. Sand, and A. Lent. Morphological image segmentation by local granulometric size distributions. *Journal of Electronic Imaging*, 1(1), Jan. 1992.
5. R. M. Haralick, S. Chen, and T. Kanungo. Recursive opening transform. In *IEEE Int. Computer Vision and Pattern Recog. Conference*, pages 560–565, Champaign IL, June 1992.
6. B. Laÿ. Recursive algorithms in mathematical morphology. In *Acta Stereologica Vol. 6/III*, pages 691–696, Caen, France, Sept. 1987. 7th International Congress For Stereology.
7. F. Maisonneuve. Extrema régionaux: Algorithme parallèle. Technical Report 781, Ecole des Mines, CGMM, Paris, 1982.
8. P. Maragos. Pattern spectrum and multiscale shape representation. *IEEE Trans. Pattern Anal. Machine Intell.*, 11(7):701–716, July 1989.
9. G. Matheron. *Eléments pour une Théorie des Milieux Poreux*. Masson, Paris, 1967.
10. G. Matheron. *Random Sets and Integral Geometry*. John Wiley and Sons, New York, 1975.
11. L. Vincent. Morphological area openings and closings for grayscale images. In *NATO Shape in Picture Workshop*, pages 197–208, Driebergen, The Netherlands, Sept. 1992.
12. L. Vincent. Fast opening functions and morphological granulometries. In *SPIE Image Algebra and Morphological Image Processing V*, San Diego, CA, July 1994.
13. L. Vincent. Grayscale granulometries: Fast algorithms and new image analysis applications. manuscript, to be published, June 1994.
14. L.-P. Yuan. A fast algorithm for size analysis of irregular pore areas. In *SPIE/SPSE Vol. 1451, Nonlinear Image Processing II*, pages 125–136, San Jose, CA, Feb. 1991.

AN EFFICIENT IMPLEMENTATION TECHNIQUE OF ADAPTIVE MORPHOLOGICAL OPERATIONS*

S. FEJES and F. VAJDA
Department of Information Technology,
KFKI Research Institute for Measurement and Computing Techniques
of the Hungarian Academy of Sciences,
P.O.Box 49, 1525 Budapest, Hungary.

Abstract. In the paper the implementation aspects of mathematical morphology based on a new formalization of the window operation is presented. The proposed technique called the Reverse Window Operation (RWO) can also be applied to adaptive morphological operations. In order to reduce the control complexity an algorithm is proposed, which uses a region-based parameter modification for the structuring element adaptation. Finally, an application of a data-dependent processing technique using the adaptive filter scheme is demonstrated.

Key words: Mathematical morphology, Adaptive filtering, Reverse window-operation, Envelope scan method, Control region optimization, Region-based parameter adaptation.

1. Introduction

Facing with challenges related to image processing the problems are multifold. Even if an efficient algorithm is already available, an efficient implementation has to be also used in many applications. Due to the large amount of data to be processed and the often strict time constraints (real time applications) only dedicated architectures can count. Therefore, the special relationship between the algorithms and the architectures needs a totally new approach and technology of the design phase.

In the first section of the paper a brief overview is given on the dominant elements of adaptive filtering and its applications to morphological operations. The next section presents an efficient implementation for morphological operations. Based on a novel alternative of the window operation (*Reverse Window Operation*, RWO [1]) and a technique called the *Envelope Scan Method* (ESM, [2]) an architecture is proposed for both binary and gray scale operations. The proposed architecture can directly support flexible adaptation of the Structuring Element (SE). It is discussed in the fourth section in details. In this section an algorithm is also introduced providing a reduction method of the number of control parameters ("filter taps"). In the last section an input data-driven filter scheme is demonstrated.

2. Adaptive Techniques in Morphological Processing

Adaptive filtering is a favorable tool for advanced data processing. The adaptive approach is able to deal with unknown statistics of the signal, which can be very

* This work was partly supported by OTKA Grant No. T4044.

J.Serra and P. Soille (eds.), Mathematical Morphology and Its Applications to Image Processing, 273-280

useful when dealing with extremely variant signal/image environment, such as noise filtering, image enhancement, etc. Nonlinear filters (*stack filters*, such as *median filters*, *rank-order filters* or *morphological filters*, etc.) with adaptive features has been becoming a new area in addition to the traditional adaptive linear filtering.

Morphological filters belong to a special class of *stack filters*. They can be characterized by the properties of *threshold decomposition*, *stacking*, *idempotence* and *increasing operators* [3, 4, 5, 6].

Adaptive approach in morphological processing can be defined on several levels. The elementary adaptation step may refer to individual pixels, regions or even pictures, as well. Each form of adaptivity provides different grade of adaptive behavior.

On the other hand, as far as the adaptation process is concerned there are two main approaches. According to the first one, a *training set* is used to get the optimal filtering for a given type of data. In this case the input is supposed to be stationary, which may be a strong restriction to many applications. In contrast, the second method is applied to *run-time* data, i.e., the filter is continuously optimized to the current statistics of the input.

In addition, *data-driven* techniques can also be interpreted as special cases of adaptive processing. According to this scheme, the parameter is not adjusted by the error signal deduced from the difference between the output and a reference signal, but by the input itself.

3. Implementation of Morphological Operations

3.1. Alternative Formulation of the Window Operations

Many image manipulation techniques are based on *window operations* [7], in which a certain region of pixels is scanned and according to a window function one output pixel is generated. As an alternative form of the window operation, the *Reverse Window Operation* (RWO, [1]) scans only *one central* pixel, upon which the new value of a whole *region* is defined taking into account the template (window) function β (see Fig. 1). Although, the two methods are not equivalent in a stricter sense, both can be applied to morphological operations. Considering e.g. the *Minkowski addition* (dilation)

$$X \oplus B = max\{x_{i-j} + b_j,\ j \in B\}, \tag{1}$$

which can be directly represented by Fig. 1a, if the window function represents the $\{max\}$ operation. In contrast, using the RWO-scheme the $\{max\}$ operation becomes unnecessary. It is due to the fact, that the consecutive write operations superimpose each other in the sense that a smaller value cannot overwrite a greater one. The same principle can be applied to the Minkowski subtraction (erosion) considering the duality principle of erosion and dilation.

3.2. Implementation of the Binary Morphological Operations

Using a systolic array [8] an efficient implementation of morphological operations can be obtained based on the RWO-principle. In binary case, the function of the flat SE is represented by OR-gates (at dilation) or AND-gates (at erosion) inserted into the data-path according to the binary template of the SE (see Fig. 2).

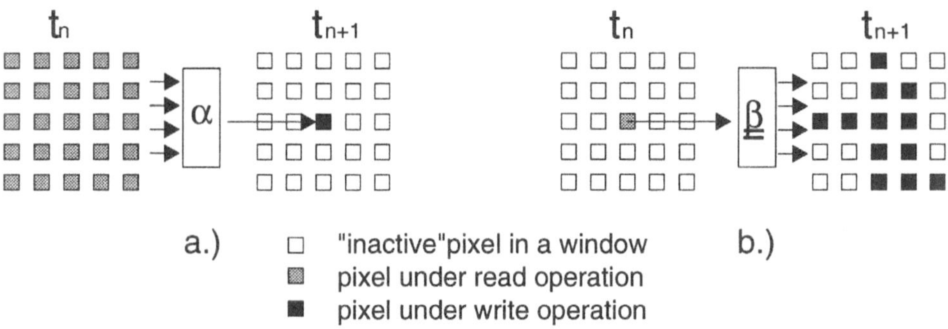

Fig. 1. Window operations: the traditional scheme (a) and the Reverse Window Operation (RWO) (b).

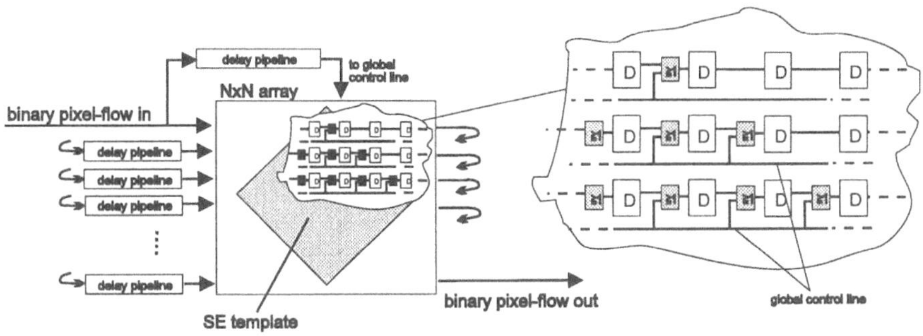

Fig. 2. The proposed systolic array based on the RWO-principle. The operation is a Minkowski addition (dilation) using flat SE.

3.3. Gray Scale Operations

The *threshold decomposition* of morphological operations can make it feasible to define an architecture for gray scales by combining several layers of the binary array. Applying the *Envelope Scan Method* (ESM, [1, 2]) the number of elementary operations can be strongly reduced. This method is based on the fact that the operations have to be calculated only on the *envelope* of the gray scales. It can be proved, that the operations on internal (lower) gray levels, i.e., not on the top surface, have no effect on the output.

To force the SE hover on the top gray level a *template control unit* has to be connected to the file of binary systolic arrays. On each layer the *cross section* of the SE's template (or *umbra* under a given altitude) is partitioned into *regions*. Each region corresponds to a given gray level of the 3D SE. They have to be activated on every layer by one according to the required "altitude", which is defined by the *top surface* of the pixel currently being read. This pixel position should correspond to the *reference point* of the SE. When dealing with several gray levels the *global control line* of a binary layer (Fig. 2) is split into several *region activation lines* (see also Section 4.3) to achieve the proper template control.

4. Adaptation of the Structuring Element

According to the general scheme the adaptive approach tries to optimize the filter parameters to minimize the given error criterion (e.g., Mean Square Error (MSE) or Mean Absolute Error (MAE), [9, 3]). At morphological operations the most obvious way of adaptation is the optimization of the Structuring Element (SE). Let us investigate the algorithm of the Least Mean Squares (LMS),

$$b_i' = b_i + 2\mu(d_i - y_i)\frac{dy_i}{db_j}, \tag{2}$$

where b_j stands for the parameter to be optimized, b_j' represents the new value, μ is the convergence parameter, y_i and d_i denote the output and the reference signal, respectively. Foe example at the Minkowski addition (Eq.1) the gradient $\frac{dy_i}{db_j}$ has to be computed for the $max\{\}$ operation, which in turn, cannot be directly applied.

In order to solve this problem the relationship between the input and the output of a morphological processing scheme has to be investigated in terms of a gradient. Using the definition of the Equation 1 with a small modification:

$$y_i = x_{i-m} + b_m, \text{ where } \; m \in B, \tag{3}$$

where m is the index of the element, which causes the summation term to reach its *maximum*, it can be concluded, that

$$\frac{dy_i}{db_j} = \begin{cases} 1 \text{ if } j = m \\ 0 \text{ otherwise} \end{cases}$$

An exact mathematical proof of the problem can be found in [9]. Finally, from Equations 2 and 3 it is obvious, that

$$b_m' = b_m + 2\mu(d_i - y_i) \text{ and } b_i' = b_i, \text{ where } m \neq i. \tag{4}$$

It shows, that the application of the LMS for morphological operation can be expressed in a very simple form. Referring to [9] again, an algorithm is proposed for the adaptation of flat SE. According to this method the adaptation of the flat SE can be treated the similar way as that of the 3D, but the parameters have to be normed to binary values "0" or "1".

4.1. The Adaptation Algorithm using the RWO

The architecture proposed in Section 3 can be extended to adaptive operations, however, the RWO-principle does not support individual parameter adaptation. On the contrary, the adaptation based on a RWO-scheme should be applied rather to *regions* introduced in Section 3.3. The use of regions can be useful to reduce the control complexity of the adaptation algorithm. Therefore, a systematic method has to be found to define the parameter control regions of the given adaptive morphological operation.

4.2. Reducing Control Complexity of Morphological Operations

In order to reduce the degree of freedom of the filter parameter control a training set of the input data has to be investigated. During the adaptation process the individually, but "nearly" identically controlled filter parameters could be adjusted as a whole. Before defining an algorithm for the parameter partitions the basic notations have to be introduced.

Let B be the support of the SE with N*N individual parameters. I order to assemble all important data about the parameter modification the variations of the SEs templates have to be investigated. Therefore, the parameter settings of the "fundamental" structuring elements that can be the most important from the adaptation point of view are recorded. Let $\mathcal{B}$ be denote the set of these SE'. Furthermore, the row vector b_i^T consists of the individual parameter settings of each SE in the following way:

$$b_i^T = (b_{i,1}, \ldots, b_{i,N^2}), \text{ where } b_i^T \in \mathcal{B} \text{ and } i = 1, \ldots, n. \tag{5}$$

Our final goal is to define the set $\mathcal{P}$ of partitions $\mathcal{R}_k$ in a way, that if

$$\mathcal{R}_k \in B, \text{ then } \mathcal{R}_k \cap \mathcal{R}_l = \emptyset \text{ ,if } k \neq l, \text{ where } k, l = 1, \ldots, n_R, \tag{6}$$

i.e., the regions (partitions) have to be disjunct sets included by the support. n_R denotes the number of regions obtained by the partitioning process.

In order to unify individual filter parameters into a region their activation, i.e., the coincidence of their activation has to be taken into consideration. Therefore, let us introduce the *differential matrix* D_i by the following definition:

$$D_i = [d_{kl}]_i, \text{ where } d_{kl}^i = (b_{ik} - b_{il})^2, \text{ and } k, l = 1, \ldots, N^2. \tag{7}$$

The ith differential matrix describes the coincidence of each parameter activation of the ith SE template. However, not one but all the SE templates have to be taken into consideration to obtain the region partitioning valid for the whole adaptation process. Consequently, of each element of the set $\{D_i\}$ the maximum has to be selected at a parameter position to get a statistics for the series of the SE templates considering the deviation of the activation of the given parameter pair:

$$\Delta = [\delta_{kl}] = [\delta_k^T], \text{ where } \delta_{kl} = max\{d_{kl}^i\}, \; i = 1, \ldots, n. \tag{8}$$

Taking Equations 5-8 the rule of the region partitioning can be formalized. Let p and q be two parameter locations in the support B. In addition, $\mathcal{P}^\lambda = \{\mathcal{R}_k^\lambda\}$ denotes the region distribution at an error limit of λ. Then

$$\forall p, q \in \mathcal{R}_k^\lambda, \text{ if and only if } \delta_{pq} < \lambda. \tag{9}$$

According to Equation 9 a simple algorithm can be constructed to partition the parameter locations (the individual supports) into regions. As far as the optimal distribution of the regions is concerned, there seems to be no analytical guarantee to reach the optimum concerning the possible least number of regions that meets the error criterion λ. In order to get better results special techniques, such as e.g. simulated annealing could also by applied.

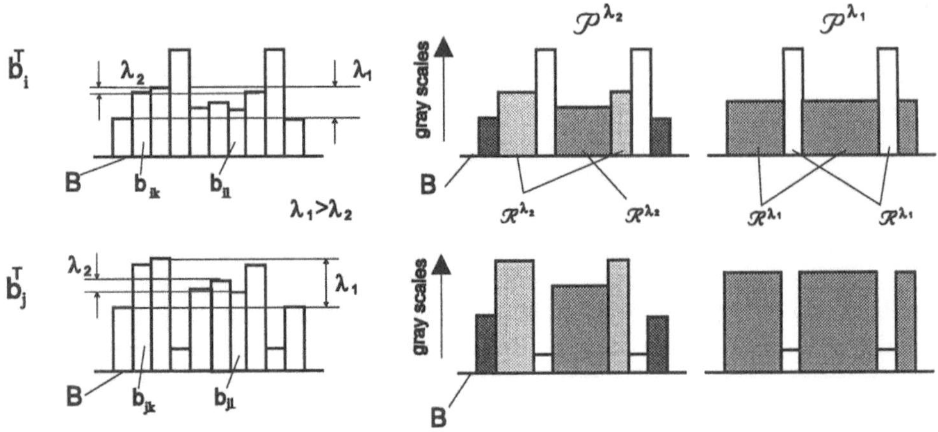

Fig. 3. The region optimization process of 3D SE. The individual SE parameters (on the left) have been merged into regions according to error limits λ_1 and λ_2, respectively.

The scheme of the partitioning for 3D SEs is showed in Fig. 3. The error level λ determines the granularity of the regions. The higher the error limit is the less number of regions can be created, but of course, with less accuracy and convergency of the adaptation process. As far as the stability of the region-controlled adaptation is concerned the study of the convergency behaviour in terms of the error limit is currently in the focus of further researches.

4.3. An Architecture for Adaptive Morphological Operations

The architecture proposed in Section 3 can be applied to adaptive operations with special care. The relationship between the output and the input of an operation based on the RWO-principle is not known. Therefore, additional identical arrays called *region activation pipelines* have to be added to the original scheme (see Fig. 4). Each activation pipeline is assigned to *one* control region of the flat SE or to that of a cross section in case of a 3D SE. The pipelines have no pixel input, their outputs are determined solely by the activation of the region they have been assigned to. Receiving a pixel at the output of the *processor array* the current value(s) of the binary *region activation pipeline(s)* signalize the region(s), by which the current pixel was resulted (see also Equation 3). These outputs are then processed by the adaptation unit, which activates the selected regions by feeding back the error signal to close the adaptation loop.

Extending the architecture to 3D SE the output becomes a vector $\overline{y}_i$ of the individual decision values of each binary layer according to the threshold decomposition principle. In this case, however, the output must obey the *stacking constraint*, therefore, the adaptation algorithm supervises each individual output bit. In [3] an operation called *Swap* is proposed to enforce the output according to the constraint. If an output bit violates the rule, i.e., $y_i^k < y_i^l$, if $k > l$, then a *swap* operation is executed. It is continued until no output bit violates the constraint. Unfortunately, this algorithm can be complex and time consuming in case of large number of gray levels. Therefore, more simple methods (e.g. correction of the constraint violation

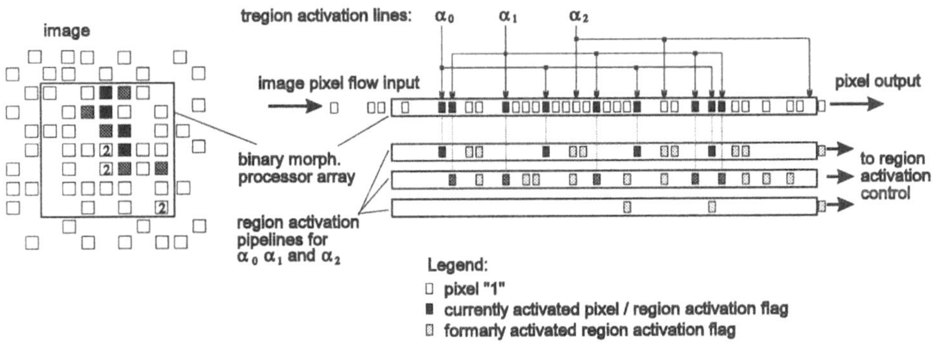

Fig. 4. The basic binary processor array is extended with 3 region activation pipelines to book-keep the source of the current output. α_0 and α_1 are currently being activated, while α_2 is inactive.

by simple overwrite operation) could also be applied. However, in these cases a strongly decreased convergency may have to be considered.

5. Applications on Images

In Fig. 5 a special application of adaptive filters (it can also be referred to as *open loop adaptation scheme*) is presented. A camera picture sequence of street traffic (left top) has been recorded. Following the extraction of the foreground (i.e., vehicles in the selected traffic lane) a sophisticated segmentation can be obtained by a mask-driven "open loop adaptation" [10]. The modification of the size of the SE (disc) is performed by a region-controlled adaptive filter using an input mask. The size of the applied SE has to correspond to the sizes of the objets decreasing by the distance to obtain optimal solution. In contrast, elementary operations would need a number of steps to gain the same result.

6. Conclusions

Adaptive morphological operations have been studied concerning implementation aspects. A new implementation and adaptation scheme has been proposed using the principle of the Reverse Window Operation. This alternative formulation of the window operation provides not only an efficient implementation for "stationary" morphological operations or operation sequences, but it can also support adaptive applications. In order to reduce the control complexity of the adaptation process a systematic method has been presented for the reduction of the parameter space. According to this method a region-based parameter control is applied. Finally, an application of a data-driven morphological operation is demonstrated using the proposed region-based filter scheme.

References

1. S. Fejes and F. Vajda. New pipelined image processor for morphological operations. In *Proceedings of the Workshop on Design Methodologies for microelectronics and signal processing,*

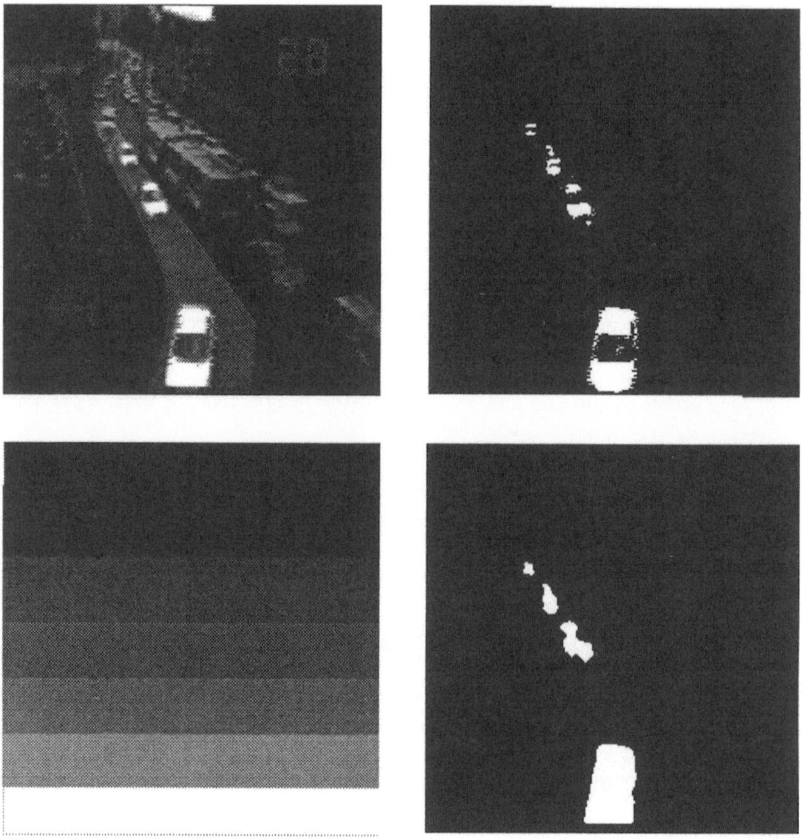

Fig. 5. Input data-driven application of an adaptive filter based on region-based parameter control. The input image (top left), the extracted foreground (top right), the input mask (bottom left) for the size-control of the SE (closing) and the properly segmented vehicles (bottom right).

pages 63–71, Gliwice-Cracow, Poland, October 20-23 1993.

2. F. Vajda and S. Fejes. An efficient morphology architecture. Orlando, Florida, April 4-8 1994. Signal Processing, Sensor Fusion and Target Recognition III of the SPIE's International Symposium on Optical Engineering and Photonics in Aerospace Sensing.
3. T.M. Sellke J.H. Lin and E.J. Coyle. Adaptive stack filtering under the mean absolute error criterion. *IEEE Trans. Acoust., Speech, Signal Processing*, ASSP-38(6):938–954, June 1992.
4. J. Serra. *Image analysis and mathematical morphology*, volume 1. Academic Press, 1982.
5. J. Serra, editor. *Image analysis and mathematical morphology*, volume 2. Academic Press, 1988. Theoretical advances.
6. P. Maragos and R.W. Schafer. Morphological filters - part I and part II. *IEEE Trans. Acoust., Speech, Signal Processing*, ASSP-35:1153–1184, 1987.
7. F. Vajda. Application and implementation of window-based image processing algorithms. *Microprocessing and Microprogramming*, 30:447–454, 1990.
8. S.Y. Kung. *VLSI array processors*. Academic Press, 1988.
9. P. Salembier. Structuring element adaptation for morphological filters. *Journal of Visual Communication and Image Representation*, 3(2):115–136, June 1992.
10. S. Fejes and Z.Fazekas. *Digital image processing in traffic control*. KFKI Internal Report, March 1994.

IMPLEMENTATION OF A DISTRIBUTED WATERSHED ALGORITHM

ALINA N. MOGA, TIMO VIERO, BOGDAN P. DOBRIN and MONCEF GABBOUJ
Tampere University of Technology, Signal Processing Laboratory
P.O. Box 553, FIN-33101 Tampere
Finland

Abstract. In this paper a parallel implementation of Meyer watershed algorithm, which does not construct watersheds between catchment basins [2, 10], is developed. A single program multiple data (SPMD) approach is used. Although the watershed algorithm is highly sequential, we have found that much parallelism can be exploited in a loosely coupled system by dividing the task to a set of processes supervised by a master process. Specialized flooding and communication methods have been developed for an efficient parallel computation of watersheds.

Key words: parallel processing, watershed algorithm, segmentation, communication in distributed systems, efficiency, running time

1. Introduction

The watershed transformation has been widely and successfully applied in different domains (e.g., in biology, medicine, computer vision). In some applications, the computation of watersheds for large image data sets may exceed the capability of a single processor computer. Due to the growing availability and cost effectiveness of multiprocessor and distributed systems, parallel computation of watersheds is becoming increasingly attractive. Parallel approach offers several advantages. First, it reduces the running time for large images. However, due to an intensive communication among processes, distribution of the computation of watersheds to n processes will not decrease the running time by a factor of n. Second, due to the divide-and-conquer domain decomposition, parallel watershed algorithm is tractable for very large images or image sequences for which memory requirements are higher than what is commonly available on a single processor computer.

The general method of using concurrent computers is by dividing the data associated with the problem to be solved into parts or grains; one grain per node of the concurrent computer. The maximum amount of a process module that can be performed before communication with other processes is done is referred to as the granularity of the parallel algorithm. It may be quantified as the ratio of the amount of computation to the number of communication events [3]. The granularity of parallel watershed algorithm is affected by the distribution of the image data among processes, the number of processors, and the content of image data. Small grains (a fine division) implies a larger number of border pixels compared to coarse division and, thus, more communication among processes is required.

In this paper implementation of a watershed algorithm on a network of worksta-

J.Serra and P. Soille (eds.), Mathematical Morphology and Its Applications to Image Processing, 281-288

tions is discussed. A cluster of seven DEC^R Alpha AXP workstations connected by FDDI is used. The drawback of FDDI is that all the communication is done across the same channel slowing down the running time. A better multicomputer topology would be, e.g., a mesh or hypercube architecture [1]. Our parallel watershed algorithm has been implemented on the PVM (*Parallel Virtual Machine*) package [6]. PVM is a software system for network-based concurrent computing which enables explicit message-passing among heterogeneous UNIX^R machines to emulate a large distributed-memory computer.

In this paper we present a parallel version of Meyer watershed algorithm which does not create any watershed pixels between catchment basins [2, 10]. In Section 2, the algorithm is presented in detail. Speedup and efficiency of the parallel algorithm are examined in Section 3. Section 4 contains some conclusions.

2. Parallel Watershed Algorithm

Our design of the watershed algorithm consists of three consecutive stages: detection of minima pixels, labeling of minima, and the final flooding or simulated immersion. Parallel implementation of each of these stages is studied below. Most of the operations are based on the corresponding sequential algorithm [4] but new solutions have been developed in order to obtain an efficient parallel watershed algorithm. We do not describe loading, partitioning and saving of global image data at all. First, we introduce some notation used in the sequel.

Let D_f, $D_f \subset \mathbf{Z}^2$, denote the domain of a two-dimensional (2-D) digital gray scale image f. For simplicity, we consider here only 2-D images. The range of f is the finite set $R = \{0, 1, \ldots, N-1\}$, where N is a positive integer number. Thus, $f : D_f \to R$. $N_G(p)$ denotes the neighboring pixels of a pixel p with respect to a given grid $G \subset \mathbf{Z}^2 \times \mathbf{Z}^2$. Let g_i, $i = 1, \ldots, n$, denote disjoint subimages of f, where n stands for the number of grains (processes) used in domain decomposition. Thus, $D_f = D_{g_1} \cup D_{g_2} \cup \ldots \cup D_{g_n}$ and $D_{g_i} \cap D_{g_j} = \emptyset, i \neq j$. An overlapped version of a subimage g_i is $f_i = \{p \,|\, d_{D_f}(p, D_{g_i}) \leq 1\}$, where $d_{D_f}(p, D_{g_i})$ stands for the geodesic distance between the pixel p and the subimage g_i inside the image f [8]. Each process P_i operates on the subimage f_i. Subimages are rectangular pieces of data of an arbitrary size. Each process maps the input subimage f_i into the non-overlapping output subimage o_i, the global output image having the domain $D_o = D_{o_1} \cup D_{o_2} \cup \ldots \cup D_{o_n}$, $o : D_o \to \mathbf{Z}^+$, $D_{o_i} \cap D_{o_j} = \emptyset, i \neq j$. The o_i subimages are framed such that they have the same size as f_i. A frame of a subimage o_i is denoted by $F(o_i)$ and $B(o_i, o_j) = \{p \,|\, p \in D_{o_i} \text{ and } \exists p' \in N_G(p) \text{ s.t. } p' \in D_{o_j}\}$ defines the border between subimages o_i and o_j. Note that $B(o_i, o_j) \neq B(o_j, o_i), i \neq j$.

Since the processes are software mapped using PVM onto a grid of virtual processors, it is necessary to define neighborhood relations between subimages. The neighboring subimages $N_f(g_i)$ of a subimage g_i are those subimages which contain pixels belonging to the neighborhoods $N_G(p)$ of any pixel $p \in D_{g_i}$ in D_f. Two processes are called neighbors if they operate on neighboring subimages.

In the SPMD scheme, each process P_i executes the same program asynchronously. Communication is needed since the watershed is a global transformation. The processes run at different speed, but they are synchronized by messages to and from a

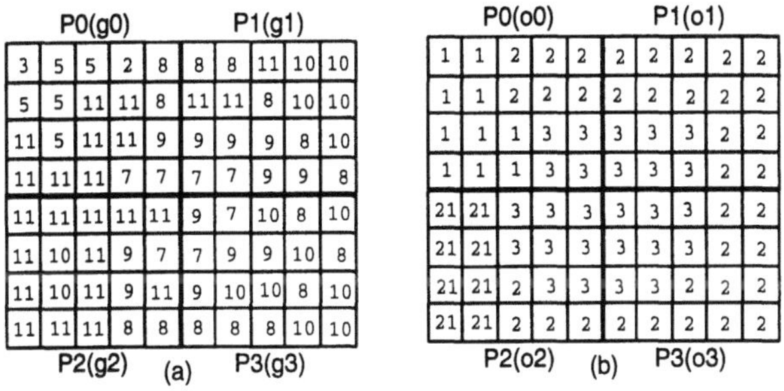

Fig. 1. (a)Input image f and its four subimages g_i (b)Output image o and its four subimages o_i (8-connectivity)

master process. Our SPMD model consists of one master process which supervises $m \times n$ processes which cooperate in solving the given problem. m and n represent the number of processes in rows and columns, respectively, in the grid configuration. Their values are defined by the user at each run. Default values can also be used (here $m = 2$, $n = 2$). Fig. 1 illustrates the input and the output images of the algorithm, supposing that each process P_i starts labeling minima from label $i \times 10 + 1$.

2.1. Detection of Minima Pixels

In this stage the master process and its $m \times n$ worker processes are designed to operate as follows: each process P_i starts with the output subimage o_i initialized with INIT value in all locations and performs a raster scan in the input subimage g_i to detect and label as Not A Regional Minima (NARM) the pixels p which have a lower gray level value in their neighborhood (non-minima pixels). When NARM pixel p is detected, breadth-first scan is done to propagate NARM label over a plateau of neighboring pixels of equal luminance with p (see [4]). Note that the breadth-first scans cannot extend across the frame $F(o_i)$. Propagations over the frames of subimages are essential in the detection of NARM pixels. Consider a plateau which is part of multiple subimages and has neighboring pixels of lower altitude only in one of the subimages. Obviously a wrong result is obtained if the whole plateau is not labeled with NARM value by a breadth-first scan. Therefore, communication among processes is needed.

After non-minima pixels are detected, each process P_i scans its borders $B(o_i, o_j)$, $o_j \in N_o(o_i)$, to see if there are NARM pixels $p \in B(o_i, o_j)$ with at least one remote neighbor $p' \in B(o_j, o_i)$ of equal luminance ($f_i(p) = f_i(p')$) (see Fig. 2a). Recall that f_i is an overlapped subimage, so no information exchange about gray level values of the original image f is needed between neighboring processes. All these pixel locations p of NARM pixels are stored in different vectors, one for each neighboring process P_j, and then sent to the corresponding neighbor. When receiving such a message, process P_j labels NARM all those INIT pixels $p' \in D_{o_j}$, which are neighbors to pixels $p \in B(o_i, o_j)$ whose locations are contained in the message and $f_j(p') = f_j(p)$. Then it resumes the breadth-first propagation of the NARM label inside o_j starting from these new NARM border pixels (Fig. 2b). Some flag vectors

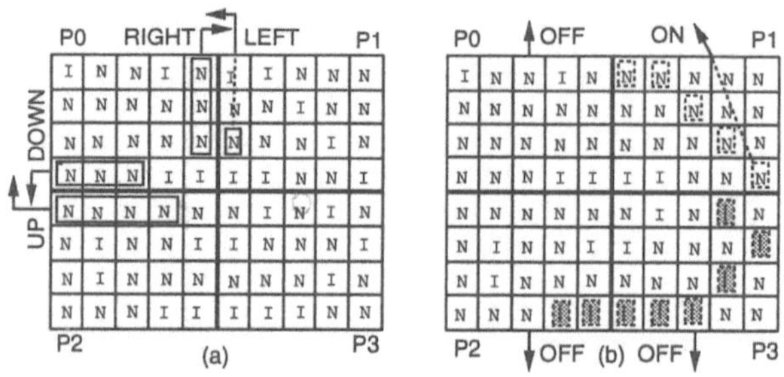

Fig. 2. (a)Image o after detection of minima inside each o_i (N = NARM, I = INIT, 8-connectivity is used). (b)Image o after the first communication step and breadth-first propagation of changes in 8-connectivity (pixels marked by a dashed rectangle). Shaded rectangles mark changes to NARM in the next two communication steps.

are used to avoid multiple sending of the same pixels. A change in the border of a subimage o_j can cause multiple changes in neighboring subimages. Thus, in many cases, a single exchange of data is not enough. A state variable is used in each process to detect the termination of the communication. Unfortunately, one process P_i cannot decide solely based on its current state when to stop, because even if its state is OFF (no change in the borders after the last communication step was detected), a non-adjacent neighbor P_j whose state is ON (at least one change in the borders was recorded) can incur changes to P_i along a path of immediate neighbors ($P_j = P_{j_1}, P_{j_2}, \ldots, P_{j_k} = P_i$ such that P_{j_m} and $P_{j_{m+1}}$ are neighbors, $m = 1, \ldots, k-1$). In Fig. 2b processes in the OFF state will switch to ON because of P_1 which incurs changes to P_3 and then to P_2 in the next two communication steps. The termination moment must be decided according to the states of all worker processes $P_i, i = 1, \ldots, m \times n$. This is done by the master process and the decision is multicasted then to the worker processes. A process P_i will switch from OFF to ON state if the master process decides to keep it active. Every worker P_i notifies the master process about its state (ON/OFF) after each data exchange. If all the processes are in OFF state, the master decides that all processes will terminate. A single ON process keeps all the other processes alive.

2.2. Labeling the Minima Pixels

In this stage, first, each process P_i gives a unique label to the minima of its local subimage o_i by a raster scan combined with breadth-first scans (Fig. 3a) [4]. Every worker uses a disjoint set of labels in this phase. Thus, the algorithm exhibits a high degree of parallelism, even though minima will be labeled with different values than in the sequential algorithm.

As in the previous stage, the assignment of labels cannot be performed only on the basis of local information. Communication among neighboring processes is needed again. Otherwise, areas which belong to the same minimum, but which are part of different subimages will have different labels. The algorithm has been designed to assure the propagation of the smallest label when two labels meet inside a minimum. Each process P_i sends to all its neighbors P_j (in 4- or 8-connectivity) a message consisting of all the labels $o_i(p)$ from the corresponding border $B(o_i, o_j)$

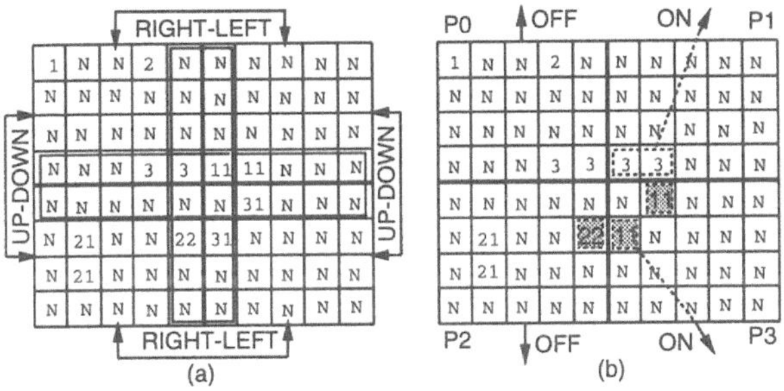

Fig. 3. (a)Image o after labeling INIT pixels inside each o_i in 8-connectivity. (b)Image o after the first communication step and breadth-first propagation of changes in 8-connectivity(pixels marked by a dashed rectangle). Shaded rectangles mark pixels which will get label 3 in the next two communication steps.

(Fig. 3a). A process P_j which receives such a message from P_i performs the following operation $\forall p' \in B(o_j, o_i)$: if $o_j(p') \neq$ NARM and it has a neighbor $p \in B(o_i, o_j)$ such that $o_i(p) \neq$ NARM and $o_j(p') > o_i(p)$, then $o_j(p') \leftarrow o_i(p)$. In order to propagate the changes inside the subimage o_j, all p' pixels from every border which have been relabeled are inserted into a queue Q_j. Thus, after all messages have been received and all changes in the borders done, a propagation of these new labels can be made in the neighborhood of each relabeled pixel by breadth-first scan (Fig. 3b). As in the detection of minima, one data exchange is not always enough. Consider a catchment basin spread over many subimages (see the plateau of altitude 7 in Fig. 1). Changes must be propagated throughout the minimum. (P_1 will propagate label 3 to P_3 and then to P_2; in Fig. 3b the shaded pixels mark these changes). If a process records no changes in its borders its state is OFF, and ON, otherwise. The communication is stopped by the master process following the same scheme as before.

2.3. Simulated Immersion

In the sequential implementation of Meyer watershed algorithm, the flooding process is performed according to the ordering relation[2, 9]. Thus, pixel x is flooded before pixel y if x lies at lower altitude than y on the relief or if they both belong to a plateau X of constant luminance, but the "geodesic" distance within X to the points of lower altitude is smaller for x than for y. An ordered queue OQ consisting on N FIFO queues provides this ordering relation, where N stands for the number of gray levels of an image. The n-th queue is associated with gray level n. Pixels are always extracted from the lowest level queue of the ordered queue. A pixel removed from the queue, assigns its label to neighboring NARM pixels and puts them into the ordered queue. Once the queue of the current level is empty, the flooding is continued with pixels from the next level queue.

In parallel watershed computation, flooding according to the above definition is not a trivial task. In our implementation, each process P_i maintains a local ordered queue OQ_i which is initialized with pixels p belonging to minima M and which have a non-minima pixel in their neighborhood $N_G(p)$. These boundary pixels are denoted by $\alpha(M)$. In the parallel environment, the flooding is hampered by the boundaries of the local data. Every time when the propagation of labels hits a border, flooding should be continued in the corresponding neighboring process.

In our approach, at each gray level, flooding is first done inside each subimage and is then followed by message passing to extend flooding across the borders. This flooding and communication cycle is iterated until no changes are detected. Processes are synchronized at as few gray levels as possible, in order to perform a proper flooding and to obtain a fast algorithm. The selection of the synchronization levels consists of two steps. First, each process P_i stores the gray levels of pixels p from each border $B(o_i, o_j)$ such that $o_i(p) =$ NARM or $p \in \alpha(M)$ in the corresponding vector V_{ij} and sends V_{ij} to P_j. In the second step, each process P_j which receives a V_{ij} vector from P_i computes the synchronization levels with the process P_i by $SL_{ji} = V_{ji} \cup V_{ij}$, but levels strictly larger than $\min(\max(V_{ji}), \max(V_{ij}))$ are not included in SL_{ji}. Now, the synchronization levels of process P_j are $SL^j = \bigcup_i SL_{ji}$. In the example, $SL^0 = SL^2 = \{7, 8, 9, 11\}$ and $SL^1 = SL^3 = \{7, 8, 9\}$.

Synchronization is done as before by the master process. In order to achieve this, it receives the synchronization levels SL^i from each process P_i, computes the global synchronization levels $SL = \bigcup_i SL^i$, and stores into a table each synchronization gray level $h \in SL$ (barrier) and the cluster C_h of process ID's which synchronize at level h (all P_i's such that $h \in SL^i$). Then, the master process starts synchronizing every cluster C_h of processes according to the order provided by the table.

Each process P_i starts flooding from the global minimum gray level $hmin = \min_{p \in D_f} f(p)$. Flooding is performed for each gray level hc following the same basic principles as in the sequential implementation (see the following pseudo-code). If hc is a synchronization level for P_i ($hc \in SL^i$), P_i notifies the master that it has reached the barrier h_i (after initial flooding inside o_i was completed) at level hc ($h_i \leftarrow hc$), and then waits for permission to go on. The master process accepts only notifications equal of the current synchronization level ($h_i = h$). After it has received such messages from all processes in C_h, it broadcasts them back the permission to continue. Then, communication among the processes in the cluster C_h is initiated. The messages contain addresses of border pixels, their labels, and their lower-complete values (further details are below). Every process receiving this information updates its border pixels and its ordered queue according to the same assignment rules given in the following pseudo-code. Then, the flooding is resumed. When the queue of level h is empty, the process checks its state. If new border pixels of level h were labeled by the last flooding, the state is ON, and OFF, otherwise. The termination of the flooding at level h is detected by the master process using the states of the processes in the cluster C_h. Processes P_i for which $h \in SL^i$, but $h \notin \bigcup_j V_{ij}$ just receive messages from neighboring processes and update their ordered queue. When flooding at level h is completed, the next gray level is processed in every process in C_h and the master process starts synchronizing the next cluster, if any. If hc is not a synchronization level for P_i, the next gray level is flooded.The flooding stage terminates when all the gray levels have been immersed.

After the first flooding step inside each subimage, plateaus distributed over many subimages are not split into geodesic influence zones [8]. Therefore, a mechanism for reflooding them is needed. A lower-complete image l is used. In this image, each pixel has a lower neighbor, except pixels belonging to minima [9]. If $l(x) < l(y)$, then pixel

x will be flooded before y. If $l(x) = l(y)$, then the parallel flooding of these pixels may depend on the scanning order. Before starting to flood, every process P_i initializes a lower-complete image l_i to ∞, except pixels p which lie in the minima of the image. For these pixels the lower-complete values are $l_i(p) \leftarrow MaxHisto \times f_i(p) + 1$, where $MaxHisto$ stands for the largest number of pixels having the same gray level value in the global image f. When starting to flood a plateau, the lower border pixels of the plateau have the lower-complete values of the pixels which labeled them. Therefore, the lower-complete values must be corrected. The algorithm and the assignment rules which perform the progressive immersion at level h are given below.

```
while(oq_empty(OQ_i, h) = FALSE){ /* flooding at level h */
    p ← oq_get(OQ_i);
    if(l_i(p) < MaxHisto × f_i(p)) l_i(p) ← MaxHisto × f_i(p) + 1;
    for each p' ∈ N_G(p), p' ∈ D_{o_i}{
        if(f_i(p') > f_i(p) and o_i(p') = NARM)
        /* floods higher levels */
        o_i(p') ← o_i(p); l_i(p') ← l_i(p); oq_add(OQ_i, p', f_i(p'));
        else if(f_i(p') > f_i(p) and o_i(p') ≠ NARM and o_i(p') ≠ o_i(p) and l_i(p') > l_i(p))
        /* refloods pixels at the lower border of a neighboring higher plateau */
        o_i(p') ← o_i(p); l_i(p') ← l_i(p);
        else if(f_i(p') = f_i(p) and l_i(p') > l_i(p) + 1)
        /* controls flooding inside plateaus */
        l_i(p') ← l_i(p) + 1; o_i(p') ← o_i(p); oq_add(OQ_i, p', f_i(p'));
    }
}
```

The proposed parallel watershed algorithm gives a very closed estimate of the output of the sequential algorithm [10]. However, differences may occur, because of the scanning order dependency of the original algorithm. In addition, the use of a distributed ordered queue causes a loss of the flooding order of plateaus at the border of subimages.

3. Simulations

Both domain decomposition and number of processors used affect the running time, speedup and efficiency. The running time is the time elapsed between the moment the first process starts computing and the moment the last process ends computing. A well known indication of the quality of the parallel algorithm is the speedup. The absolute speedup of a N-processor parallel computation is defined as $S_P = T(1)/T(N)$ [7], where $T(1)$ denotes the running time of the parallel algorithm on a single processor, and $T(N)$ the running time of the parallel algorithm using N processors. The corresponding relative parallel efficiency is defined as $E(N) = S_P/N$ [7]. These values are tabulated next for a 512×512 input image (lenna), including the loading, distribution and saving.

TABLE I
Performance Evaluation.

N	$m \times n$	$T(N)$	S_P	$E(N)(\%)$
1	2 x 2	7.41		
2	2 x 2	7.27	1.01	50.9
3	2 x 2	6.86	1.08	36.0
4	2 x 2	7.05	1.05	26.2
5	2 x 2	6.47	1.14	22.9
6	2 x 2	5.85	1.26	21.1
7	2 x 2	5.25	1.41	20.1

4. Concluding Remarks

A distributed watershed algorithm has been implemented and tested on a loosely coupled system of workstations using PVM package. An evaluation of the average execution times (idle, communication, computation, and the total time) proved that the idle time is a significant part of the total running time. This is partly due to the insufficient number of available processors and the slow communication rate. Thus, it is well justified to transport the algorithm to a more suitable system,e.g., a transputer network, that allows a higher degree of parallelism and a faster communication. This is a topic of current research and results will be published elsewhere. However, even the current algorithm issues good performances for large images. More work remains to be done in the optimization of the current algorithm.

References

1. S. G. Akl, *The design and Analysis of Parallel Algorithms*, Prentice-Hall International, Inc., pp. 3–29, 1989.
2. S. Beucher and F. Meyer, "The morphological approach to segmentation: The watershed transformation," in *Mathematical Morphology in Image Processing*, E. R. Dougherty, Editor, pp. 433–481, Marcel Dekker Inc., New York, 1993.
3. P. Chaudhuri, *Parallel Algorithms-Design and Analysis*, Prentice-Hall International Inc., pp. 37–39, 45–60, Sydney, Australia, 1992.
4. B. P. Dobrin, T. Viero, and M. Gabbouj, "Fast Watershed Algorithms: Analysis and Extensions," in *IS&T/SPIE Proc. of the Symposium on Electronic Imaging: Science and Technology*, vol. 2180, pp. 209–220, San Jose, California, February, 1994.
5. B. P. Dobrin, T. Viero, and M. Gabbouj, "An Improved Split-and-Merge Watershed Algorithm," accepted to *ISMM*, Fontainebleau, France, September, 1994.
6. A. Geist et al., *PVM 3.0 User's Guide and Reference Manual*, Technical Report ORNL/TM-12187, Oak Ridge National Laboratory, Feb. 1993.
7. K. H. Hoffman and Jun Zou, "Parallel efficiency of domain decomposition methods," *Parallel Computing*, vol. 19, pp. 1375–1391, North-Holland, Dec. 1993.
8. C. Lantuejoul and F. Maisonneuve, "Geodesic methods in quantitative image analysis," *Pattern Recognition*, vol. 17, no. 2, pp. 177–187, 1984.
9. F. Meyer and S. Beucher, "Morphological segmentation," *Journal of Visual Communication and Image Representation*, vol. 1, no. 1, pp. 21–46, Sept. 1990.
10. F. Meyer, "Un algorithme optimal de ligne de partage des eaux," in *Proc.* 8^e *Congres Reconnaissance des Formes et Intelligence Artificielle*, pp. 847–857, Lyon, France, Nov. 1991.

VISUALIZATION OF MINKOWSKI OPERATIONS BY COMPUTER GRAPHICS TECHNIQUES

J.B.T.M. ROERDINK and G.S.M. BLAAUWGEERS
Dept. of Mathematics and Computing Science, University of Groningen,
P.O. Box 800, 9700 AV Groningen, The Netherlands
Tel. +31-50-633931; Fax +31-50-633800; Email: roe@cs.rug.nl

Abstract. We consider the problem of visualizing 3D objects defined as a Minkowski addition or subtraction of elementary objects. It is shown that such visualizations can be obtained by using techniques from computer graphics such as ray tracing and Constructive Solid Geometry. Applications of the method are found in solid modelling and shape description.

Key words: visualization of Minkowski operations, ray tracing, Constructive Solid Geometry

1. Introduction

The problem of visualizing 3D objects defined as a Minkowski addition or subtraction of elementary objects — referred to as *Minkowski objects* below — is not a trivial one. Even when the elementary objects are very simple, such as spheres, boxes, cylinders, etc., the composite objects can become very complicated higher order surfaces with not even an explicit functional or parametric representation.

The present approach uses techniques from computer graphics to visualize these objects. The basis is the *ray tracing* technique, which is an established method in computer graphics to visualize 3D objects by simulating the physical processes of ray propagation, reflection and transmission [1,4]. To visualize *composite* objects, the ray tracing technique uses Constructive Solid Geometry (CSG) methods, in which it is possible to ray trace objects formed by elementary set operations, such as union, intersection and set difference (called *CSG objects* from now on) [5].

We establish a mapping between 3D Minkowski objects and objects defined in terms of CSG operations, which can subsequently be visualized by the standard ray tracing technique. In particular, we use a basic set of *elementary shapes*, and derive a decomposition of a Minkowski sum of any number of objects, chosen from the basic set, into CSG objects. Even for a small basic set the number of decomposition rules can become very large. So we use various preprocessing steps to reduce this number. Various examples of 3D visualizations will be shown.

Applications of the technique presented are twofold: first, it constitutes an extension of standard CSG methods in computer graphics. Second, we mention morphological image processing, where the basic image transforms — dilations and erosions — are based upon the Minkowski operations [3,6]. Visualization of the results of such operations on 3D images might be a useful research tool. Also in shape description and solid modelling the use of Minkowski operations has already proved to be fruitful, see e.g. Ghosh [2].

J.Serra and P. Soille (eds.), Mathematical Morphology and Its Applications to Image Processing, 289-296

2. Preliminaries

In this section we first present the basics of ray tracing and Constructive Solid Geometry.

2.1. Ray tracing

Ray tracing is a technique for image synthesis: creating 2-D pictures of a 3-D world. The first step in simulating such an image will be a projection of the scene on the screen. We assume we only have one eye through which we look at the screen. The location of the eye in the 3-D world is referred to as the *eye position*. In front of the eye we place the screen, and behind it we build the scene from which we want to generate an image. The color of a pixel on the screen is determined by all light rays — emitted by one or more light sources — that strike that pixel and the average color of all these rays is assigned to it.

Since many of the rays emitted from the light source(s) never hit the screen, one uses *backward ray tracing*: for every pixel on the screen, follow back the light ray from the eye through the given pixel, and see where it first hits an object. The intersection point thus found in principle determines the color at the pixel. From this intersection point, a line (called a *shadow ray*) is traced towards every light source in the scene. When such a line intersects an object in front of the light source, the point lies in the shadow of this object — unless the object is (partially) transparent — and the rays of that light source play no role in the color of the pixel. Otherwise the amount of light (of each color component) that is reflected is calculated and averaged with the colors of the rays coming from other light sources. The amount of light that is reflected depends on the angle between the normal vector at the intersection point on the surface of the object, and the line connecting it with the light source. But this is not the only light that strikes the object. As a result of reflection it is possible that rays strike the object via an indirect path. This part must also be accounted for. The standard way to achieve this, is by pretending that the eye is moved to the intersection point, and starting the whole process from there again. In this way we can implement the ray tracing technique *recursively*. For objects which are both transparent and reflective, we also have to find the colors of the light it transmits and reflects: such light arrived along *reflection* or *transmission rays*, whose directions are determined by the laws of (specular or diffuse) reflection and transmission (Snell's law). Finally we include an *ambient* term, to account for diffuse light arriving via indirect paths.

2.1.1. *Ray/Quadric intersection*

A general class of objects which are relatively simple to intersect with a ray are the quadrics: cylinders, cones, ellipsoids, paraboloids, hyperboloids, spheres, planes, etc. For reasons of efficiency, such simple objects are often given their own intersection routines.

2.2. Constructive Solid Geometry

In order to compute the intersection point of a ray and an object, we need a mathematical description of the ray and the object. However, we generally do not have such a description of all the objects. To solve this problem, a technique called *constructive solid geometry* (CSG) has been developed. In CSG, simple primitives (like polygons) are combined by means of set operators. A composite object can be represented as a binary tree where each node contains a set operation and two child nodes, which may also be composite solids. The leaves of this tree are primitive objects such as quadrics or polygons. Evaluation of set operations usually reduces to classification whether a point p lies on the inside or outside of the composite object.

3. Visualization of 3D Minkowski objects

3.1. Terminology

Before describing the process of transforming 3D Minkowski objects into objects which are defined in terms of CSG operations and therefore can be visualized via standard ray tracing techniques, we shall present some terminology.

We introduce a basic set of primitive shapes, referred to as *primary Minkowski primitives*, consisting of the following elementary geometric objects: *point, xline, yline, zline, xdisc, ydisc, zdisc, sphere.* Here an `xline` is a line segment in the x-direction, and an `xdisc` is a disc with thickness zero in the plane through the origin with normal in the x-direction, etc. All Minkowski primitives are solid objects.

As with the ordinary boolean set operators *union, intersection* and *difference*, one can define terms — referred to as *Minkowski terms* — consisting of multiple operands (primary Minkowski primitives) separated by Minkowski operators.

Processing Minkowski terms may lead to new Minkowski objects, which can be regarded as elementary for further calculations, although they are (Minkowski-) reducible. We refer to this kind of primitives as *secondary Minkowski primitives.* Examples are *rectangles, blocks, cylinders, toroidal discs* (discs of which the edge consists of the outer half of a torus, a bit like a discus) and a *cyclohedron* (the Minkowski sum of two perpendicular flat discs).

Our goal is to decompose 3D Minkowski objects into elementary objects, representing the original shape, that can be visualized through ray tracing techniques by means of CSG. These objects will be referred to as *ray tracing primitives.* Examples of such ray tracing primitives are: *blocks, spheres, cylinders, tori,* and *polycircles* (we define a polycircle to be the Minkowski sum of two perpendicular circles).

3.2. Decomposition of Minkowski terms

Let us consider Minkowski sums of the form

$$A_1 \oplus A_2 \oplus \ldots \oplus A_n \tag{1}$$

where each A_j is chosen from the set of primary Minkowski primitives. Such sums may be of a simple form, such as `xline` $\oplus$ `yline`, leading to a `zrectangle`, which is a rectangle with normal in the z-direction. The Minkowski sum of a circle and a sphere is a torus, which is a *quartic* (fourth order surface). The Minkowski sum of two orthogonal circles leads to a somewhat unfamiliar object which we call a *polycircle*, which is also quartic, shown in Fig. 1.

Now our goal is to decompose sums of the form (1) into a *union* of objects B_j, where each B_j can be visualized by standard ray tracing techniques. The union of

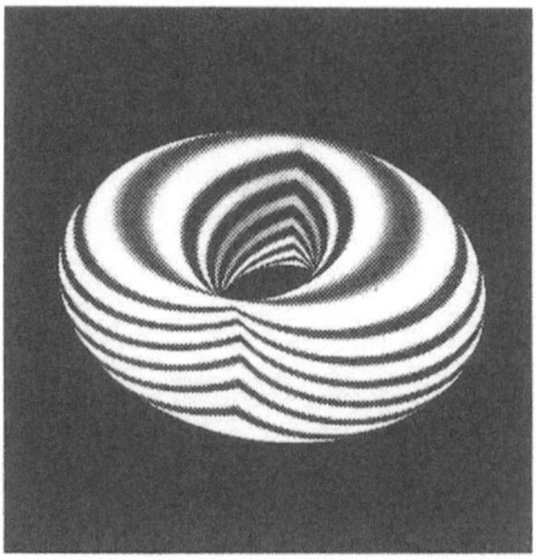

Fig. 1. Visualization of the Minkowski sum of two perpendicular circles (a polycircle).

the B_j's can then be handled by using CSG operations, as explained above. For this reason we refer to the B_j as *ray tracing primitives.*

Thus, the purpose is to derive a list of replacement rules for every sum of two Minkowski primitives. With these rules and using properties of the $\oplus$-operator like commutativity, associativity and distributivity over union, every Minkowski sum term can be reduced to a set of objects which, united, represent the whole Minkowski sum.

Addition of two primary Minkowski primitives of the same type yields a primitive of the same type. Thus, given a Minkowski term of arbitrary length, we may group together operands of the same type and then, using the associativity of the Minkowski addition, reduce every group to precisely one element of this type. The set of secondary Minkowski primitives that can arise with the current set of primary Minkowski primitives consists of thirteen objects: *xrectangle, yrectangle, zrectangle, block, xcylinder, ycylinder, zcylinder, xdiscus, ydiscus, zdiscus, xcyclohedron, ycyclohedron, zcyclohedron.*

3.3. Representation of Minkowski primitives

We introduce following representation of the primary Minkowski primitives:

point(x, y, z) : point with coordinates (x, y, z).

xline(x, y, z, lx) : line starting at (x, y, z) and ending at $(x + lx, y, z)$.

yline(x, y, z, lx) : line starting at (x, y, z) and ending at $(x, y + ly, z)$.

zline(x, y, z, lz) : line starting at (x, y, z) and ending at $(x, y, z + lz)$.

xdisc(rx) : disc of radius rx in the YZ-plane centered at the origin.

ydisc(ry) : disc of radius ry in the XZ-plane centered at the origin.

zdisc(rz) : disc of radius rz in the XY-plane centered at the origin.

sphere(r) : sphere with center at the origin and radius r.

3.4. Reduction to CSG objects

There are a total of 21 primary and secondary Minkowski primitives. This means that there are 21 x 21 = 441 different combinations possible for the pairwise Minkowski addition. Because of commutativity this number can immediately be reduced to 21 + (441 - 21)/2 = 231 combinations. This still is an awful lot. So we shall try to decrease this number.

One of the first things we notice is that several combinations may lead to the same result. This phenomenon arises in combinations where at least one of the operands is a secondary Minkowski primitive. To exclude this kind of non-uniqueness, sorting the primary Minkowski primitives in a Minkowski term of any length in a specific order before carrying out the reduction process does the trick. For example the following order is very suitable: `point`, `xline`, `yline`, `zline`, `xdisc`, `ydisc`, `zdisc`, `sphere`.

Next, using distributivity, we can recursively reduce left-to-right the reordered Minkowski term. First we split up the set of primary Minkowski primitives into two groups. In the first group we put the line primitives plus the point primitive. In the second group we put the disc primitives and the sphere primitive. After reordering the initial Minkowski term so primitives of the same type are put together and then reduced easily, we divide the resulting primitives over the two groups and make reductions for both groups separately. The last step is then to reduce the outcome of the reductions of both groups.

3.5. Reduction formulas

Minkowski terms are being reduced using a list of reduction formulas we have to determine by hand. Consider for example the following Minkowski sum:

```
point(a0,b0,c0) ⊕ ydisc(a1,b1,c1,r1) ⊕ sphere(a2,b2,c2,r2)
        ⊕ xline(a3,b3,c3,l3) ⊕ zline(a4,b4,c4,l4)
```

To carry out these reductions the following reduction formulas are required:

$$\textbf{point}\,(x1, y1, z1) \oplus \textbf{xline}\,(x2, y2, z2, l) \longmapsto \textbf{xline}\,(x1 + x2, y1 + y2, z1 + z2, l)$$

$$\textbf{xline}\,(x1, y1, z1, lx) \oplus \textbf{zline}\,(x2, y2, z2, ly) \longmapsto \textbf{yrectangle}\,(x1 + x2, y1 + y2, z1 + z2, lx, ly)$$

$$\textbf{ydisc}\,(x1, y1, z1, ry) \oplus \textbf{sphere}\,(x2, y2, z2, r) \longmapsto \textbf{ydiscus}\,(x1 + x2, y1 + y2, z1 + z2, r, ry)$$

Next we have to reduce a `yrectangle` and a `ydiscus`, which leads to an object that can be viewed as a union of several secondary Minkowski primitives. As an example we demonstrate in Fig. 2 a sketch of the Minkowski term just discussed.

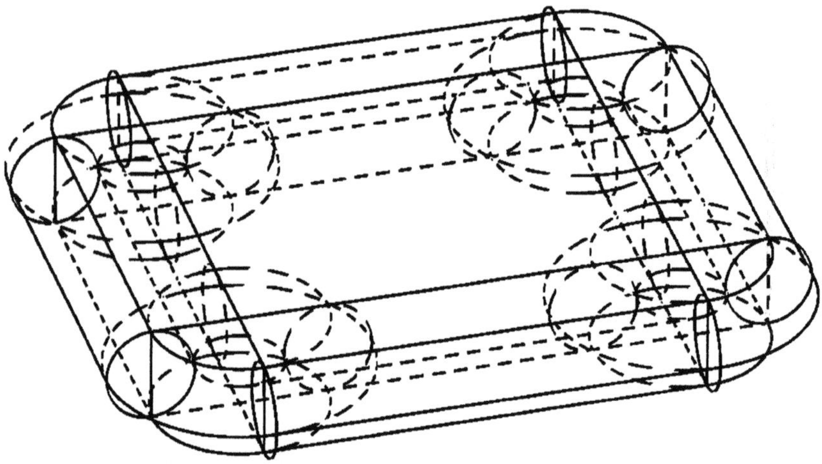

Fig. 2. Sketch of a Minkowski sum of a `point`, a `xline`, a `zline`, a `ydisc` and a `sphere`, from which the various primitives can be derived.

3.6. Optimizations

The first optimization we could make is to postpone reductions involving `point` primitives. Since Minkowski addition with points comes down to shift operations we effectuate these not until the final step in the process of decomposition: the translation of the Minkowski primitives into ray tracer primitives.

Another optimization is to insert unions of ray tracer primitives instead of disci and cyclohedra. This way we are able to prevent the generation of redundant cylinders.

Finally we present an adaptation which will reduce the number of reduction formulas drastically. Many ray tracer primitives exist in three variants (x, y, and z), that differ only in orientation. We can exploit this by transforming all akin reduction formulas to one particular variant, applying an inverse transformation to the set of produced ray tracer primitives to get the right rotational forms.

3.7. Implementation

To implement the method a *preprocessor* routine was developed which takes a file containing a scene description as input. This description contains: positions of light sources and objects; descriptions of the composite objects in terms of unions, intersections, or Minkowski sums of elementary objects; and also, properties of the elementary objects (reflection and transmission coefficients, smoothness parameters). Also some texture may be applied to the surface of the objects to give more shape clues.

Output of the preprocessor is a file in which the Minkowski operations have been replaced by a union of ray tracer primitives, using the reduction process sketched above. This file is then itself used as input file for an ordinary ray tracer.

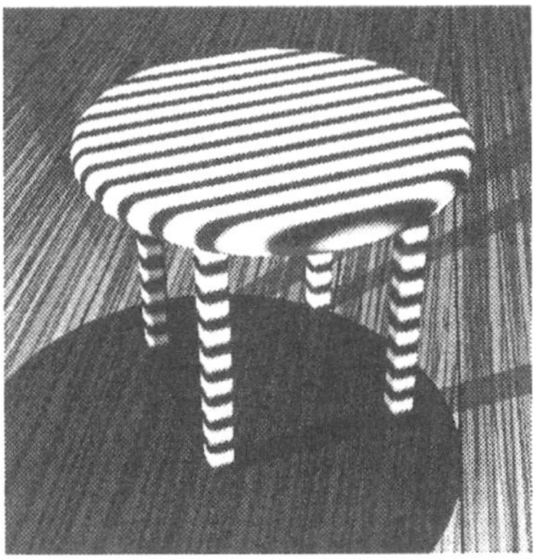

Fig. 3. Legs and top of the table are modelled by Minkowski sums.

As an example Fig. 3 shows a scene of a table on a floor where the legs and top of the table have been modelled by Minkowski sums.

Preprocessors for the ray tracers "DKBTrace v. 2.12" and POV-Ray v. 1.0 were developed. The pictures in this paper have been ray traced with "POV-Ray v. 1.0", an excellent ray tracer which offers many advanced features.

4. Summary

In this article we outlined a method of decomposing Minkowski operations into unions of elementary objects, that can be visualized through ray tracing techniques by means of Constructive Solid Geometry. To bring about the decomposition of Minkowski terms we contrived a series of reduction formulas, endeavouring to keep their number as low as possible and keeping the result of the various reductions compact.

To implement the method a preprocessor routine was developed which takes a scene description as input and delivers an output file in which the Minkowski operations have been replaced by a union of ray tracer primitives. This file is then itself used as input file for an ordinary ray tracer.

Some remarks about extensions of this method are in order. First, when the use of Minkowski *subtraction* is permitted in Minkowski terms also, then the decomposition of these terms is a lot more complicated, requiring a huge number of reduction formulas and yielding a much larger variety of primitive ray tracer objects, whether tractable or not.

Secondly, one may wonder to what extent we can adapt this method in order to handle Minkowski sums of *arbitrary* objects. So far we have chosen to consider only a well-defined class of primitive objects, the Minkowski sums of which can be decomposed into ray tracer objects. In fact what we would need for arbitrary objects is a direct method to derive the intersection equations of a Minkowski sum from the equations of the individual objects. Perhaps methods used for sweep representations can be adapted to our situation [4,Ch.3]. A minimum requirement still is that the operands of the Minkowski sum themselves are described in terms of explicit mathematical equations.

5. References

[1] Foley, J. D., Dam, A. Van & Feiner, S. K., *Computer Graphics : Principles and Practice*, Addison Wesley, Reading, MA, 1990.

[2] Ghosh, P.K., "A mathematical model for shape description using Minkowski operators," *Comp. Vis. Graph. Im. Proc.* 44 (1988), 239—269.

[3] Giardina, C.R. & Dougherty, E.R., *Morphological Methods in Image and Signal Processing*, Prentice-Hall, Englewood Cliffs, NJ, 1988.

[4] Glassner, A.S., ed., *An Introduction to Ray Tracing*, Academic Press, New York, 1989.

[5] Roth, S., "Ray casting for modeling solids," *Comp. Graph. Im. Proc.* 18 (1982), 109–144.

[6] Serra, J., *Image Analysis and Mathematical Morphology*, Academic Press, New York, 1982.

MORPHOGENESIS SIMULATIONS WITH LATTICE GAS

R. BRÉMOND
*Ecole des Mines de Paris, Centre de Morphologie Mathématique,
35, rue Saint-Honoré, F-77305 Fontainebleau Cedex, France*

and

D. JEULIN
*Ecole des Mines de Paris, Centre de Géostatistique,
35, rue Saint-Honoré, F-77305 Fontainebleau Cedex, France*

Abstract. Some possibilities of morphogenesis simulations using lattice gas models are illustrated. Starting from a lattice, the model, initially developed in statistical physics, generates random walks of a population of particles in mechanical interactions, respecting basic physical conservation laws (mass and momentum). The behaviour of this model reproduces viscous flows obeying the Navier-Stokes equations. When considering different types of particles, it is possible to introduce rules of interaction that mimic processes, based on transport phenomena, that generate multiphasis random media on a lattice. This physical approach of simulations is illustrated by constructing random aggregates obtained by diffusion, nucleation and growth.

Key words: Morphogenesis , cellular automata , lattice gas , DLA , cluster , multi-species

1. Introduction

Many structures are the result of complex interactions between various components. A simple way to simulate these interactions is to build a physical model such as the lattice gas proposed in statistical physics (Frish, Hasslacher & Pomeau1986): the motion of particles on a lattice is constrained by basic conservation laws, such as the conservation of mass and momentum. This enables us to simulate the flow of a fluid obeying the Navier Stokes equations (Frish, d'Humières, Hasslacher, Lallemand, Pomeau & Rivet1987). Starting with the lattice gas model, complex situations may be simulated by introducing new rules: two fluid flows accounting for surface tension (Rothman & Keller1989), liquid-gas mixtures to simulate the evaporation process (Appert, Rothman & Zaleski1990), chemical reactions, phase separation, deposition or cluster morphogenesis (Brémond & Jeulin1994).

This last class of phenomena occurs in many fields, such as the solidification from a melt including various surface tension effects, the filtration of suspensions by a porous medium, or the deposition of sediments. Thus, many fields in experimental and physical sciences require simulation tools in order to have a better understanding of the processes involving the clustering of particles in suspension in a fluid. Many models, among which we should mention the DLA (Meakin & Sanders1985), allow the description and the simulation of various clustering processes with the help of a diffusion model. The lattice gas, which is a cellular automaton with hydrodynamical

J.Serra and P. Soille (eds.), Mathematical Morphology and Its Applications to Image Processing, 297-304

behaviour was used to present a new clustering model (Brémond & Jeulin1994) suitable for more complex hydrodynamical conditions. In this paper we suggest to extend this lattice gas clustering model to fluids containing several populations of suspensions, as it may occur in the physical world in sedimentation or in solidification for instance. This enlarges the fields of the physical applications with which the model is relevant.

2. Algorithmics

We first present the lattice gas algorithm and its use for morphogenesis. Then we describe the new algorithm that simulates the clustering with several species. Finally we show the interest of this kind of simulations for a better understanding of some clustering processes, through several didactic simulations in order to point out the main properties of this kind of simulation.

The lattice gas model is a recent method to simulate hydrodynamics (Hardy, Pomeau & de Pazzis1976)(Frish et al.1986). It is a discrete version that is free of inherent defects of classical numerical methods (boundary conditions, round-off errors), and that is easily implemented on general purpose computers. In addition, the physical boundary conditions are easily taken into account, even if they change with time as it occurs in morphogenesis.

Principle. Consider a periodic lattice on a hexagonal graph. Each vertex of the graph is connected to its six nearest neighbours, and may contain between 0 and 6 particles with a mass and a velocity one (but at most one particle per velocity, corresponding to the six velocities of the grid). Every time step, the location of particles is changed according to the following local operations: a propagation of particles to the nearest neighbour in the direction of their velocity (Fig. 1.b), and a collision redistributing the velocities as shown in Fig. 1.c.

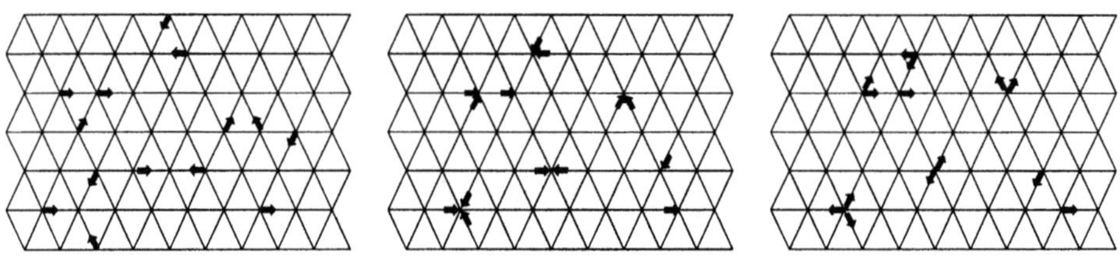

(a) initial step (b) Translations (c) Collisions

Fig. 1. Lattice gas on a hexagonal grid, elementary step.

Collisions. The collisions are local operations that preserve the total mass and momentum (and consequently the kinetics energy) on each node. Fig. 1.c shows two configurations changed according to this transformation. Frish et al. (1987) shown that this kind of automaton follows the Naviers-Stokes equation on a macroscopic scale. Therefore, the simulation of complex flows is possible from a lattice gas.

2.1. AGGREGATION.

We proposed in a previous work (Brémond1993) to add an aggregation step to the "translation-collision" loop of the cellular automaton in order to let some particles, pointing towards the solid phasis, to stick to it. Other aggregation rules can be defined based on geometrical or physical criteria. It is also possible to give an *aggregation probability* p^+ to each moving suspension and a *disaggregation probability* p^- to each particle trapped in a cluster. Fig. 2 gives an example of the aggregation step, where the only marked particle pointing towards the cluster (in black) sticks to it.

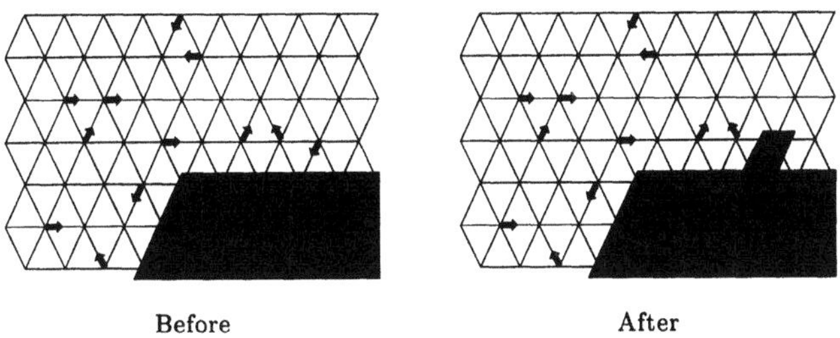

Fig. 2. Rule of aggregation.

2.2. MULTI-SPECIES CLUSTERS

From this algorithm, in which the fluid particles are marked with *Liquid* or *Suspension* labels, it is possible to build a new algorithm , more general, in which the fluid particles can be marked with one color among a set of markers. The resulting simulations are closer to real physical experiments, in which several kinds of suspensions are involved. If the aggregation rule remains unchanged, no global effect will be noticed on the cluster geometries, or on the dynamic of the morphogenesis either. The interest of our proposal is that the aggregation and disaggregation rules can be made dependant on the markers. The rules can this way be linked with the physical meaning of each marker.

Self-aggregation. One extremely simple rule, that we call *self-aggregation*, is that a particle of type T can only stick to another type T. At first sight, one may guess that this would not change much of the final geometries, at least when the whole labelled population follows this rule. Further simulations will show that this it not the case, and that new interesting geometries can be simulated this way. More complicated aggregation rules can be imagined, and the combinatory leads to a large range of morphologies. Our aim in this paper is to prove the feasibility of the simulation method, hoping that physicists may find it convenient for their particular case, for which specific aggregation rules should be defined. Therefore, we will not simulate other aggregation rules in this paper. Nevertheless, we would like to indicate some directions where to search. When several populations of suspensions, say A, B and C, are available in a fluid, they will probably differ in the aggregation probability p^+ (probability to stick together): this leads to p_A^+, p_B^+ and p_C^+ probabilities. In some cases, depending on the physical or chemical meaning of each specy, it will be necessary to define inter-species aggregation probabilities, like for instance the probability $p_{AB}^{+} = p_{BA}^{+}$ that particles of type A and B stick together. All these distinctions are, of course, relevant for the disaggregation rules. One may imagine, for instance, an aggregation process involving two populations, one of which can leave the clusters and go back to the fluid, the other being crystallized forever.

3. Simulations of random aggregates

3.1. Mono-specy simulation

In order to visualize the effect of the aggregation rule for a single specy fluid, a simulation is made on a periodic system of size 200×200. Starting with a solid seed in the middle of the field (Fig. 3.a) or from a set of Poisson seeds (Fig. 3.b), the clusters grow by diffusion for a zero average velocity, as in the case of the DLA model (Meakin1986)(Witten & Sanders1981). In the lattice gas simulation, the change in the local density of particles and the perturbation of the velocity field by the aggregate are automatically satisfied.

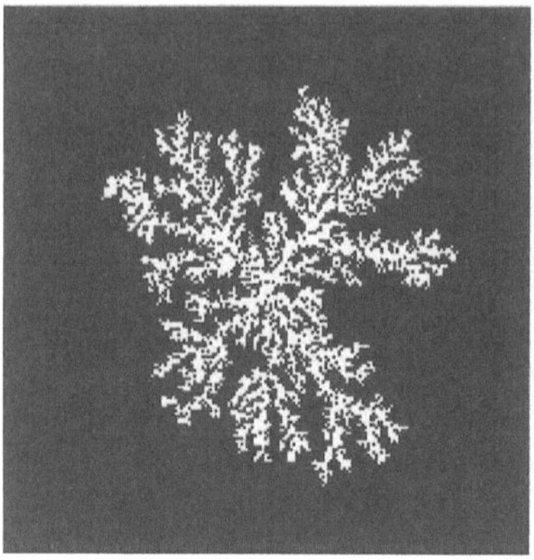

(a) Central seed

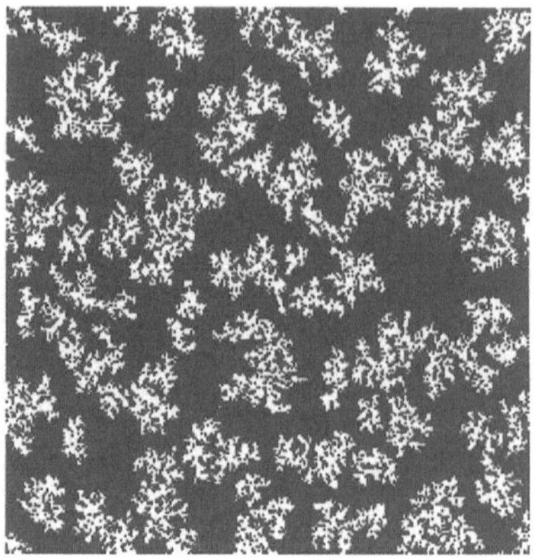

(b) Poisson seeds

Fig. 3. Morphogenesis with one population of suspensions.

3.2. Two species simulations

Principle. We present here two sets of simulations with two populations of suspensions, that use 256×256 images with periodic boundary conditions. The aggregation rule is the self-aggregation one explained before: If we call A and B the two species, an A particle can stick to another A, a B to another B (with the same probability), but A and B cannot stick together.

Poisson seeds. In a first set of simulations, we drop seeds of type A and B following a Poisson process at the beginning of the simulations, and we observe the growth of clusters A and B with time, using various density conditions. The A and B particles' density ρ_A and ρ_B are set equal. If the seeds' densities g_A and g_B are also equal, the resulting clusters are, from a morphological point of view, the same as clusters grown up with a single suspension specy. The differences concerns the dynamic of the process, because the incompatibility $A - B$ slows down the cluster's growth rate when there are two species. This is illustrated on Fig. 4, which plots the total mass of the clusters as a function of time, for a one-specy and for a two-species simulation.

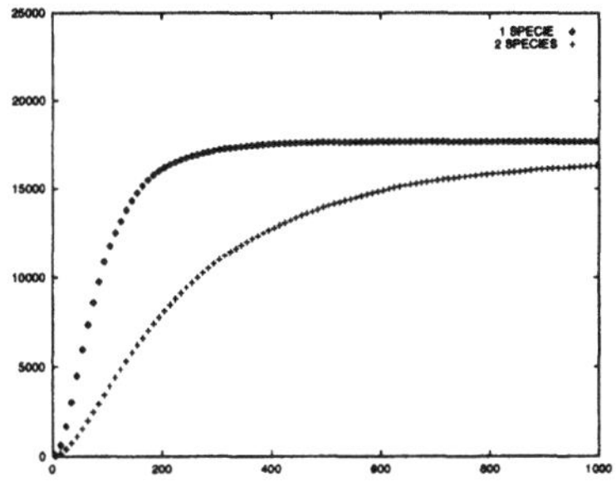

Fig. 4. Evolution of the cluster's mass as a function of time.

Keeping ρ_A and ρ_B equal, it is possible to obtain A and B clusters quite different from each other by changing the seed's density g_A and g_B. This is illustrated on Fig. 5 with $g_B = 9g_A$ and different suspension densities. A clusters are grey, while B clusters are black in the images. These simulations differ from the previous one because the B seeds are 10% of the total seed population instead of 50%. We observe a large range of different geometries, depending on $\rho = \rho_A = \rho_B$, and a strong difference between the geometry of the A and B cluster in each simulation as well.

This can be quantified for instance through the number of connected components plotted in Fig. 6.a as a function of the density ρ for both A and B clusters, or more accurately through covariances:

$$C_{AB}(h) = P[X = A, X + h = B] \tag{1}$$

$$C_A(h) = P[X = A, X + h = A] \tag{2}$$

$$C_B(h) = P[X = B, X + h = B] \tag{3}$$

These 3 measurements are plotted on Fig. 6.b and 7. Fig. 6.a shows that the ratio $1/9$ between g_A and g_B is not kept in the cluster's connected components, because the largest components (type A) coalesce first. In Fig. 6.b, the slope $C'_{AB}(0)$ increases with ρ as the length of contact between A and B, while the range[1] is nearly constant.

From Fig. 7, the range is almost constant for A clusters, but increases with ρ for B clusters. This can be explained by the fact that A clusters are constrained to stay in a certain area that depends on the position of the surrounding B clusters (wall effect). This area does not depend on the suspension densities. On the contrary, the growth of B clusters is not disturbed, so that their range increases with ρ.

[1] Length h for which $C_{AB}(h)$ reaches its plateau.

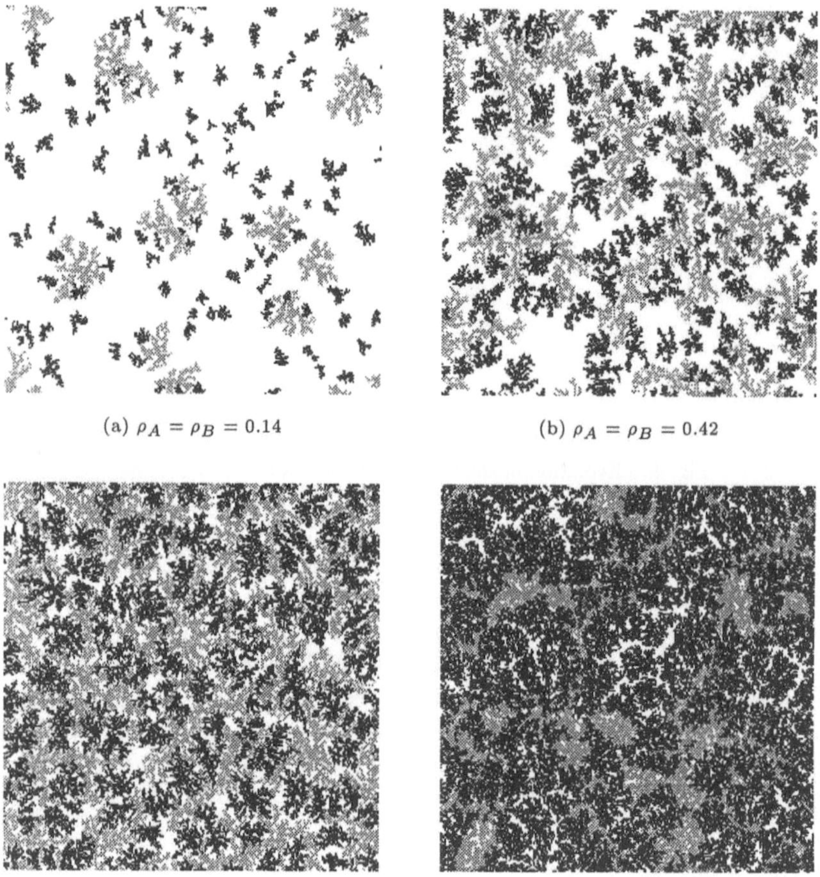

(a) $\rho_A = \rho_B = 0.14$ (b) $\rho_A = \rho_B = 0.42$

(c) $\rho_A = \rho_B = 0.7$ (d) $\rho_A = \rho_B = 1.4$

Fig. 5. Clusters obtained with solid seeds in proportion 1/10 for various densities.

Precipitation. The front between two phases after solidification can be, in some cases, simulated with a small change in the model. Instead of dropping the seeds at the beginning of the simulations, we may give to each suspension a probability p_P for precipitating in the surrounding fluid.

This process produces seeds continuously with time, the seeds of each specy appearing more frequently in places where this specy has a higher density. As a didactic example, we start the simulations with the species A and B split in two half parts of the system.

The two species melt into each other, and the slower the solidification happens, the more irregular the interfacial front is. In this set of simulations we observe the influence of the aggregation probability p^+ on the interfacial front: a high value speeds up the solidification process and leads to flatter fronts, as we can see in

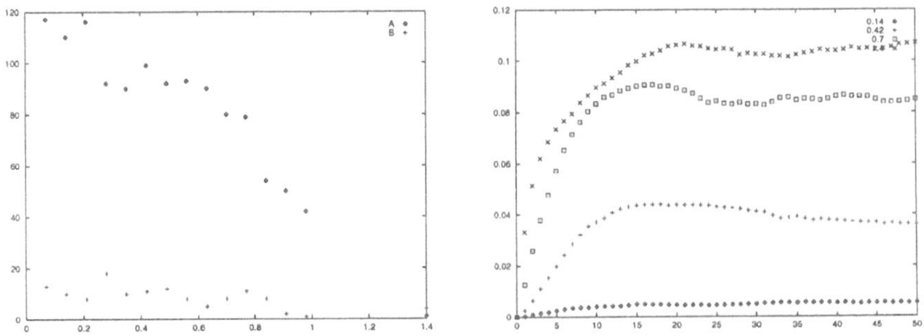

(a) Number of connected components (b) Crossed covariance

Fig. 6. Measurements on the clusters obtained with solid seeds in proportion 1/10.

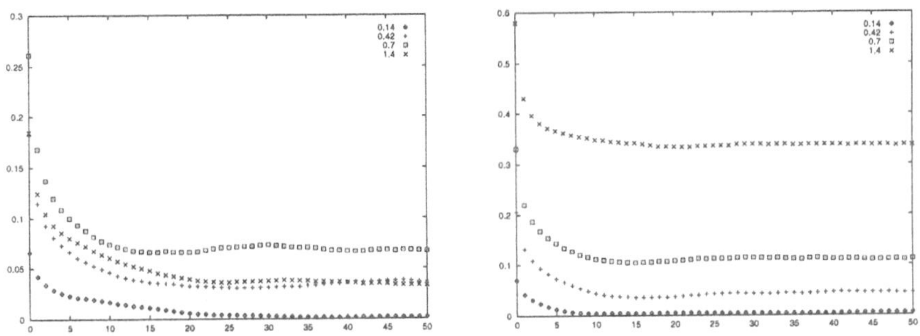

A clusters B clusters

Fig. 7. Covariances of the clusters obtained with solid seeds in proportion 1/10, for 4 values of ρ.

Fig. 8. The interfacial width is brought into evidence in the mass profiles of the final clusters, and is less and less important with the increasing of p^+ (Fig. 9).

(a) $p^+ = 0.01$ (b) $p^+ = 0.03$ (c) $p^+ = 0.1$

Fig. 8. Clusters obtained by precipitation and aggregation with several values of p^+. Separation fronts between A and B.

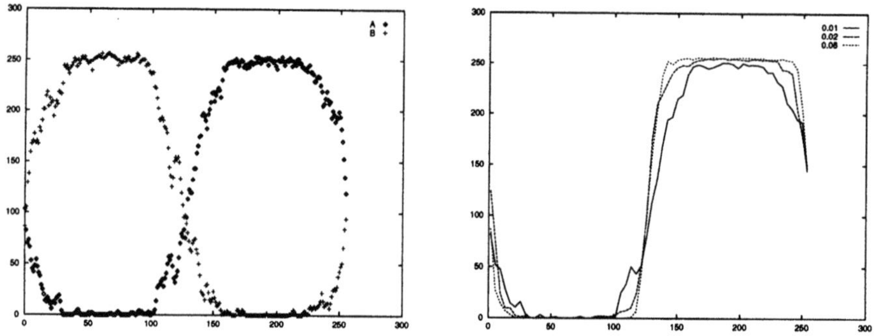

(a) A and B profiles, $p^+ = 0.01$ (b) A profile, depending on p^+.

Fig. 9. Clusters obtained by precipitation and aggregation, mass profiles.

4. Conclusion

The flexibility of the lattice gas model enables us to simulate the generation of media regulated by hydrodynamical rules. This was illustrated here by the formation of random clusters with two physical species. Two simple examples give a first idea of the diversity of the physical processes available through this modelization. The large range of geometrical structures obtained with this new class of models allows us to use them in many physical contexts, such as solidification, sedimentation and crystallization. In addition, the strong coupling between the velocity field and the geometry is satisfied with these simulations, unlike other methods. This fact allows us to perform the simulations in complex hydrodynamical flows.

References

Appert, C., Rothman, D. & Zaleski, S. (1990), *A liquid-gas model on a lattice*, G.D. Doolen, Physica D, pp. 85-96.

Brémond, R. (1993), Modélisation de la filtration par gaz sur réseau, PhD thesis, Ecole des Mines de Paris.

Brémond, R. & Jeulin, D. (1994), *Random media and lattice gas simulations*, in M. Armstrong & P. Dowd editors, Geostatistical Simulations, Kluwer academic publisher, pp. 89-105.

Frish, U., d'Humières, D., Hasslacher, B., Lallemand, P., Pomeau, Y. & Rivet, J. (1987), *Lattice gas hydrodynamics in 2 and 3 dimensions*, Complex Svstem 1, pp.75-136.

Frish, U., Hasslacher, B. & Pomeau, Y. (1986), *Lattice-gas automata for the Navier-Stokes equation*, Phys. Rev. Lett, pp. 11-18.

Hardy, J., Pomeau, Y. & de Pazzis, O. (1976), *Molecular dynamics of a classical lattice gas : transport properties and time correlation functions*, Phys. Rev. A, 13, pp. 1949-1961.

Meakin, P. (1986), *Computer simulation of growth and aggregation processes*, On growth and forms, fractal and non-fractal patterns in physics. Martinus Nijhoff publishers, pp.111-135.

Meakin, P. & Sanders, L. (1985), Phys. Rev. Lett, vol 54, p. 2053.

Rothman, D. & Keller, J. (1989), *Immiscible cellular automaton fluids*, Lattice gas methods for PDE, Addison-Wesley, pp.275-282.

Witten, T. & Sanders, L. (1981), Phys. Rev. Lett, vol 47, p. 1400.

SINGLE OBJECT GEOMETRY — THE STEREOLOGY OF REGISTERED SERIAL SECTIONS

C. VYVYAN HOWARD
Department of Fetal & Infant Pathology, University of Liverpool
PO Box 147, Liverpool L69 3BX, U.K.

1. Introduction

The advent of the confocal microscope has stimulated the development of a series of new design-based stereological estimators that require perfectly registered serial sections. Most classical first order stereological estimators, which do not employ registered serial sections, deliver estimates that are an average over all features in the reference volume. This approach is very efficient and remains the most expedient way of obtaining such data. However the collection of data from an 'unbiased brick' (Howard *et al.*, 1995) made up of perfectly registered serial sections opens the way for the accurate stereological measurement of geometrical features of a single object. It also provides a sampling mechanism for the measurement of second order stereological properties.

For some estimators, notably volume and 0-dimensional features such as number, spatial distribution and connectivity, the orientation of the 'unbiased brick' is of no consequence for the unbiasedness of the estimate, although it can have an effect on estimator variance. Estimators of feature length and/or surface however do require randomisation of orientation, according to protocols mentioned below. Each of the possible estimators will now be mentioned, giving references to the published literature.

2. Unbiased Stereological Estimators

Volume The Cavalieri Principle can be applied to a stack of arbitrarily oriented registered serial sections that are uniform random in position (Gundersen & Jensen, 1987). This has been applied to a single nerve cell by Howard et al. (1991).

Number estimation In arbitrarily oriented unbiased bricks particle number has been estimated by Howard et al (1985) using a sweeping optical section in the confocal microscope.

Spatial distribution 3-D spatial distribution functions have been demonstrated on x, y, z coordinate data for biological cells collected from unbiased bricks in confocal microscopy (Baddeley *et al.*, 1987; Konig *et al.*, 1991; Baddeley *et al.* 1993).

J.Serra and P. Soille (eds.), Mathematical Morphology and Its Applications to Image Processing, 305-307

Length estimation The length density of a space curve in 3-D can be estimated from the number of intersections of a projection of the curve, within a 'vertical' (Baddeley *et al.*, 1986) slab of known thickness, onto a cycloidal test system whose long axis is parallel to the 'vertical' direction (Gokhale, 1990).

If the whole curve is contained within a 'vertical slab' then its total length can be estimated without knowing the thickness of the slab (Cruz Orive & Howard, 1991). This has been applied to the estimation of nerve cell dendritic length (Howard *et al.*, 1992; Howard *et al.* 1993)

Surface estimation The surface of a single object can be estimated from an isotropic stack of perfectly registered sections by the method of the spatial grid (Sandau, 1987; Howard and Sandau, 1992). This method has been applied to a single nerve cell by Howard *et al.* (1993).

A major drawback is that, until recently, everything except the surface of a single object could be measured from an unbiased 'vertical' brick. Now an implementation of the 'vertical spatial grid' has been conceived by Cruz Orive & Howard (1994) in which it is possible to unbiasedly measure surface from a uniformly positioned and vertically rotated brick. This technique will be discussed in detail.

A summary of requirements for estimators using optical sections is given in Table I. 'IUR' means isotropic uniform random orientation and 'REGIST' indicates whether or not perfectly registered sections are required. Note that all the features listed can be estimated from a vertical brick.

TABLE I
Estimators using unbiased 'optical' bricks

Feature	Estimator	orientation Arbitrary	orientation Vertical	orientation IUR	REGIST
volume	Cavalieri	x	x	x	
surface	isotropic spatial grid			x	x
	vertical spatial grid		x		x
length	total vertical projections		x		x
number	Unbiased 'optical' brick	x	x	x	x
particle size	Unbiased 'optical' brick	x	x	x	x
spatial distribution	Unbiased 'optical' brick	x	x	x	x

3. Discussion

The advantage of the stereological approach currently is that they can be applied directly to live images where the eye can make the segmentation. In most of biological microscopy reliable segmentation is the major problem in any automatic image analysis application. The combination of interactive computer technology with the power of the eye for segmentation has already been proposed (Moss *et al.*, 1989) and an example of its implementation for single object stereology is given by Howard *et al.* (1993).

Commercial software has been produced by Kinetic Imaging Ltd[1] (formerly Confocal Technologies Ltd) which makes these and other standard stereological ratio estimator measurements automatically on binarised images or interactively on grey scale images.

If the whole 3-D data set can be reliably segmented then all these measurements become completely available and automatic techniques then become the approach of choice. An example of such an approach on a confocal data set is given by Conan *et al.* (1992).

References

Baddeley A., Gundersen H.J.G. & Cruz Orive L.M. (1986). Estimation of surface area from vertical sections. *J. Microsc.* 142: 259-276.

Baddeley, A., Howard, C.V., Boyde, A. & Reid, S. (1987). 3-D spatial statistical analysis of osteocyte lacunae, using Tandem Scanning Reflected Light Microscopy. *Acta Stereologica*, 6(Suppl II), 87-100

Baddeley A.J., Moyeed R.A., Howard CV & Boyde A. (1993). Analysis of a three dimensional point pattern with replication. *Appl. Statist.* 42: 461-668.

Conan V., Gesbert S., Howard C.V., Jeulin D. Meyer F. & Renard D. (1992). Geostatistical and morphological methods applied to three-dimensional microscopy. *J. Microsc.* 166: 169-185.

Cruz Orive, L.M., & Howard, C.V. (1991). Estimating the length of a bounded curve in 3D using total vertical projections. *J. Microsc.* 163: 101-114.

Cruz Orive, L.M., & Howard, C.V. (1994). Estimation of individual feature surface area with the vertical spatial grid. *J. Microsc.* (submitted)

Gokhale A.M. (1990). Unbiased estimation of curve length in 3D using vertical slices. *J. Microsc.* 159: 133-141.

Gundersen H.J.G. & Jensen E.B. (1987). The efficiency of systematic sampling in stereology and its prediction. *J. Microsc.* 147: 229-263.

Howard C.V., Cruz Orive L.M. & Yaegashi H. (1992). Estimating neuron dendritic length in 3-D from total vertical projections and from vertical slices. *Acta Neurologica Scandinavica* 137: 14-19.

Howard, C.V. & Sandau, K. (1992). Measuring the surface area of a cell by the method of the spatial grid with a CSLM - a demonstration. *J. Microsc.* 162: 183-188.

Howard, C.V., Reid, S., Baddeley, A. & Boyde, A. (1985). Unbiased estimation of particle density in th Tandem Scanning Reflected Light Microscope. *J. Microsc.* 138, 203- 212

Howard, C.V., Jolleys G., Stacey D., Fowler A., Wallen P., & Browne M (1993). Measurement of total neuronal volume, surface area and dendritic length following intracellular physiological recording. *Neuroprotocols* 2: 113-120.

Konig D., Caravajal-Gonzalez S., Downs A.M., Vassy J. & Rigaut J.P. (1991). Modelling and analysis of 3D arrangements of particles by point processes with examples of application to biological data obtained by confocal scanning light microscopy. *J. Microscopy* 161: 405-433.

Moss, M.C., Browne, M.A., Howard, C.V. & Joyner, D. (1989). An interactive image analysis system for measuring mean particle volume. *J. Microscopy.* 156: 79-90

Sandau K. (1987). How to estimate the area of a surface using the spatial grid. *Acta Stereol.* 6/III: 31-36.

[1] Kinetic Imaging Ltd, South Harrington Building, Sefton St, Liverpool L3 4BQ UK Fax int+ 44 51 709 6466.

TEXTURE CLASSIFICATION USING NEURAL NETWORKS AND LOCAL GRANULOMETRIES

C. GRATIN and J. VITRIÀ
Departament d'Informàtica, Universitat Autónoma de Barcelona, 08193 Bellaterra (Barcelona).

and

F. MORESO and D. SERÓN
Department of Nephrology, Hospital Príncipes de España, Barcelona.

Abstract. This paper presents a method for segmenting interstitium and tubules in images of kidneys' biopsies. Openings by structuring elements of increasing size, forming a *granulometry*, were performed on the entire image. For every pixel x and for each size of the structuring element the volume over a small window centered at x was measured (a *local* Granulometry). The vectors defined as the volume gradient served as an entry to a neural network (NN). The NN was taught to discriminate between vectors corresponding to pixels of the interstitium (textured region) and vectors corresponding to pixels of the tubules (non-textured region). The correlation factor between the area of the interstitium and the renal function was computed and compared to the results obtained with the manual procedure and two other automatic procedures.

Key words: Neural Networks, Granulometry, Kidney, Texture, Classification

1. Introduction

It was shown in [2] that there exists a strong correlation ($R^2 = 0.54$, for the set of data used in this study) between the interstitial surface measured in kidneys biopsies and the Renal Function (RF). Interstitial surface was measured by stereological methods, i.e. by superimposing a grid of points to the image and counting manually the number of points falling into the interstitium (Fig. 1a). Results of these measures, obtained for 202 images taken from 35 biopsies, are shown in Fig. 1b. The main disadvantages of this method are that it is time consuming and may vary depending on the observer.

Colomé-Serra [4] proposed an alternative approach which constisted of treating the image as a whole and not trying to segment it. A grey level granulometry was used which involved openings by hexagons of increasing size computed over the entire image. The result of this granulometry is a curve associated with each image. A multilinear regression was then obtained to establish a correlation with the renal function and to build an estimator. However, the approach proposed herein relies on segmentation of the images. Since it is impossible to decide whether a pixel belongs to a tubule or to the interstitium by considering only its grey level, textural information was used by computing a local granulometry over a small square window

J.Serra and P. Soille (eds.), Mathematical Morphology and Its Applications to Image Processing, 309-316

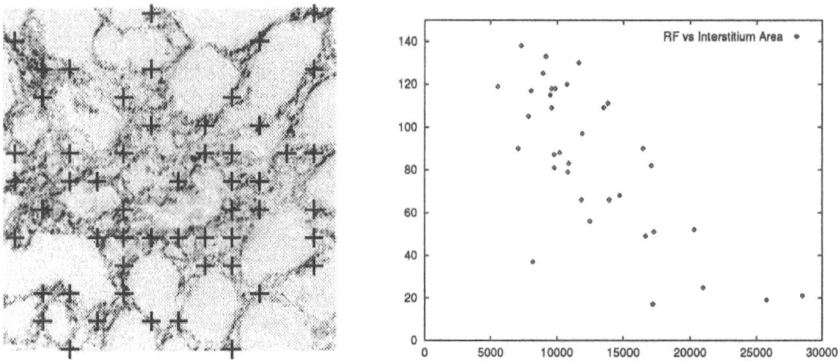

a b

Fig. 1. Measure of intersticial surface using point counting.

centered on each pixel. This granulometry forms vectors which were classified using a two (hidden) layer neural network.

2. Materials

The data set used consists of 202 images of size 256×256 pixels taken from 35 biopsies (4 to 6 fields for each biopsy) with different degrees of renal damage. Biopsies were stained with sirius red and digitized under polarized light. Images obtained with this technique are nearly binary, as can be seen in Fig. 2. Here tubules appear as white, non-textured and rather convex regions, while interstitium is limited to fine dark lines separating the tubules in the sanest biopsies (Fig. 2a). *Progression of tubulo-interstitial chronic renal damage is characterized by interstitial fibrosis, tubular atrophy and a decrease in the number of peritubular capillary* [3]. As damage increases, interstitium area tends to increase. Interstitial structures appear as textured regions, with no privileged orientation, in which it is not always easy to distinguish between interstitium and small size tubules or tubules in phase of decomposition (Fig. 2b and Fig. 2c).

3. Method

3.1. GRANULOMETRY

A series of openings γ [10] with a family of structuring elements $B_1, B_2, \ldots, B_n$, is a granulometry if it satisfies the following axiom [8]:

$$\forall(i,j) \;\; i \leq j \Rightarrow \gamma_{B_i} \geq \gamma_{B_j}.$$

As the size of the structuring element increases, more and more details in the image are suppressed. Small structures present in the interstitium disappear after the first openings, whereas large structures such as tubules remain nearly unchanged until large structuring elements are used. This phenomenon is illustrated in Fig. 3. Since

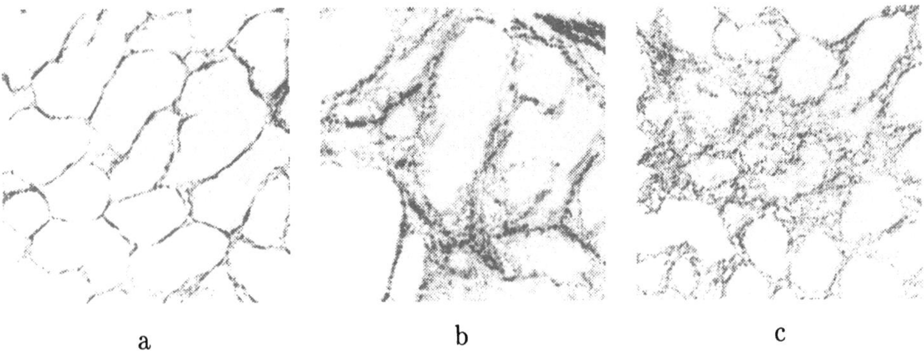

Fig. 2. Images presenting an increasing renal damage: (a) sane, (b) & (c): pathological.

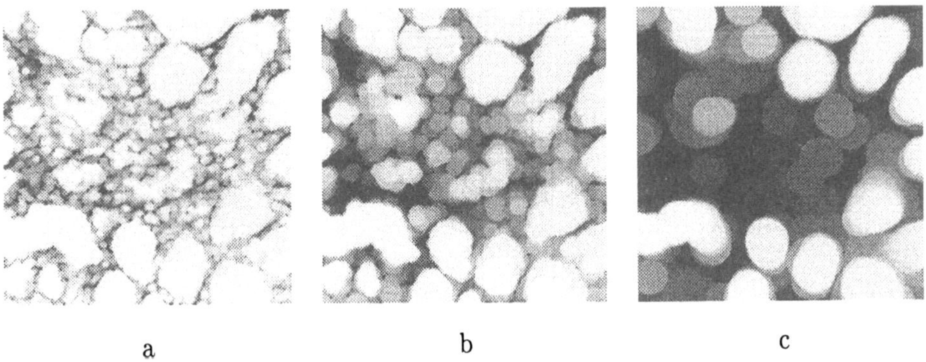

Fig. 3. Openings by disks of increasing radius: (a) 2, (b) 6 & (c) 15.

interstitial texture is isotropic, isotropic structuring elements were chosen. These were digital approximations of disks (B_i) satisfying:

$$\forall(i,j) \;\; i \leq j \Rightarrow \gamma_{B_i}(B_j) = B_j.$$

This property ensures that the granulometric axiom is fulfilled (note that $\gamma_{B_i}(B_{i+1}) = B_{i+1}$ is a sufficient condition as well).

Interstitium texture is characterized by structures of small size, typically almost completely erased after an opening by a disk of radius 6. Therefore more importance was given to small size structures by putting in the granulometry (γ_i) more openings of small size. ($\gamma_1 \; \gamma_2 \; \gamma_3 \; \gamma_4 \; \gamma_6 \; \gamma_{10} \; \gamma_{15} \; \gamma_{25}$) was the family of closings chosen.

3.2. Local Granulometry

In contrast to what was done in [4], the volume of the successive openings was not measured over the whole image. For each pixel x the volume $V_i(x)$ was measured over a 17×17 pixels window centered on x. The volume $(V_i(x))_{i=1,\dots,n}$ is an n-dimensional vector at x, called here a local granulometry (LG). In the following we will only consider the *granulometric spectrum* of the image at x, i.e. the differential of the LG defined as

$$dV_i(x) = V_i(x) - V_{i-1}(x),$$

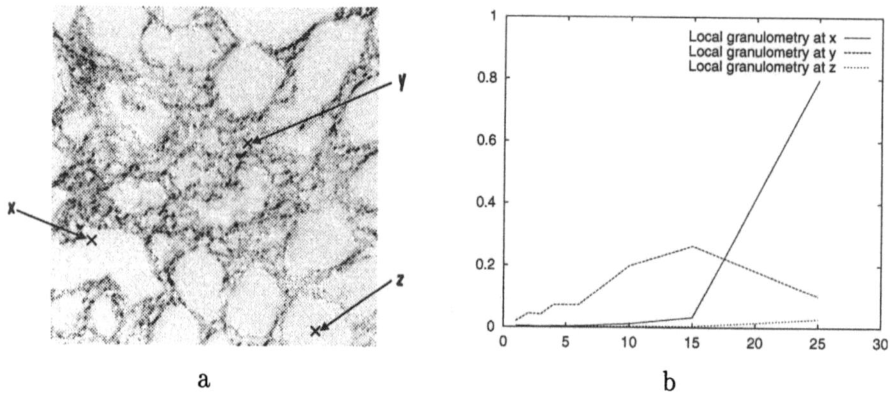

Fig. 4. Local Granulometries of points situated in a tubule (x and z) and in the interstitium (y).

with $V_0(x)$ being the volume measured on the initial image. Figure 4b shows the granulometric curves $dV_i(x)$ corresponding to the three points selected in Fig. 4a.

We considered a 17×17 window large enough to contain textural information and small enough to remain "local". However, two neighboring pixels will have similar granulometric curves. Therefore, transitions from textured regions to non-textured regions tend to be smooth (and progressively smoother as the size of the window used increases).

LG's are an efficient tool to discriminate between textured and non-textured regions but it has a major disadvantage: only using this information usually makes it impossible to detect the fine dark interstitial lines that appear in normal biopsies between two tubules. Therefore, the grey level of pixel x was added to vector $dV_i(x)$. The resulting $n+1$ dimensional vector constituted the input to the neural network.

3.3. Neural Network

A fully connected neural network with 9 input neurons, 10 neurons in a first layer, 3 in a second layer and 1 neuron in the output layer, was formulated in the Aspirin language [7]. A C program was generated using Aspirin's compiler. A description of the network in Aspirin and it's graphical representation is shown in Fig. 5.

We limited the dimension of the input space to 9 in order to reduce the number of examples necessary for the network to generalize. In fact, as noted in [6], if there are less examples than weights (i.e. connections), then the network tends only to memorize and reproduce these examples. A first attempt was made with a one (hidden) layer network, but results improved significantly by adding a second layer.

The dimension of the input space also influences the number of neurons of the first hidden layer. For example, a neuron calculating only the sign of the weighted sum of its inputs (i.e. the sigmoid function is replaced by a simple threshold) is in fact partitioning the space with a hyperplane into two half-spaces [9]. It follows that 10 $(9+1)$ is the minimum number of neurons necessary to delineate a bounded region in the 9-dimensional input space.

In this study about 150 points, taken from 8 images, were selected, classified manually and introduced in the network. A zero output value was assigned to

```
DefineBlackBox Kidney {
  OutputLayer-> OUTPUT
  InputSize-> [9 x 1]
  Components-> {
     PdpNode OUTPUT [1 x 1] {
       InputsFrom-> Layer2
     }
     PdpNode Layer2 [3 x 1] {
       InputsFrom-> Layer1
     }
     PdpNode Layer1 [10 x 1] {
       InputsFrom-> $INPUTS
     }
  }
}
```

a

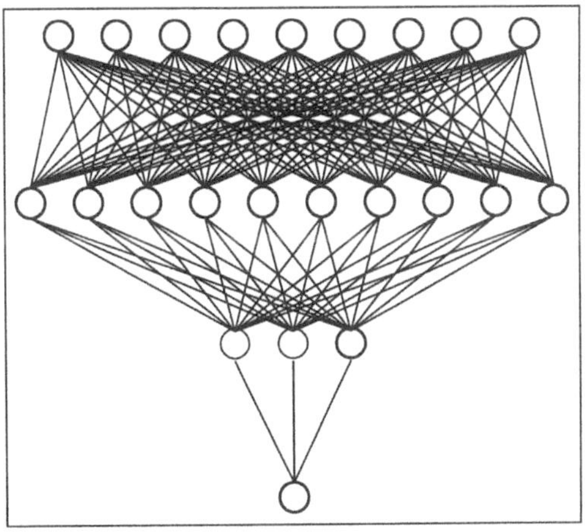

b

Fig. 5. Aspirin description (a) and graphical representation (b) of the NN.

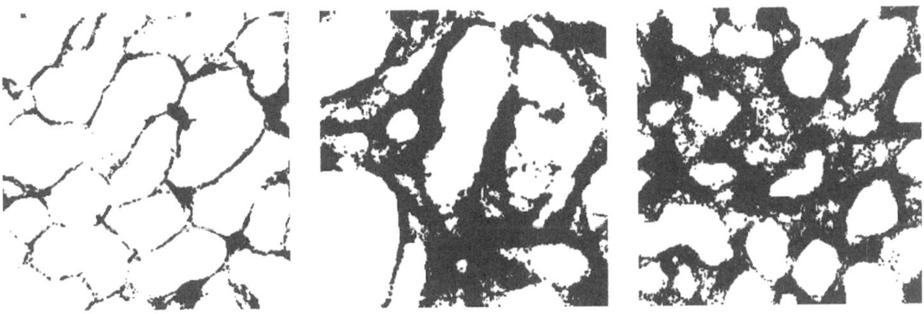

Fig. 6. Classification obtained for the images presented in Fig. 2.

interstitium while value of one was assigned to tubules. Weights were computed using a backpropagation learning algorithm with a 10 % output error.

4. Results

Local granulometries for all the points of the 202 images were achieved with the help of ViLi software [1]. The output of the neural network was then computed and results were reassembled to form an image whose values were contained between 0 and 100. Pixels whose values were lower than 49 were classified as interstitium and pixels whose values were greater than 50 were classified as tubule. Figure 6 illustrates the results obtained for the 3 images in Fig. 2.

More interesting are the correlation factors between the interstitium area measured on all the images and the area determined manually, and between the mean of the interstitium area for all the images of a same biopsy and renal function.

- Automatic measure vs manual measure: $R^2 = 0.85$,
- Mean of interstitium area (automatic) vs renal function: $R^2 = 0.53$,

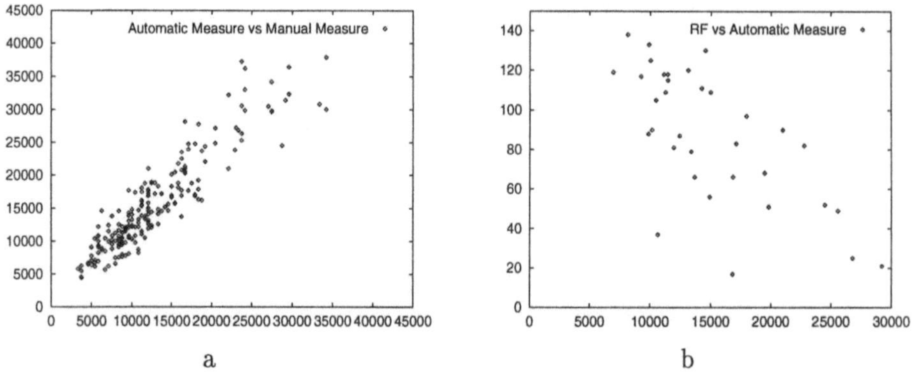

Fig. 7. Results plotted as a function of the areas measured manually (a) and as a function of renal function.

– Mean of interstitium area (manual) vs renal function: $R^2 = 0.54$.

Figure 7 shows the distributions of these measures as a function of the areas measured manually (a) and as a function of renal function (b).

These diagrams indicate that the proposed classification method reproduces the human process ($R^2 = 0.85$) rather well and that it is nearly as accurate in the estimation of the renal function ($R^2 = 0.53$ vs 0.54).

5. Comparison with other methods

Neural Networks were not the only method investigated to segment interstitium. Two other more conventional methods, based on mathematical morphology operators, were also tried. They are described briefly below and their results can be compared with the results shown above.

5.1. Method using a simple threshold

As we noted earlier, images are nearly binary although some variations of the grey level's dynamic can be observed between two images taken from two distinct biopsies. The main issue is that interstitium does not restrict to dark regions but also includes textured regions where white small structures alternate with dark ones. The solution that we adopted was simply to threshold each image between 0 and $N\%$ of the mean and apply a morphological closing to the result using as a disk structuring element. The best result (in terms of maximum correlation with renal function) was obtained by setting N to 96% and the radius of the disk to 4.

Figure 8 shows the segmentation obtained with this method for the image of Fig. 2c (a) and renal function plotted as a function of the measures obtained for the 35 biopsies (b). The correlation factor was $R^2 = 0.52$, which we consider to be a good result (although area tends to be over-estimated).

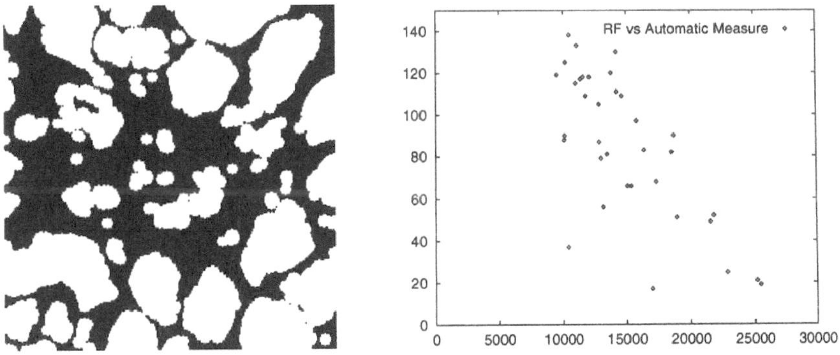

a b

Fig. 8. Results of the threshold based method.

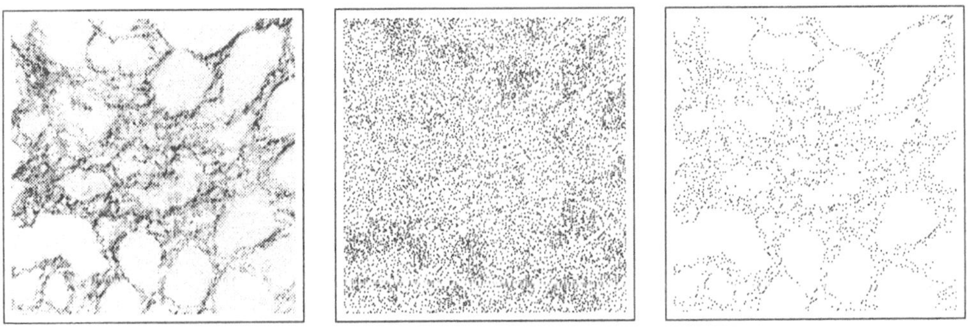

a b c

Fig. 9. Original Image (a), Regional Minima (b), Regional Minima whose dynamic is greater than 13 (c).

5.2. Method based on the dynamic of the minima

The second method is based on the observation that interstitial regions are regions containing many regional minima. Due to acquisition noise, there are also many minima inside the tubules but the former and the latter can be easily discriminated using a criteria of dynamic [5]. Figure 9 illustrates this phenomena: In (b) tubules contain many minima but in (c) none of dynamics greater than 13.

The solution retained was thus to compute the dynamic of the minima and threshold the resulting image between N and 255 (the maximum grey level value). Interstitium was then reconstructed by applying a morphological closing using a disk as structuring element. The best result (in terms of maximum correlation with the renal function) was obtained by setting N to 13 and the radius of the disk to 5.

Figure 10 shows the segmentation obtained with this method for the image of Fig. 2c (a) and the renal function plotted as a function of the measures obtained for the 35 biopsies (b). The correlation factor was $R^2 = 0.54$. This is equivalent to the correlation obtained with the manual method.

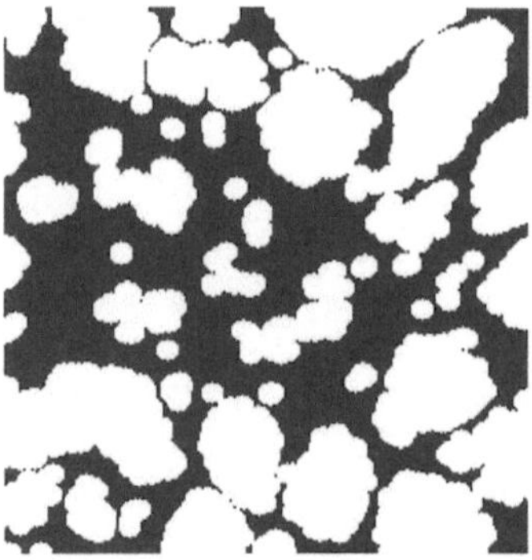

a

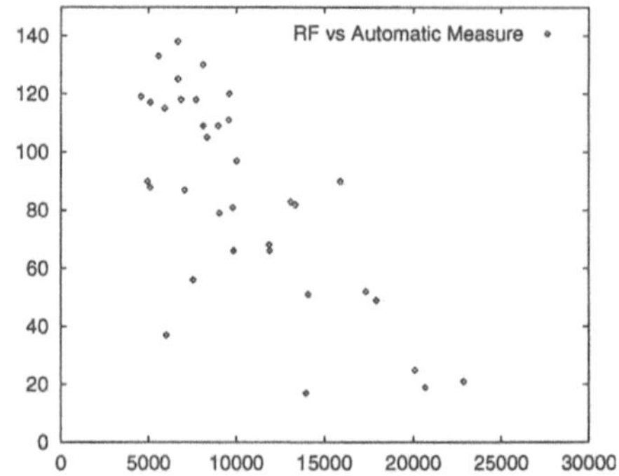

b

Fig. 10. Results of the dynamic based method.

6. Conclusion

Three methods for the automatic segmentation of interstitium in images of kidneys' biopsies have been presented, with particular emphasis on a method achieving pixel classification through the use of a Neural Network. All three methods reproduce the results obtained by manual classification rather well. The use of a neural network seems promising since it does not require any size or threshold parameter. Moreover it is a "dynamic" system that can be modified through learning if it appears to give unsatisfactory results for some images. Clinical implementation of the three methods is in progress and should provide data to validate or invalidate the results presented here.

References

1. Vili (vision lisp). Image Processing Functions. User & Programmer Manual. Technical report, Universitat Autònoma de Barcelona, 1993.
2. D. Serón et al. Relationship between donor renal interstitial surface and post-transplant function. *Nephrol Dial Transplant*, 8:539–543, 1993.
3. F. Moreso et al. Quantification of interstitial chronic renal damage by means of image analysis. *Submitted*, 1994.
4. M.F. Colomé-Serra et al. Image analysis: utility of grey level granulometry to measure renal intersticial chronic damage. In *Proc. IEEE Int. Conf. Medicine*, pages 1934–1935, 1993.
5. M. Grimaud. *La géodésie numérique en morphologie mathématique. Application à la détection automatique de microcalcifications en mammographies numériques.* PhD thesis, Ecole des Mines de Paris, Décembre 1991.
6. K.J. Lang, A.H. Waibel, and G.E. Hinton. A time-delay neural network architecture for isolated word recognition. *Neural Networks*, 3:23–44, 1990.
7. Russel R. Leighton. The aspirin/migraines neural network software. User's Manual. Release V6.0. Technical report, MITRE Corporation, 1992.
8. G. Matheron. *Random Sets and Integral Geometry.* New York: Wiley, 1975.
9. L.I. Perlovsky. Computational concepts in classification: Neural networks, statistical pattern recognition, and model-based vision. *Journal of Mathematical Imaging and Vision*, 4:81–110, 1994.
10. J. Serra. *Image analysis and mathematical morphology.* Academic Press, 1982.

FUSION OF MR AND CT IMAGES OF THE HUMAN BRAIN USING MULTIRESOLUTION MORPHOLOGY

S. MARSHALL and G. K. MATSOPOULOS
Department of Electronic and Electrical Eng.
University of Strathclyde,
204 George St, Glasgow, U.K.

and

J.N.H. BRUNT
Department of Medical Physics,
Clatterbridge Centre for Oncology,
Wirral, Merseyside, U.K.

Abstract. A hierarchical image fusion scheme is presented which preserves the details of the input images regardless of their scale. The technique is demonstrated by fusing images of the human brain derived from magnetic resonance (MR) and computed tomography (CT) scanners. Results are given to show that fused images preserve a more complete representation of anatomical and pathological structures, providing information that cannot be obtained by processing the images at a single scale. The use of different morphological filters for pyramid construction and reconstruction is investigated and the variations in results are highlighted.

Key words: Medical Imaging, Morphology, Pyramids, Magnetic Resonance, Computed Tomography

1. Introduction

This paper describes an application of multiresolution morphological pyramids to the fusion of a stack of CT and MR data from the same patient. The patient was specially scanned to allow registration of images. In management of patients undergoing radiotherapy or skull based surgery, the information provided by magnetic resonance imaging (MR) and X-ray computed tomography (CT) is complementary. Normal and pathological soft tissue are better visualised by MR, whilst the structure of bone is better visualised by CT. This paper describes a fusion scheme to combine information from different modalities which is based on Morphological Multiresolution Image Representation and Decomposition, Haralick [1] and Toet [2]. Existing multiresolution image representation and decomposition schemes, Burt [3], have used linear filters with progressively increasing spatial extent to generate a sequence of images with decreasing resolution, called a pyramid. More recently, morphological filters have been applied to generate a resolution hierarchy. The pyramid is produced by low-pass filtering the image and then sampling to generate the next lower resolution level of the hierarchy. The basis for a morphological pyramid requires a morphological sampling theorem, Haralick [4], which explains how an appropriately morphologically filtered and sampled image relates to the unsampled image. The use of the scheme is illustrated by images from a cancer patient for whom radiotherapy

J.Serra and P. Soille (eds.), Mathematical Morphology and Its Applications to Image Processing, 317-324

was being planned.

Why use non linear rather than linear pyramid techniques? Non linear filters have certain advantages over their linear equivalents for this type of analysis, such as speed of computation and edge- and feature-preserving properties. It has long since been claimed that non linear filtering preserves edge features and that linear filtering blurs them. Bangham [5, 6] has made some detailed studies of the behaviour of specific features, such as edges, under both linear and non linear filtering. He concludes that under linear filtering, edge features decompose into a wide range of scales. This is to be expected, as linear decomposition is closely related to frequency analysis and we know that edge features contain many frequencies. However, under non linear filtering, edge features tend to 'drop out' at a single scale under decomposition and are not present at the other scales. It is for this reason that an approach based on non linear filtering has been used in this paper.

2. Image Acquisition

The patient wore a radiotherapy planning mask during both CT and MR imaging. In both modalities, 'survey' scans were initially performed for use in planning the main scans and, in both modalities, the main scans were transverse to the (head to foot) axis of the patient. The CT images were obtained on a General Electric Pace scanner using a 512×512 pixel matrix. The MR images were obtained using a Philips Gyroscan T5-II scanner (0.5T). The size of the MR field of view was selected so that the linear dimension of the pixels (on a 256×256 matrix) was double that in the CT scans, and the separation distance between centres of slices in MR and CT was made equal. The MR sequence used for this fusion study was Spin Echo, with repetition time and echo time values (450 ms, 25ms) chosen to cause the imaging to be weighted by the longitudinal relaxation time T1. Attached to the mask were lengths of tubing of diameter approximately 3 mm. The wall of the tubing incorporated an X-ray opaque stripe visible on CT, and the tubing contained vegetable fat, melted for filling, and producing a strong signal on MR. The use of these markers confirmed the accuracy of the registration between CT and MR scans.

3. Morphological Pyramid construction

The overall fusion strategy is shown in Figure 1. According to this strategy a morphological pyramid is first produced for each of the input images. Then a morphological difference pyramid is constructed, for each of the above pyramids. This is achieved by taking the differences between the morphological images residing at successive levels in the original pyramid. An intermediate pyramid is constructed combining information from the two difference pyramids at each level. Finally, reconstruction of the intermediate pyramid, using appropriate morphological operations, produces the required fused image.

The morphological pyramid construction scheme, Matsopoulos *et al.* [7], is applied to each input image. The process which generates each image from its predecessor is called a Pyramid Construction (PC) operation, which is known as a reducing operation, since both resolution and sampling density are decreased. After the PC operation is applied, the new morphological image is sampled to generate the next level of the pyramid. This process is repeated to construct two pyramids, one for the MR data and one for the CT data. As well as being flat, the structuring element, K, is also symmetric and it is used at each level during the pyramid construction process. S_t is the sampling lattice corresponding to the level t of the pyramid . The pyramid is constructed such that $(S_i > S_j)$ for $(i < j)$. Let I_t be the representation of the image at level t of the pyramid, then I_0, I_1 and I_N represent, respectively, the original image I, the bottom level and the top level of the pyramid. i.e. I_N has the coarsest level of sampling and I_1 has the finest. The iterative pyramid generation scheme, using the PC operation, is given by:

$$P_t = PC(I_{t-1}) = \{MF_k(I_{t-1})\}|_{S_t} \tag{1}$$

where MF_k is the general result of applying a morphological filter to image I at level t. The precise choice of filter is discussed later.

3.1. Morphological Difference Pyramid construction

The difference pyramid D is a group of difference images in which each image contains only details within a restricted range of scales and therefore contains only those image features lost from one filter step to the next. The difference pyramid can be computed as the difference between successive levels of P, using an inverse morphological operation, called Pyramid ReConstruction (PRC), which is an expanding operation. The difference pyramid is produced by the following operation:

$$D(P_t) = \begin{cases} P_t - PRC(P_{t+1}) & \text{when } t < N \\ P_N & \text{when } t = N \end{cases} \tag{2}$$

where PRC is a morphological filtering operation by a binary structuring element, M, at level t, following a resampling operation. Effectively, each level of the pyramid is expanded to have the same number of points as the one beneath, smoothed and then subtracted from it.

3.2. Intermediate Pyramid Construction - Reconstruction

After a difference pyramid is constructed for both of the input images, a new intermediate pyramid, ID, is produced. The new pyramid combines information from the two difference pyramids at each level. A fusing function is defined which determines how the values from each image are combined and results in the construction of the intermediate pyramid. Various fusing functions could be applicable but the one used in this paper took the absolute point by point maximum, i.e. in the case of the fusion of two input images A and B into a single output image C, then:

$$ID(C)_t(i,j) = \begin{cases} D(A)_t(i,j) & \text{when } (\|D(A)_t(i,j)\| > \|D(B)_t(i,j)\|) \\ D(B)_t(i,j) & \text{otherwise} \end{cases} \tag{3}$$

where $D(A), D(B)$ represent the difference pyramids for the two source images and $ID(C)$ represents the intermediate difference pyramid for the fused output image. Finally, the fused image was recovered from its difference pyramid representation through the reconstruction procedure, as follows:

$$R_t = \begin{cases} ID_t + PRC(ID_{t+1}) & \text{when } t < N \\ ID_N & \text{when } t = N \end{cases} \tag{4}$$

where the ID_t is the intermediate difference image at level t.

The final reconstructed image contains details of both input images regardless of scale. This method was applied to real data, derived from MR and CT images of the human brain and the results are presented in the next section.

4. Results

The morphological data fusion scheme was applied to the MR and CT images of a patient scanned at Clatterbridge. Figures 2a and b show the data pyramid for the CT and MR scans. The original CT and MR scans are the images shown at the bottom level of these two pyramids. The morphological filter used in both the construction and reconstruction of these data structures was an open-close by a 3×3 flat structuring element. The sampling ratio was 2:1. The intermediate difference pyramid is shown in Figure 2c and the reconstructed pyramid in Figure 2d. The final fused image is at the bottom level of this pyramid. Notice how the details from each modality appear in the fused image.

To compare different types of filter, the process was repeated using an opening operation for pyramid construction (equation 1) and a closing for reconstruction (equations 2 and 4). In order to identify the places where the resulting images differed, the two were subtracted and the resulting difference image was overlayed on the results of Figure 2d. The result is shown in Figure 3, where the differences have been exaggerated to highlight their effect. Note that the differences are isolated and are thought to correspond to valleys in the original intensity profile which were not sufficiently smoothed prior to sampling, due to the asymmetric effect of the opening operator.

5. Discussion

An application of morphological pyramids, as introduced by Haralick [1] and Toet [2] has been presented. Figure 2d suggests that the morphological fusion scheme is of value for fusing data sets from different modalities. The fused images appear to preserve the regions of interest presented in both modalities, regardless of their size. As well as showing the details from each image, they are able to show their relative positions. This is useful in viewing MR and CT images of a patient where the position of bone is visualised relative to normal and pathological soft tissue.

The present work is intended for application in the field of radiotherapy treatment planning. In this field, the dose distribution from therapy radiation beams can be mapped onto images obtained by conventional projection X-ray techniques and by CT. Fusing MR imagery, which provides further information about the extent of malignant tissue, with CT would allow improved visualisation of the spatial relationship of dose distribution to tumour. Another field of application would be in planning plastic reconstructive surgery.

There are may combinations of filters which can be used to create the pyramids. It seems intuitively correct to employ a balanced operator such as open-close for both construction and reconstruction. The use of an asymmetric operator such as an opening for construction smooths the peaks but not the valleys within the intensity profile. This makes the sampling operation for the next level of the pyramid invalid and can lead to unpredictable effects.

Where a single pyramid is constructed and reconstructed from one image it will be recovered fully, as no information is lost. Even when the smoothing is insufficient, the difference pyramid will encode all differences from level to level. But in these cases the image features no longer decompose in a predictable and graceful way. The difference image can contain signals which bear little correlation to the image features.

During the data fusion stage these difference signals are combined with the difference signals from the other modality and they can lead to artifacts within the final image. It is therefore recommended that a balanced operator such as an open-close be used for both pyramid construction and reconstruction.

6. Conclusions

A medical image fusion scheme was presented in this paper. The method was based on a morphological multiresolution image representation and decomposition technique. The method was successfully applied for fusing pairs of images from different modalities; magnetic resonance (MR) and computed tomography (CT). The morphological fusion scheme seemed the most appropriate, since morphological filters preserve local contrast (i.e. edges) in comparison with linear filters, which blur these features. Results were presented to show that the fused images provided a more complete representation of the anatomy and pathology than was available from either individual modality or from simple single scale fusion techniques. The results also supported the hypothesis that it is preferable to use symmetric operators such as open-close rather than an opening or closing alone.

References

1. R.M. Haralick, C. Lin, J.S.J. Lee, and X. Zhuang, "Multiresolution Morphology", in Proc. 1st Intern. Confer. in Computer Vision, London, England, pp. 516-520, June 1987.
2. A. Toet, "A morphological pyramid image decomposition", Pattern Recognition Letters, vol. 9, No. 4, pp.255-261, 1989.
3. J. Burt, "The pyramid as a structure for efficient computation.", In: A Rosenfeld (ed) Multiresolution Image Processing and Analysis. Springer Verlag, Berlin, pp. 6-35, 1984.
4. R.M. Haralick, X. Zhuang, C. Lin, J.S.J. Lee, "The Digital Morphological Sampling Theorem", IEEE Trans. on Acoustics, Speech and Signal Process., vol. 37, No. 12, pp. 2067-2089, December 1989.
5. J.A. Bangham, "Properties of a series of nested median filters, namely the data sieve", IEEE Trans. on Signal Processing, vol. 41, No 1, pp. 31-42 January 1993.
6. J.A. Bangham, T.G. Campbell, "Sieves and wavelets: Multiscale transforms for pattern recognition", IEEE Workshop on Non Linear Digital Signal Processing, Tampere, Finland, January 1993.
7. G.K. Matsopoulos, S. Marshall, J.N.H. Brunt , "Multiresolution Morphological Fusion of MR and CT images of the human brain", Proceedings of IEE, Vision, Image and Signal Processing, vol. 141, No. 3, pp. 137-142, June 1994.

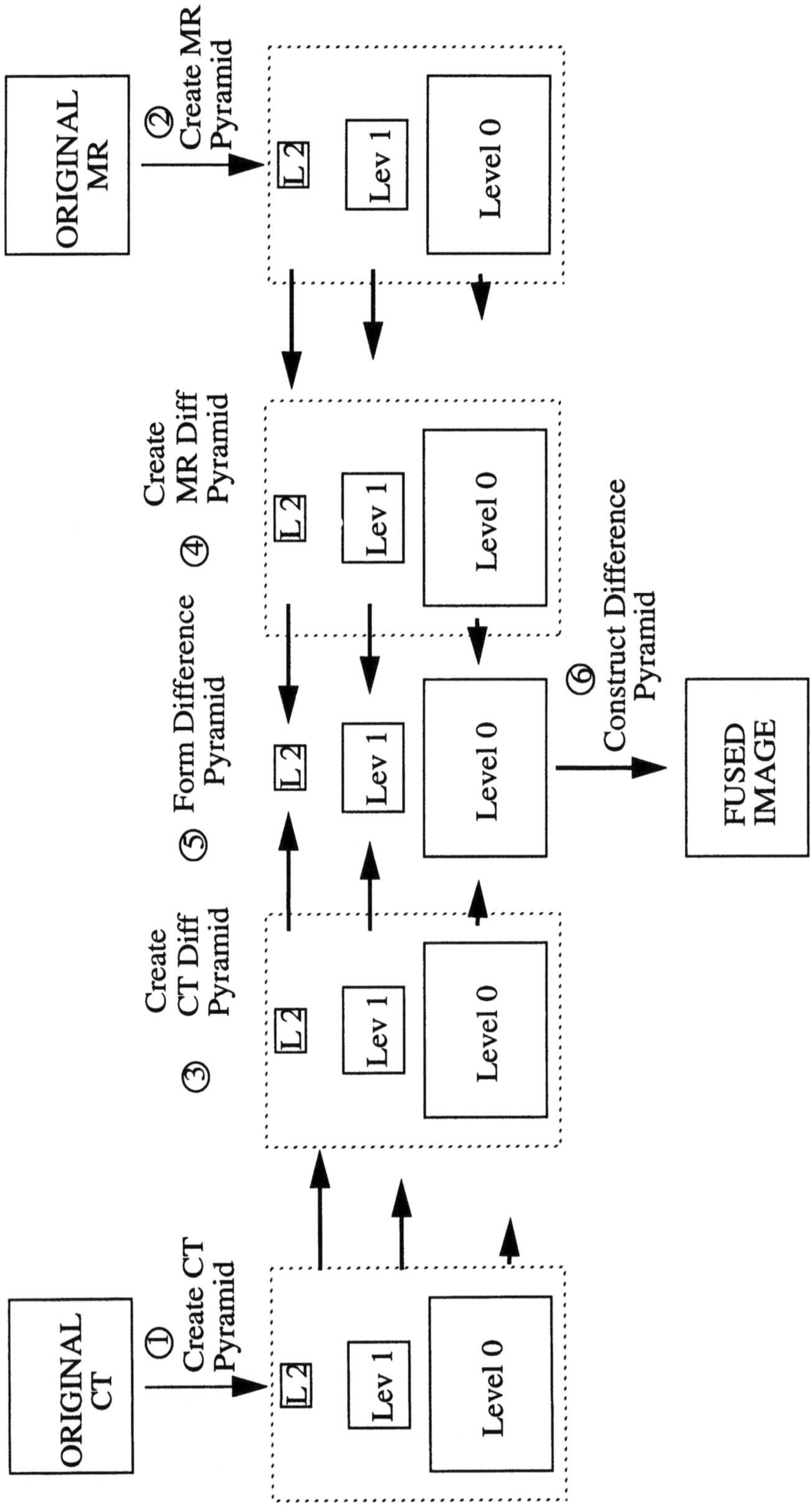

Fig. 1. Fusion Strategy

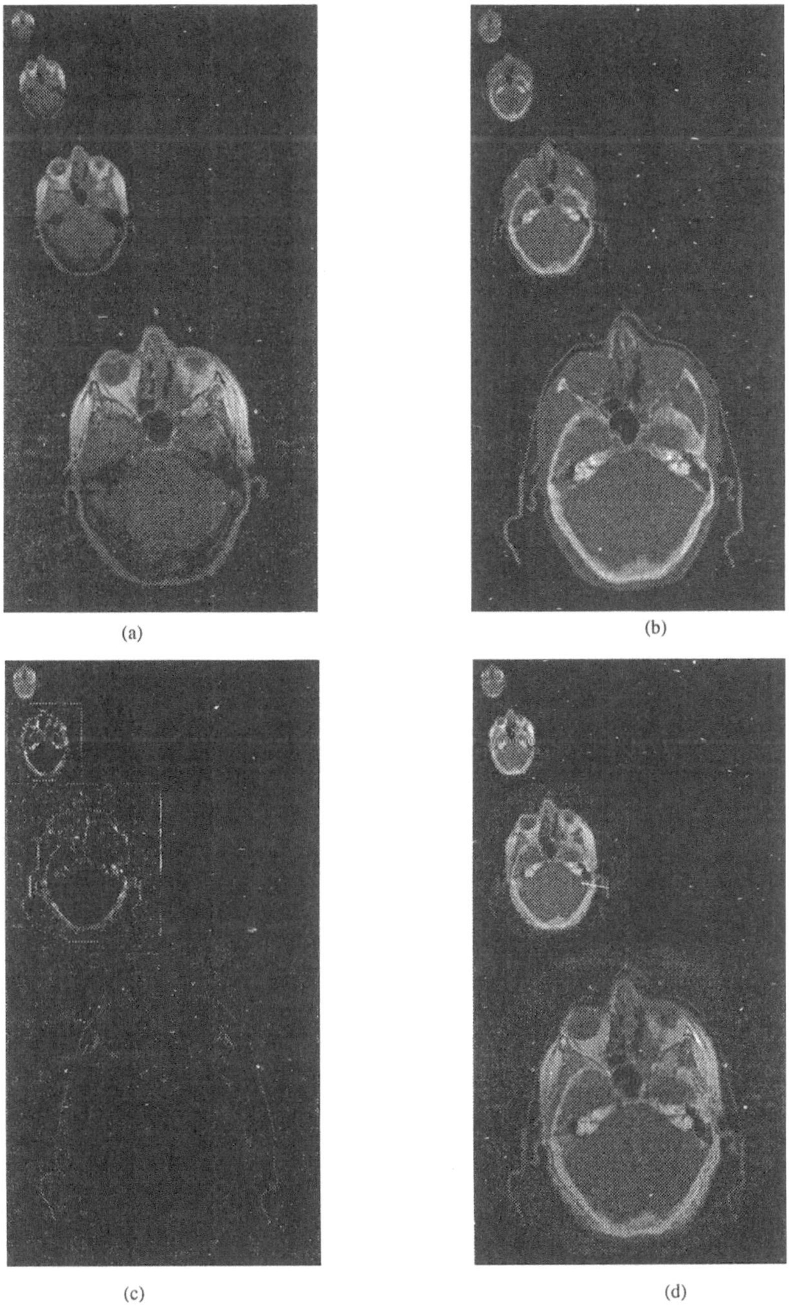

Fig. 2. Results of Fusion. The original (a) MR and (b) CT data pyramids, (c) the intermediate difference pyramid and (d) the reconstructed fused image. The original MR and CT images are at the bottom level of pyramids in (a and b) respectively and the final fused image is at the bottom level of (d). Both the pyramid construction and reconstruction operators used for these results were the open-close operation.

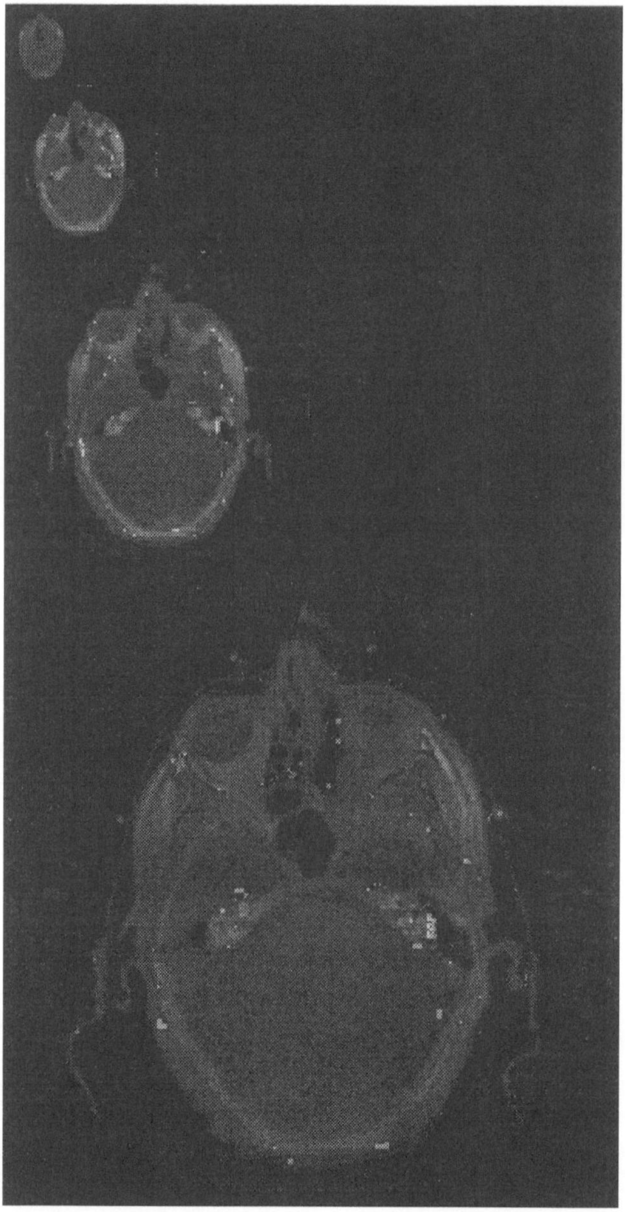

Fig. 3. Comparison of different pyramid construction/reconstruction operators. The figure shows the differences highlighted between an image fused using the open-close operator for both construction and reconstruction and an image fused using open for pyramid construction and closing for reconstruction.

MORPHOLOGICAL SCHEME FOR MORPHOMETRIC ANALYSIS OF EPIDERMAL BIOPSY IMAGES

J.R. CASAS and P. ESTEBAN
Dept. de Teoria del Senyal i Comunicacions
Universitat Politecnica de Catalunya
Apdo. 30 002, 08071 Barcelona, Spain.

and

A. MORENO and M. CARRERA
Servei d'Anatomia Patologica
Ciutat Sanitaria de Bellvitge
Feixa Llarga s/n, 08907 L'Hosp. de Llobregat, Spain.

Abstract.
This paper addresses the problem of morphometric analysis of microscope images from cutaneous biopsy samples. A morphological scheme is applied for the automatic measurement of histologic parameters of the epidermis. It consists in an unsupervised segmentation approach that is strongly based on an 'a priori' model of the images. The watershed algorithm has proven to be a very powerful tool for the introduction of such 'a priori' information, because the segmentation process can be conveniently guided by some strategic markers in order to perform the detection of the desired structures. This permits an automatic measurement of some objective parameters which are highly correlated with the evolution of some skin diseases.

Key words: Morphometric analysis, cutaneous biopsy, skin layers, segmentation

1. Introduction

Morphometric analysis of epidermal biopsies permits an objective study of several skin diseases. Skin morphology in patients under treatment can be accurately analyzed by means of image processing techniques, avoiding less reliable methods such as visual inspection. In this paper, we present a morphological scheme for the analysis of epidermal biopsy samples. The target is the detection of the main transitions that are visible on the sample. Such transitions separate the different skin layers whose associated morphometric parameters have to be measured.

The proposed technique relies on three different steps: prefiltering, detection of the transitions and the measurement itself. In the first step, alternate sequential filters are used for image simplification in order to enhance significant transitions and to remove small noisy components. The second step is performed by the watershed algorithm. The set of markers imposed to constrain the watershed algorithm allows the introduction of helpful 'a priori' information about the images being processed. Once the main transitions in the image have been detected, the morphometric mea-

J.Serra and P. Soille (eds.), Mathematical Morphology and Its Applications to Image Processing, 325-331

sures are carried out.

The paper is structured as follows: section 2 describes the application problem and the work images. In section 3, an outline of the proposed morphological scheme for morphometric analysis is discussed. Finally, section 4 presents some results and the conclusions.

2. Morphometric Analysis of Epidermal Biopsy Samples

Figure 1 shows two samples of skin biopsies. Apart from the brighter band at the top of the images, which is simply air, from top to bottom three different layers can be observed: the corneal stratum, the epidermis and the dermis. Between these last two layers, there is an extremely thin cellular tissue where epithelial cells germinate: the dermo-epidermal junction (DE-junction). From this place, epithelial cells grow and migrate outwards, through the epidermis, until they reach the corneal stratum. Once here, the cells die and come off the skin in the form of scales. Different skin diseases are associated with changes in this process. Most of them can be observed as an alteration of the morphology of the skin layers. As an example, the right image in Fig. 1 is a sample of 'psoriatic skin' at the same magnification. 'Psoriasis' is characterized by epidermal hyperplasia with elongation of the interpapillary folds. In the right image of Fig. 1 the dermis is so ripply that in some points it even touches the corneal stratum, producing bleeding wounds. The bidimensional section also produces isolated dermal lobes located inside the epidermis and apparently disconnected from the dermis.

Morphometric analysis of skin biopsies permits an objective measurement of these alterations. The usual parameters to be computed are the average thickness of the epidermis and the degree of ripple of the DE-junction. Such parameters are highly correlated with the evolution of the disease, and so, of importance for several medical applications.

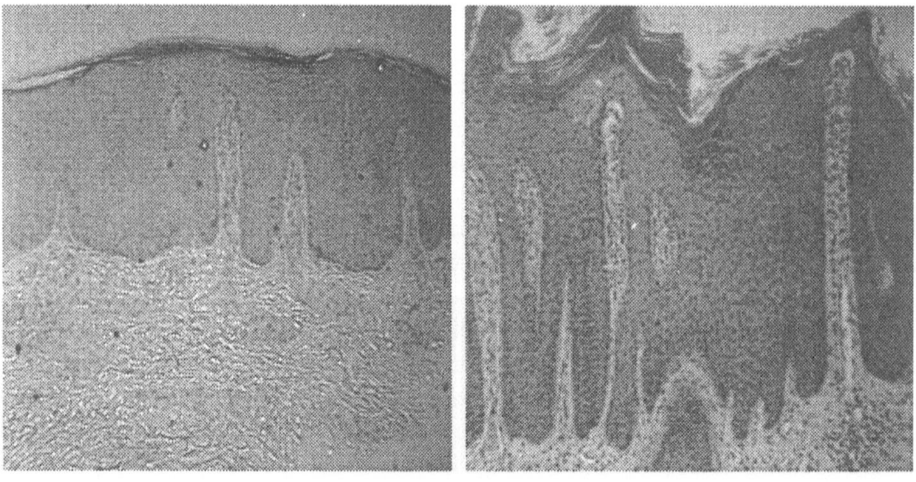

Fig. 1. Skin biopsy samples (H&Ex200). a) left: normal skin; b) right: psoriasis.

Skin biopsy images are generally noisy and low contrasted. Sometimes, even for an expert observer, the transition lines between the layers are difficult to draw. Morphometric analyses are usually performed manually, either by means of a ruler superimposed on photographic enlargements, or with the aid of a digitized tablet. This approach is extremely time-demanding and does not permit to obtain many repeated measures to ensure the reliability of the results. The automatic analysis proposed in this paper greatly simplifies this task.

3. Morphological Filtering and Segmentation

The prefiltering step is aimed at the simplification of the image. Alternate sequential filters [1] can remove both bright and dark noisy components of small size. In this application, open (close) filters by reconstruction of erosion (dilation) of increasing sizes [2] are used in the filtering sequence, in order to change as least as possible the structure of the remaining components. The results of applying these filters to the images of Fig. 1 are presented in Fig. 2.

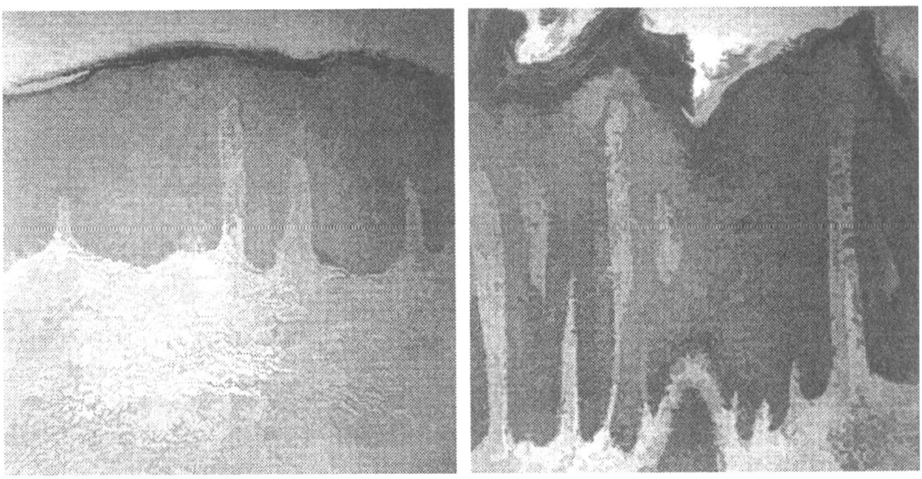

Fig. 2. Application of an alternate sequential filter by reconstruction of size 2.

The watershed algorithm [3] is then applied in three steps to detect one by one the different transitions between the above mentioned layers. This process is strongly guided by the 'a priori' model of the image, which is assumed to be crossed by three horizontal transitions among the four layers. Such a supposition imposes that biopsy samples should be upright and correctly centered for acquisition, what does not restrict very much the image acquisition process while allowing the introduction of specific markers in the segmentation step.

The first layer to be detected is the corneal stratum because it is the most outstanding feature in the image. Being darker and narrower than the others, the black top-hat transform [4] performs as an appropriate enhancement operator. The watershed of the result, with two markers placed at the bottom and top lines of the enhanced image, gives the result plotted in the left image of Fig. 3 with an axis-line locating the corneal stratum. The inner and outer contours of this layer are found by running again the watershed, this time on the morphological gradient of the enhanced image (Fig. 3, right) using the previous watershed line as a new marker.

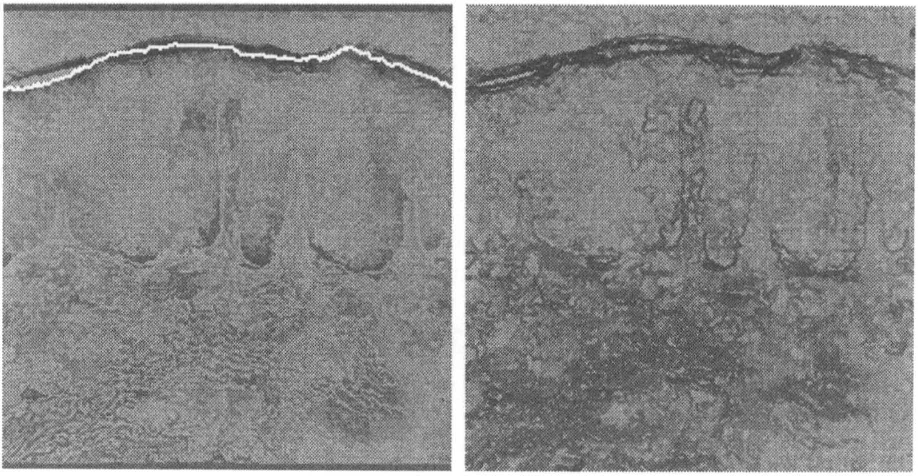

Fig. 3. Detection and segmentation of the corneal stratum for the sane skin sample. a) left: watershed on the black top-hat with 2 markers; b) morphological gradient of the top-hat.

The last transition to be detected is tinier than the former ones. The watershed algorithm is then applied on the morphological gradient of the prefiltered image, but some folds of the DE-junction may be lost, as shown in the left image of Fig. 4. There is a physiological reason that explains such a behaviour of the watershed algorithm: the inflammatory infiltrate generates noisy points (reaction points) inside the dermis, which are responsible for this wrong detection. An alternate sequential filtering of larger size is performed in order to remove this noise. The iteration of the watershed algorithm, now on the gradient of this strongly filtered image constrained by the two markers (the cornea layer and the previous approximation just obtained for the dermis) yields the final result. The right image of Fig. 4 shows this new gradient image for the second run of the watershed with the constraints imposed by the new markers.

The isolated interior lobes of the epidermis should also be detected. They are part of the dermis and their contours are also considered part of the DE-junction. A morphological contrast transform between an opening and a closing by reconstruction [5] is used for the enhancement of these components. Note that these lobes are of the same grey level than the dermis layer and darker than the surrounding epidermis. Therefore, the set of markers for the segmentation is obtained by two operations: thresholding and size selection on the enhanced image. The threshold level is estimated from the average values of the regions obtained in the previous steps, whereas the size parameter is selected according to the size of the smaller lobes that are going to be found. Finally, the application of the watershed algorithm on the gradient image with the obtained markers allows the precise location of the contours of the interior lobes.

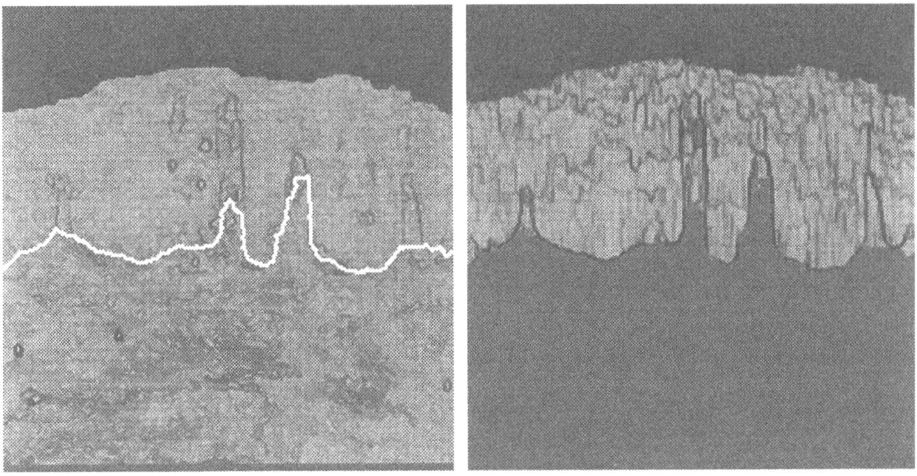

Fig. 4. Location of the DE-junction. a) left: watershed on the morphological gradient; b) right: gradient image for the second run of the watershed (with constraints).

Figure 5 presents a flow chart summarizing the methodology for the segmentation of the epidermal biopsy samples. Please note that the information about the 'a priori' model of the image is introduced by the markers in the decision step (the watershed).

4. Results and Conclusions

The results for the two images of Fig. 1 are shown in Fig. 6, with the transition lines superimposed on the original images. Notice than the transition between the corneal stratum and the air has not been very accurately located, but this is the least important transition for the morphometric analysis due to the presence of scales coming off the skin.

Two sample parameters obtained for these images are given in table I: the *equivalent thickness* of the epidermis and the *index of rugosity* of the DE-junction. Both parameters are representative of the morphology of the epidermal layer and have been defined as follows:

The equivalent thickness of the epidermis is defined as the apparent surface of this layer divided by the width of the image, expressed as a percentual ratio over the image height, i.e.,

$$thickness(\%) = \frac{dermis\_surface}{image\_width} \cdot \frac{100}{image\_height}$$

The index of rugosity of the DE-junction measures the degree of ripple of such transition. Its value should be 0% for a completely flat transition and 100% if the transition was so ripply that filled up the whole image with folds of height equal to the image height. A possible expression for this parameter is the next one:

$$ripple(\%) = \frac{transition\_length - image\_width}{dermis\_surface - image\_width} \cdot 100$$

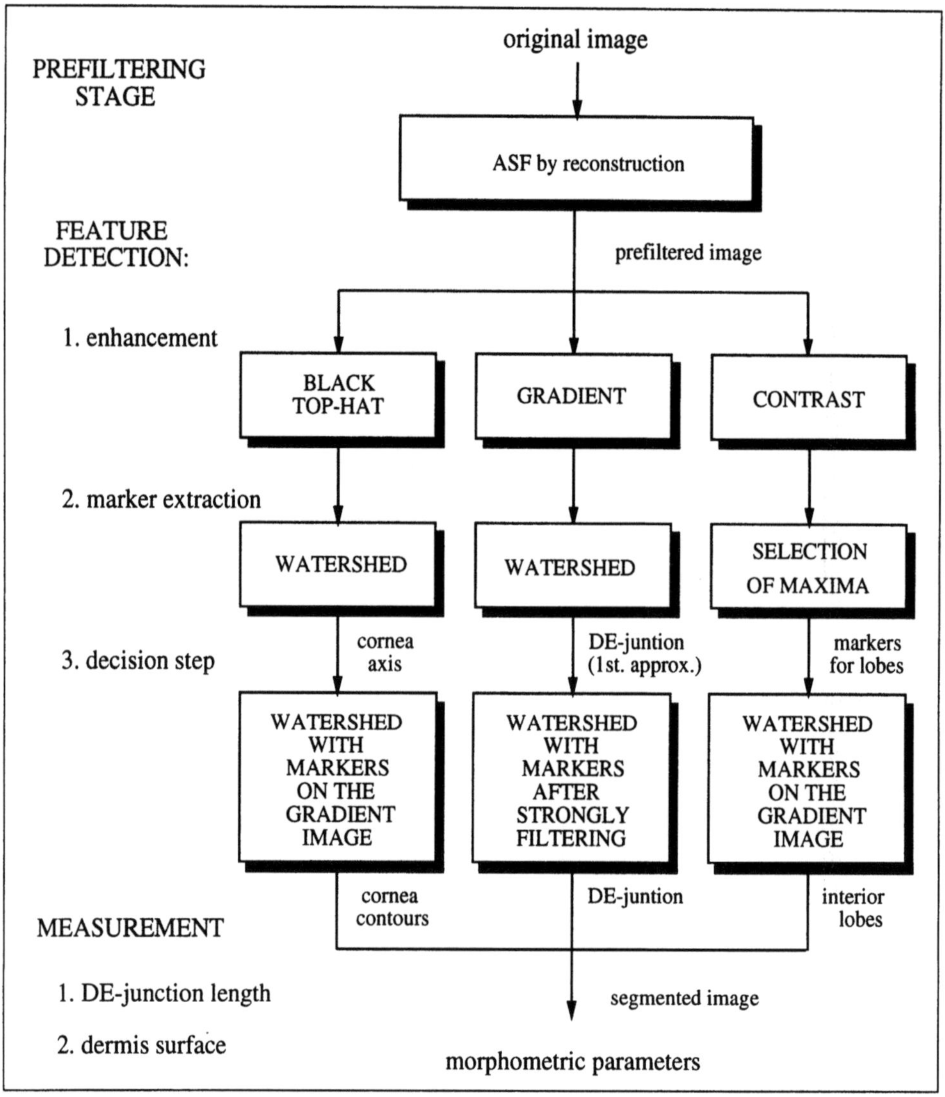

Fig. 5. Methodology for the segmentation of skin biopsy samples.

TABLE I
Morphometric parameters obtained for the images of Fig. 1

IMAGE	thickness(%)	ripple(%)
sane skin image (Fig. 1a)	35.1	1.6
'psoriasis' image (Fig. 1b)	52.6	5.1

The values shown in table I are objective measures of the morphology of the skin layers. The same parameters have been computed for a wide range of biopsy samples

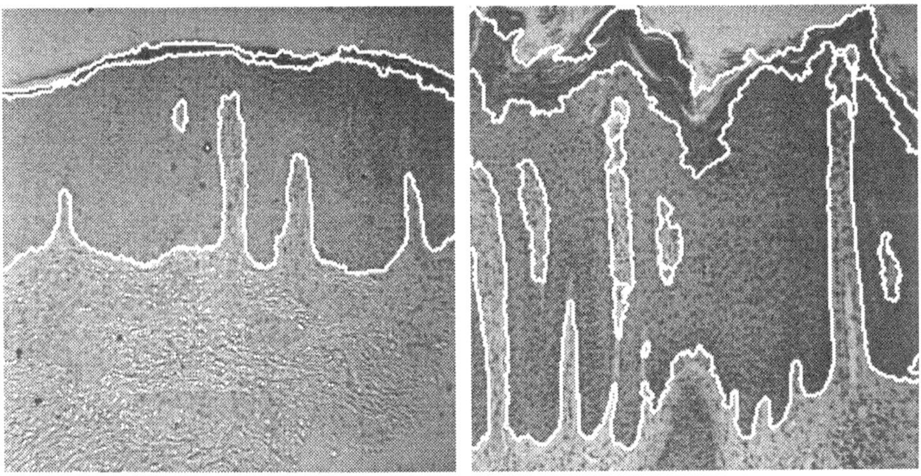

Fig. 6. Final results for the original images of Fig. 1.

and have proven to be useful in order to follow the evolution of alterations in the epidermal layer.

As a conclusion, it has been shown that the measurement of histologic parameters from epidermal biopsy samples can be efficiently performed by unsupervised morphological segmentation techniques. The watershed algorithm allows the straightforward introduction of the model of the image to be segmented, so that the available 'a priori' information can be used in order to guide the detection of the structures of interest. The degree of correlation of the values of these parameters with the usual histopathologic findings has been found to be sufficient in order to guarantee the reliability of the proposed automatic method.

References

1. J. Serra. Alternating sequential filters. In J. Serra, editor, *Image Analysis and Mathematical Morphology. Volume 2: Theoretical Advances*, chapter 10, pp. 203–214. Academic Press, 1988.
2. P. Salembier and M. Kunt. Size-sensitive multiresolution decomposition with rank order based filters. *Signal Processing*, vol. 27, pp. 205–241, 1992.
3. F. Meyer and S. Beucher. Morphological segmentation. *Journal of Visual Communication and Image Representation*, vol. 1, no. 4, pp. 21–46, 1990.
4. F. Meyer. Automatic screening of cytological specimens. *Computer Vision, Graphics and Image Processing*, vol. 35, pp. 356–369, 1986.
5. F. Meyer and J. Serra. Contrasts and activity lattice. *Signal Processing*, vol. 16, pp. 303–317, 1989.

AUTOMATIC QUANTIFICATION OF SPINE PARAMETERS FROM X-RAY IMAGES BY MEANS OF MORPHOLOGICAL TOOLS

F. MARQUÉS and T. MEGÍA
Dept. Teoria del Senyal i Comunicacions, ETSETB, UPC
Apdo. 30.002, 08080 Barcelona

and

N. JOSHI and A. NAVARRO-QUILIS
Dept. Cirugia Ortopèdica i Traumatologia
Hospital Vall d'Hebron, Barcelona

Abstract. This work presents an automatic technique for computing from an X-ray image the value of the set of parameters that characterizes the morphological structure of a human lumbar spine. To compute these parameters it is necessary to detect, in the X-ray image, each one of the vertebrae that forms the spine, as well as their relative location. Given the low quality of normal X-ray images, a direct detection cannot be performed. Thus, the proposed technique consists in five different steps: image simplification, detection of elements, decision, validation of objects and parameter computation. In order to be consistent, the validation step and the parameter computation rely on the same medical vertebra model.

Key words: Spine model, Segmentation, Geodesic distance

1. Introduction

The goal of the treatment of any vertebral fracture is to recover the morphology of the vertebral body and to normalize the biomechanics of the injured segment, as much as possible. To assess the efficiency of a treatment, either conservative or surgical, the study of the geometrical changes of the vertebral body is necessary. The vertebral morphology is defined by means of eight geometric parameters: five linear and three angular ones [1]. This set of parameters is computed from lateral radiographies of the patient.

Currently, these parameters are computed manually by measuring distances and angles with a ruler on the radiography. Hence, it is a tedious and little reliable task. Furthermore, subjectivity on the manual measures may change the results and, therefore, the assessment of the treatment. On the other hand, the automatic quantification of spine parameters is fast and precise; that is, it allows the objective study of a large number of patients while reducing the measurement error.

Images to be used for such an automatic analysis are lateral radiographies of the patient, in which usually the lumbar vertebrae are embedded in a very noisy environment. Figure 1 shows a part of an image containing two complete vertebrae. This image is used throughout this paper to illustrate the proposed technique. In

J.Serra and P. Soille (eds.), Mathematical Morphology and Its Applications to Image Processing, 333-340

spite of the low quality of these X-ray images, vertebrae can be detected relying on criteria such as local contrast, size and shape of the objects within the scene. Due to these characteristics, morphological tools [2] have been applied for the vertebra detection.

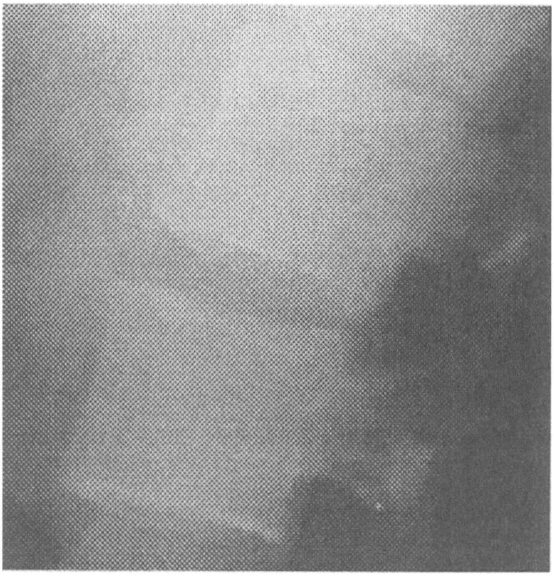

Fig. 1. Original X-ray image

The structure of this paper follows the different steps of the proposed technique. In Section 1, the image simplification is detailed. Section 2 illustrates the procedure for detecting the elements; that is, the way to obtain a set of markers from the simplified image. These markers are used in Section 3 to carry out the decision step which relies on the Watershed algorithm. Section 4 is devoted to the validation of the objects obtained after the decision step while, in Section 5, the way to compute the spine parameters is described. Finally, Section 6 contains a discussion on the results as well as a brief summary of the current research.

2. Image simplification

Objects in the image present gray level values slightly greater than the background (see Figure 1). However, the gray levels of both the background and the objects are not homogeneous but they fluctuate. These fluctuations can disturb the object detection and, therefore, they should be previously removed. To remove them, an alternating sequential filter is applied [3]. The basic filter to be used is a close_open, since the noise to be removed takes both positive and negative values:

$$\gamma_n \varphi_n(...(\gamma_2 \varphi_2(\gamma_1 \varphi_1(I)))...) \tag{1}$$

Given that the actual shape of the objects is to be preserved as much as possible, both the close and the open should imply a reconstruction process. However, when using openings and closings by total reconstruction, small connections among the different parts of the image lead to the reconstruction of unwilling structures. Therefore, such connections have to be removed previous to the reconstruction procedure. That is, the reconstruction should be performed on a simplified version of the image. This idea results in using filters by partial reconstruction [4]:

$$\textit{opening by partial reconstruction} : \gamma^{rec}(\gamma_i, \epsilon_j) \tag{2}$$

$$\textit{closing by partial reconstruction} : \varphi^{rec}(\varphi_i, \delta_j) \tag{3}$$

where i should be smaller than j. Finally, since the elements to be detected are quite large (see Figure 1), the alternating sequential filter can also use up to a large structuring element. In Figure 2, the result of applying the filter described in (1) and (2) up to size 12 is shown.

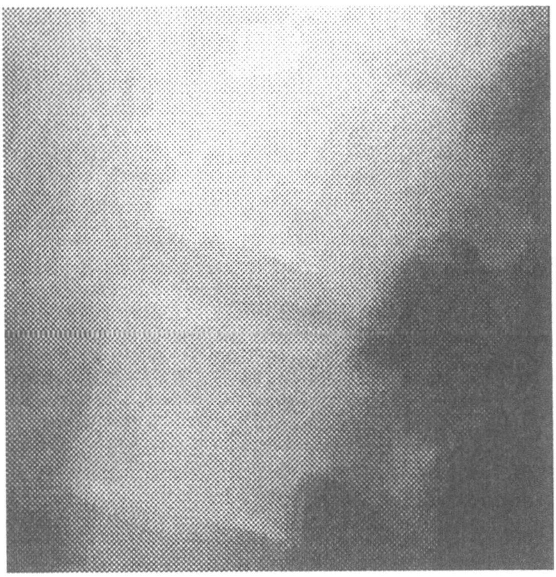

Fig. 2. Simplified image

3. Detection of elements

The goal of this step is to obtain a set of markers corresponding to each object present in the image, plus one for the background. Although the image have been simplified, its gradient cannot be used directly to mark the objects. The reason for that is that the gradient is still too noisy. Nevertheless, it has been observed that each vertebra usually contains one, and only one, relevant local maximum of the gray level function. These maxima are related to the accumulation of calcium on the extremes of the vertebrae.

This way, the local maxima of the simplified image can be used to mark the presence of a vertebra. Due to the previous simplification step, these maxima are flat zones

[5]. From this set of flat zones, the more relevant ones are kept. This selection is done relying on the fact that the number of objects to be detected is known before hand: there are five lumbar vertebrae. Following a conservative policy, the ten largest flat zones are kept for further analysis. Thus, a set of connected points marking each vertebra, as well as some artifacts, are selected.
To perform correctly the following step (decision), it is necessary to have, not only a marker for each object in the scene, but also a marker for the background. The frame of the image could be used as marker for the background: the quantification of geometrical parameters of a vertebra cannot correctly be done if its shape it is not completely represented in the image. Therefore, any object touching the frame should be withdrawn from the analysis. Nevertheless, it is more safety to obtain a marker for the background surrounding each one of the previously detected objects. To obtain such a marker for the background, the Watershed technique [6] is applied on the inverted image, setting the previous markers as minima of the function, as well as the frame of the image. The final markers are shown in Figure 3.a.

4. Decision

Once the objects and the background of the scene have been marked, the correct location of their boundaries is achieved using the Watershed technique. In this case, the image to be segmented is the gradient of the simplified image imposing minima in the points selected as markers. This segmentation yields a final result containing the sought objects (coming from the markers of the vertebrae) and some wrong ones (coming from the markers of the artifacts). This result is illustrated in Figure 3.b.

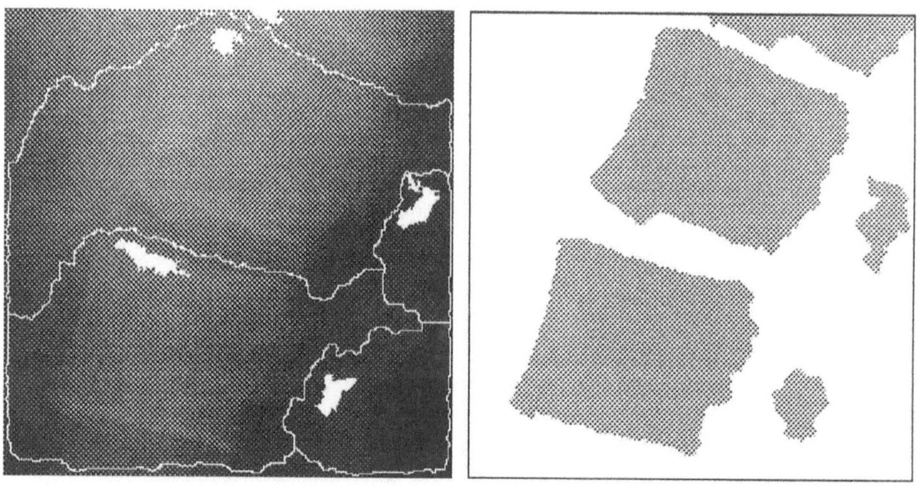

Fig. 3. a) Set of markers b) Segmentation result

5. Validation of objects

The result of the previous segmentation contains the vertebrae and also some artifacts. In order to discriminate between the sought objects and the artifacts, the shape information is used. The objects detected in the previous step are validated taking into account that the geometrical model for a vertebra is a rhombus. Since artifact shapes do not follow any pattern, only the five (two in the example) most rhombus-like objects are kept.
Thus, the approximation of each object by a rhombus is computed; that is, the main four corners of each objects are obtained. Only those objects whose representation as rhombus leads to the smallest error are accepted as vertebrae. The procedure for obtaining the main four corners of an object has been implemented by looking for the center of the object and computing the geodesic distance from this point to any other point within the object. The maxima of this distance function represent the most relevant points of the contour. The concept of relevant points is related to that of ends derived from the propagation function as explained in [7].
However, when using a unitary structuring element to compute the distance, it presents too many maxima and too many points are detected as relevant ones (see Figure 4.a). Therefore, a larger structuring element is used to compute the geodesical distance and the areas of maximum distance are taken. Within these areas, the maxima of the unitary distance function are selected as relevant points. This procedure is shown in Figure 4.b.

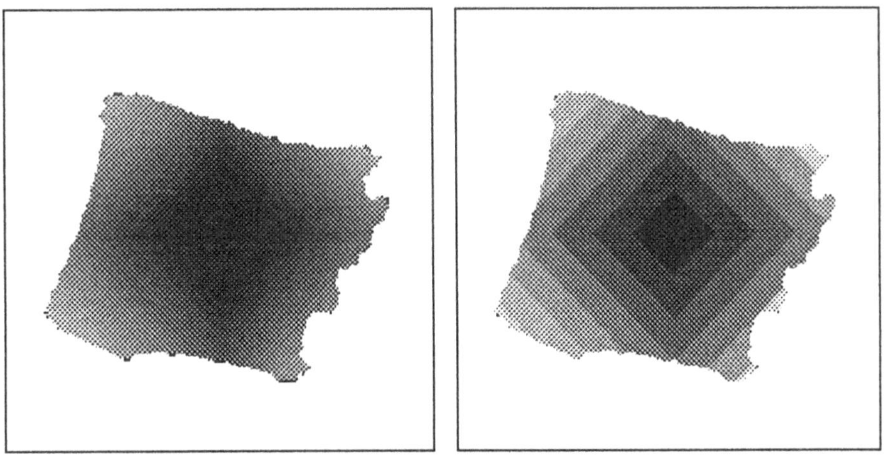

Fig. 4. a) Points detected with unitary and b) non-unitary structuring element

The kind of structure element to be used in the computation of the distance function depends on how tilted the vertebra is. For instance, in the case presented in Figure 4, the used structuring element is a cross. However, if the object was tilted 45 degrees, it would be better to use a square structuring element to detect the relevant points. Therefore, before computing the distance function, a procedure for estimating the angle between the main axes of the object and the grid is performed. Once these points have been selected, a polygonal approximation of the object is performed (see Figure 5.a). If the number of relevant points is larger than four, the above procedure is repeated on the previous result up to achieving only four points (see Figure 5.b). Finally, the error between the original object and its polygonal approximation is used to discriminate between vertebrae and artifacts.

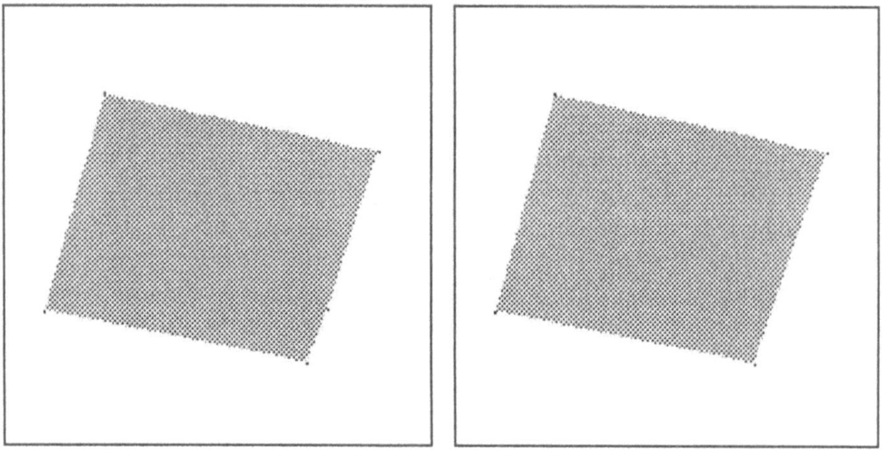

Fig. 5. a) First and b) final polygonal approximation

An example of applying the previous validation procedure on an artifact is shown in Figure 6. Since the artifact shape cannot be correctly approximated by a rhombus, the iteration of the procedure on the different polygonal approximations ends yielding a single line (only two relevant points are detected). The final polygonal approximation is, therefore, rather poor and the object is detected as an artifact.

6. Parameter computation

The reason for modeling the vertebrae as rhombi and, therefore, of detecting the four corners of each vertebra is twofold. First, it is useful for discriminating between vertebrae and artifacts given that the first ones follow this pattern, whereas artifacts do not follow any pattern. Second, this polygonal approximation is the medical model used in order to obtain the parameters describing the spine [1]. This model is quite accurate and the set of parameters that can be obtained relying on it has been recently extended [8]. That is, the geometrical spine model is totally characterized by means of the relative position between vertebrae and eight points for each vertebra. Four of these eight points are those used in the validation step and related to the four corners of the polygonal approximation, whereas the other four points should be obtained, yet. The detection of these points is an easy task since they correspond to the center of each one of the line segments of the previous polygonal approximation. As an example, Figure 7 shows the way to compute the value of the regional kyphosis, which is one of the angular parameters describing the lumbar spine which were proposed in [1]. Furthermore, Figure 8 illustrates the computation of the anterior vertebral height (AVH), which is one of the linear parameter proposed in [8].

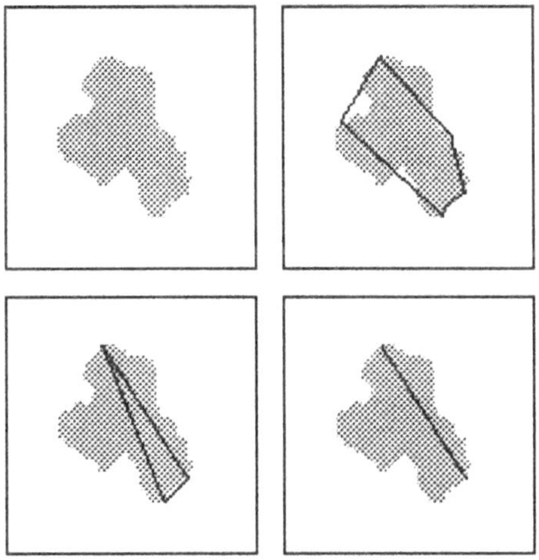

Fig. 6. a) Original shape b) first polygonal approximation c) second polygonal approximation and d) final polygonal approximation

7. Comments and current research

An algorithm for computing the lumbar spine parameters from an X-ray image has been proposed. The algorithm is able to handle images with very low quality (X-ray images that have been digitized not directly but from a radiography). The current research aims at developing a similar technique for the thoracic spine. This case is much more complicated since the thoracic cage hides, in some places, the position and shape of the vertebral bodies. To detect this new set of vertebrae, the information about the position of the lumbar vertebrae achieved in the previous detection is used. That is, the searching area is restricted by extrapolating, from the position of the lumbar vertebrae, the most like position of the torathic vertebrae.

References

1. A. White III, M. M. Panjabi (1990), Clinical Biomechanics of the Spine, J. B. Lippincott Company, Philadelfia 1990.
2. J. Serra (1982), Image analysis and mathematical morphology, Academic Press, London, 1982.
3. S. Sternberg (1986), "Grayscale morphology", Computer Graphics and Image Processing, vol. 35, pp. 333-355, 1982.
4. P. Salembier, J. Serra (1992), "Morphological multiscale image segmentation", Proc. of Visual Communications and Image Processing'92, Boston, MA, 1992.
5. J. Serra and P. Salembier (1993), "Connected operators and Pyramids", Proc. of SPIE Image Algebra and Mathematical Morphology, San Diego, Vol. 2030, pp. 65-76, 1993.
6. S. Beucher (1990), Segmentation d'images et morphologie mathématique, PhD Thesis, Paris School of Mines, Paris, June 1990.
7. C. Lantuéjoul and F. Maisonneuve (1984), Geodesic methods in image analysis", Pattern Recognition, vol. 17, pp. 177-187, 1984.
8. R. M. Lin, M. M. Panjabi, T. R. Oxland (1993) "Functional Radiographs of Acute Thoracolumbar Burst Fractures", Spine, vol. 18, Num. 16 pp. 2431-2437,J. B. Lippincott Company 1993.

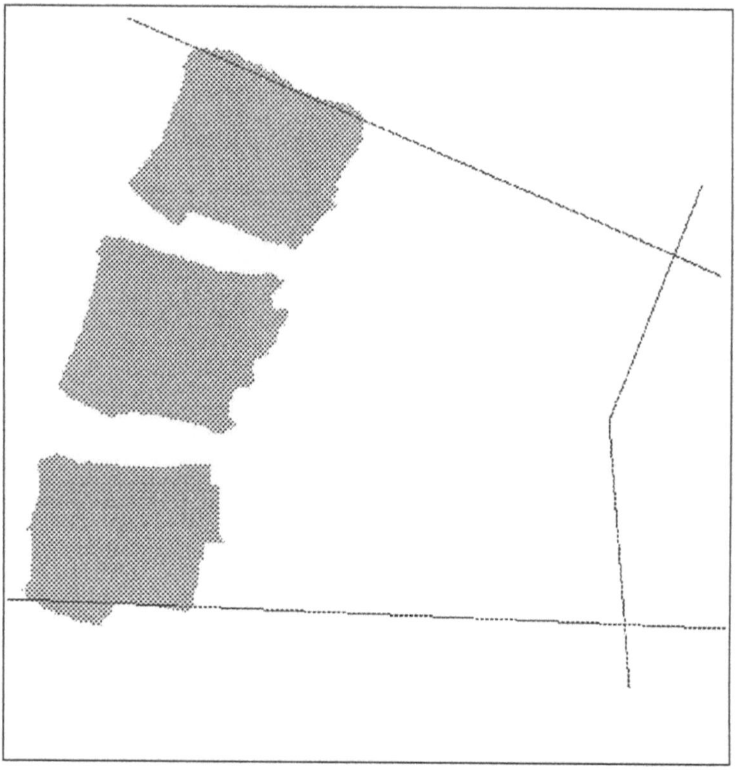

Fig. 7. Computation of the regional kyphosis

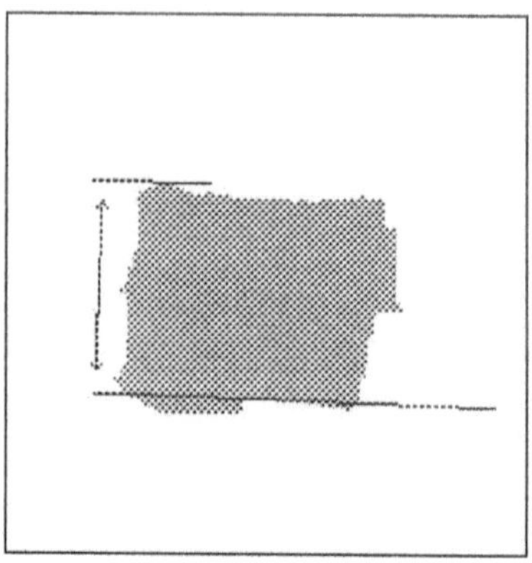

Fig. 8. Computation of the anterior vertebral height parameter (AVH)

IMAGE PROCESSING: A KEY TO SUCCESS IN INDUSTRIAL APPLICATIONS

BRUNO LAŸ
NOESIS Inc.
4, rue René Razel, F–91892 Orsay Cedex, France

Abstract. In the past, image processing techniques for quality control were mostly based on local measurements such as the computation of the histogram. Nowadays, algorithms based on morphology or complex filtering are widely used and allow us to tackle applications that were impossible to solve in the past with a standard system.

With the emergence of very sophisticated processors which can turn a standard computerized imaging system into a very high-speed system, architectured around a fast pipe-line, it is now possible to use complex image processing algorithms in real-time. This paper presents six applications involving high level algorithms.

Key words: Mathematical morphology, industrial applications, real-time image processing, 1–3D image processing

1. Introduction

An industrial application implies the control of a process such as looking for defects, or locating the presence or absence of objects. A typical example would be a bottle conveyor belt, the purpose of the vision system being to detect any kind of defects which could appear on the bottle: the positionning of a label, the detection of the liquid level or the presence of broken parts on the bottleneck. The vision system will have to process one or multiple images at the speed of the conveyor belt and eventually provide an answer: "Go/No Go".

The power of the vision system will be determined by answering the following questions:

– Can it follow the speed of the manufacturing process?
– Can it work 24 hrs a day?
– Does it find all the defects?
– Is it more reliable than a manual inspection?

If we try to decompose the typical applications, the following partial list can be given: food inspection, robot manipulation, automative quality control (wheel, painting, windscreen, etc.), paper inspection and any kind of web analysis, PCB inspection, Character recognition, Metallographic imaging, Motion analysis, 3D imaging applications, etc.

In this paper, we will describe six typical complex applications developed at NOESIS, the calibration of a speedometer, a food inspection, the detection of camshafts in a bin, the automatic detection of defects in titanium, the detection of defects on a metallic object and the 3D reconstruction of a neuron using a transmission electronic microscope.

J.Serra and P. Soille (eds.), Mathematical Morphology and Its Applications to Image Processing, 341-352

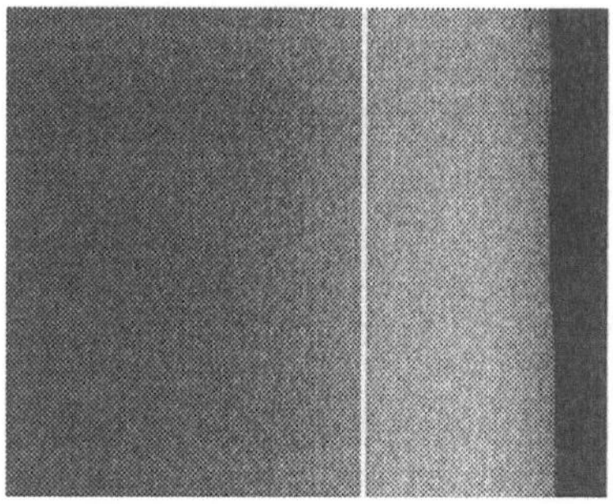

Fig. 1. X-Ray image with fold automatically detected by a linear sensor.

2. Existing systems

There are actually two ways to analyze a process. The first and simplest one is to use a linear sensor, very well adapted to any circular object or a web in motion. The second way is to use a CCD matrix camera, and to process the image as a 2D array of pixels.

2.1. Linear Sensor

There exist some very typical applications involving a 1D sensor, example of these could be the detection of defects on a circular object as a bottle or a tube, the observation of the quality of a sheet steel, the setting of a windscreen on a car, and the automatic detection of a fold on a sheet.

Due to the speed of the system, there are usually very basic algorithms involved in the imaging process. The easiest task to perform is to observe the intensity of the points along a line, and looking for the minimum, maximum grey level values and their locations. A little more complex task is to compute the gradient or Laplacian, thresholding it to get the edges, and then trying to follow those edges by some chain linking and finally performing some geometrical analysis.

The image shown in Fig. 1 is coming from the application of sheets and a linear CCD sensor was used to automatically detect the fold.

2.2. Matricial sensor

All other applications will usually involve one or more matrix camera, and will be based on the location of defects or particular objects on a 2D image. Obviously, that kind of sensor is not very well suited to any application where there is an object in motion, except if multiple mono-shot cameras are used to cover all the moving objects without losing any possible information, or if very complex algorithms are used to track the moving object.

Among the matrix applications, one may find very basic ones involving tools such as local histograms within a window, or thresholds to get a binary image on which measurements such as area, perimeter will be performed. That kind of applications requires a low-level and usually very cheap hardware including a camera, a frame grabber and a fast CPU such as a member of the Motorola 68000 family to process the pixel values. A black and white monitor may be connected to the output of the frame grabber, however its use is not obvious as the only result of such an application is "good or bad", or "Go/no go".

More complex applications will involve edge detection, morphological transformations and any kind of high level filtering able to extract in real-time the defects, or to locate with a very good precision the edges of a mechanical part.

3. Image Processing Functions in the 2D Space

Image processing transformations can be roughly decomposed in two distinct parts: the world of linear operations, mostly based on convolution, and the morphological world based on erosion and any combination of basic operations to achieve the goal of the application.

In the first group, one will find edge detectors such as Sobel, Prewitt or Roberts, and correlation which is basically the convolution of an image by another image. Usually the image processing system will stop there, and the edges or the peak of correlation will be sent to the host computer for further processing.

The second group includes all binary or grey-level morphological functions such as erosion, dilation, opening, closing, skeleton, labelling, etc. which can be performed in real-time or near real-time as usually more than one operation has to be performed. It will also include morphological filters to clean the image and new algorithms such as the watershed detection. If only a convolution or an edge detection is performed on the image, one may imagine a very fast CPU to do the computation, and then the chain linking and the approximation by segments of the edges is also done by the computer. For morphological transformations, it is absolutely mandatory to use a special hardware system with one or more morphological processors, and a particle analysis processor to do the measurements.

4. Vision architecture for quality control

4.1. Major groups

There exist four major groups of architecture to perform vision applications:

- PC-AT bus and advanced frame grabber plugged into the system.
- VME bus and very specialized and dedicated boards plugged into the system, with a real-time operating system.
- MULTI-BUS architectures very similar to the VME ones, however that kind of system is not as frequent as the VME.
- Private architecture with proprietary bus and processors.

As it is rather complex to add multiple boards in the PC, a typical vision system will usually be architectured around a VME bus with Motorola CPUs. The operating system has to allow the control of multiple processes, such as 0S9 or VMEXEC. The main advantage of the second one is that it is now possible to develop a system with multiple CPUs in the same chassis. One of the CPUs will be responsible for the user interface and will usually run with a standard, easy to use operating system such as UNIX or DOS. Obviously, the user will have the capability to develop in a multi-window environment, such as X Windows or Windows 3.0 with very well-known tools such as debugger, linker, etc. The second CPU will have the control of the image processing functions and will really take benefit of the real-time processors of the system and potential I/O boards for robot control, or any other automatic control.

The philosophy of the system is then to develop on the first CPU and to download the code of the application in the second one. Concerning the image processing systems on the VME bus, the user should be able to control the data going through the video bus and define a special path to minimize the application processing time, taking benefit of a video pipeline.

4.2. The vision processors

The vision processors can be shared in three distinct groups:

- The ASICs which can usually perform only one task such as a convolver, a morphological processor or a labelling ASIC.
- The transputers which are multi-purpose processors programmable by the user. In theory, you may have as many transputers as you want on a single board, the only problem being to program them in parallel.
- The DSPs which are also multi-purpose processors, especially good for floating-point operations such as polygonal approximation or filtering.

In all the applications described later in the paper, the vision system was based on the VME bus with two operating systems and a family of boards with convolution, morphology, histogram, labelling, arithmetic and logic operation facilities and a DSP taking the data from the bus for all tricky computations involving floating-point operations.

4.3. The I/O devices

The typical I/O devices connected to the system are:

- a camera usually 512 × 512 format, for a cost-effective problem.
- a black and white monitor.
- any programmable automaton such as a robot, an arm to reject or grab the false part.

5. Complex Vision Applications

5.1. Food inspection

This application is based on the automatic inspection of food using X-ray devices, and the detection of pieces of broken glass in bottle, uncut bones in meat products and any contamination by metallic objects, especially for baby food (see Fig. 2).

The goal of the application is to be able to detect any foreign material in about twelve samples (cans, bottle, etc.) in less than 500 ms.

The input image being an X-ray image (Fig. 2a), it is necessary to filter it using a median filter . Then, all material appearing as dark particles among a lighter surrounding, a top-hat transform is performed, as the difference between a closing and the original image (Fig. 2b) followed by a threshold (Fig. 2c) . The values of the threshold are defined using an automatic segmentation based on the shape of the histogram of the difference image.

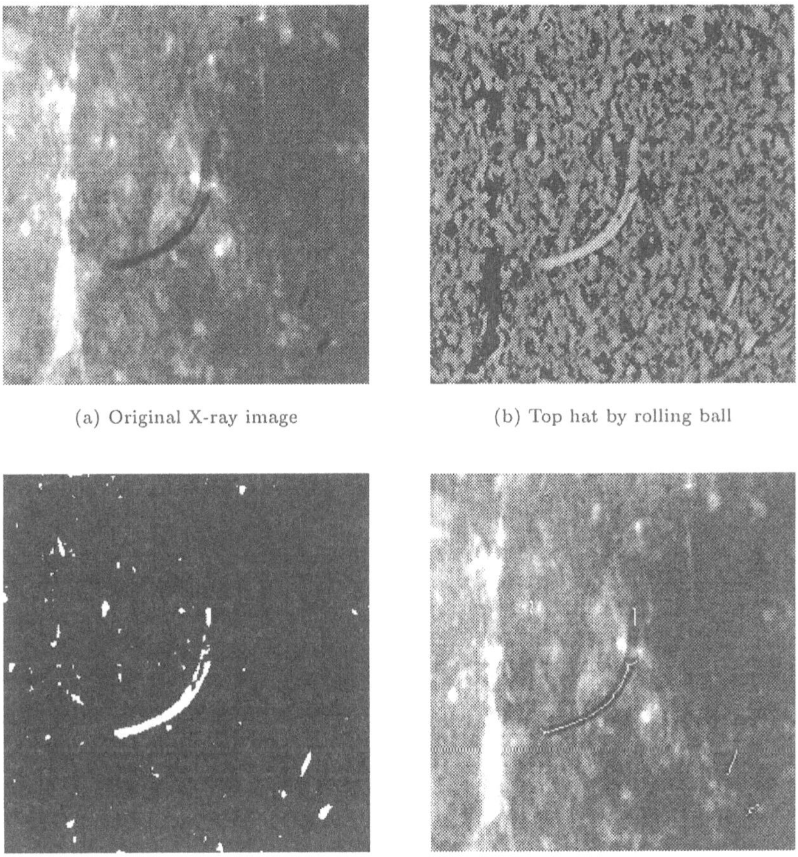

(a) Original X-ray image

(b) Top hat by rolling ball

(c) Threshold of top hat

(d) Skeletonized uncut bones on original

Fig. 2. Food inspection: detection of unwanted objects in processed food.

At this point, the processing depends on the type of objects to detect:

- for broken glass and metallic objects, all the holes of the binary image obtained after thresholding are filled and a large opening is performed to remove all non-significative particles.
- for uncut bones, which are stretched objects, a skeleton followed by a pruning is performed to retain all the objects having a given length (Fig. 2d).

The process is then completed with a surface measurement of what is left in the image, and a go/no go result.

5.2. Speedometer Calibration

All cars assembled by Fiat, Peugeot or Renault are including VEGLIA-JAEGER speedometers and other hand displays (for oil and gazoline etc.) checked by a vision system. Results obtained for each speedometer are compared with theoretical

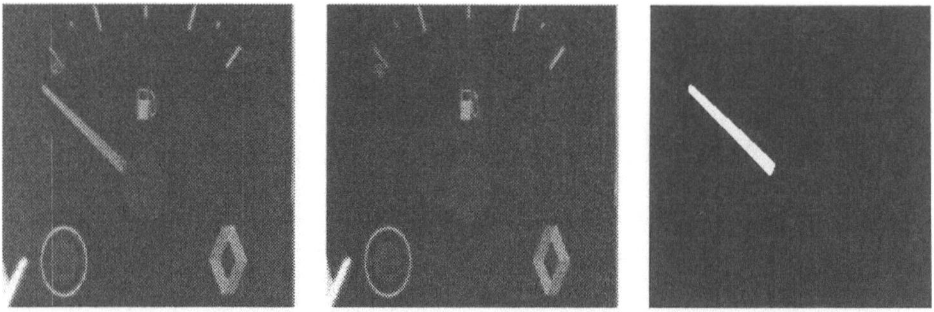

(a) Origimal image (b) Background (c) Hand

Fig. 3. Speedometer calibration.

response curve, in order to ensure that when a car is running at 50 mph on the highway, the hand actually points 50 and not 30 or 40. The ultimate goal is to verify theoretical behaviour of meters for linearity, hysteresis and response time.

The first stage of the algorithm is the difference between the incoming camera image and a reference image without hand only displaying digits (Figs. 3a and 3b). The difference is masked out with another image to eliminate unwanted areas. During the same video frame, the image is thresholded to extract the hand which may be discontinued, and sent to a DSP board which is going to process the edges of the object (Fig. 3c).

The analysis phase performed by the DSP consists in reconstructing the hand which is often cut and has holes, and to compute the exact orientation with a precision lower than 0 degree. The result is then passed through a calibration table to produce a measure in the unity of the meter.

Every 100 seconds, the results are accumulated, and plotted on the screen and on a plotter. Three curves can be plotted: result, theoretical and difference between result and theoretical. The time of the process is 40 ms between each step on a 512×512 image, meaning that the behaviour of a speedometer can be checked in real-time.

5.3. Metallographic application

This quality control application is a typical metallographic image analysis where a small defect of tungsten carbide has to be found within a titanium matrix (Fig. 4a). It is once again an X-ray image where the defect appears as a stain darker than its surroundings. The algorithm works in two steps as it is able to detect in real-time any defect larger than a size of 20 pixels, and then if nothing was found during the first step, analyzes in 200 ms the image to precisely locate the very small defects whose size can reach 2 pixels. The algorithm is based on a top-hat transform performed in 4 frames (Fig. 4b), and then a labelling, the computation of the area, and the determination of the center of gravity of each blob greater than 2 pixels (Fig. 4c) . The whole process requires 6 frames or 200 ms.

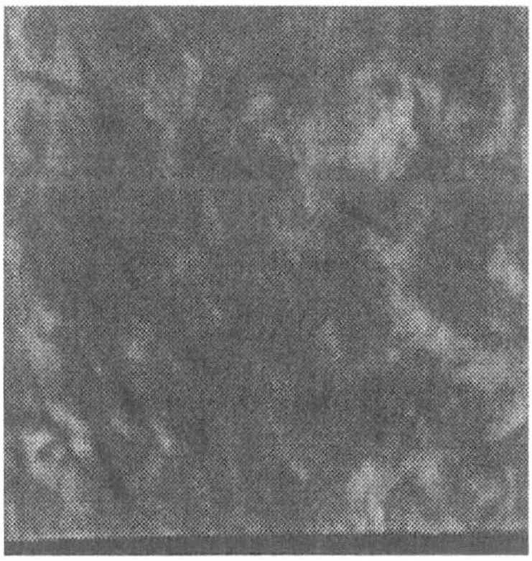

(a) X-ray image of a titanium matrix

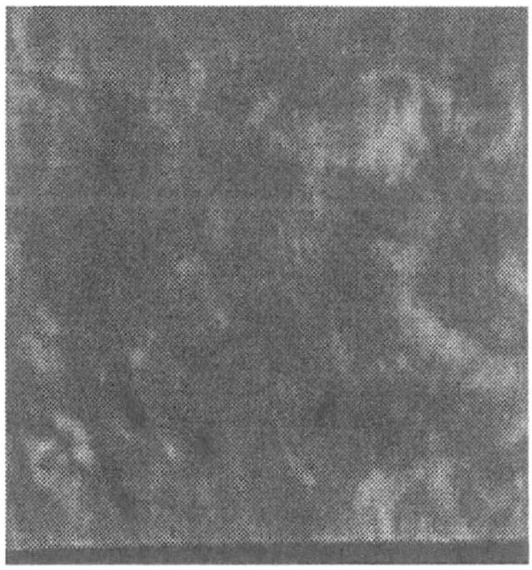

(b) Closing

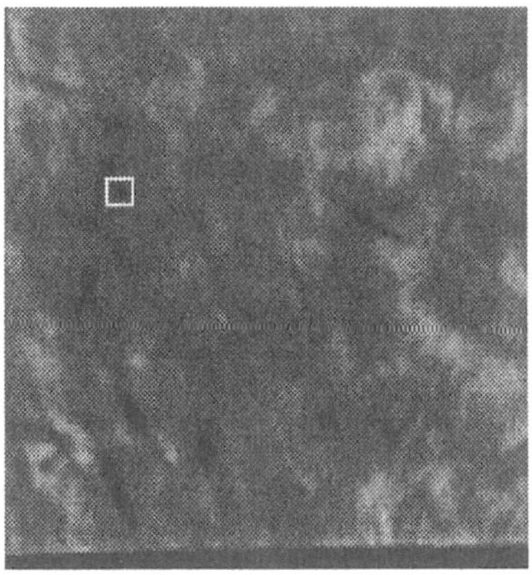

(d) Detected defect (inclusion of tungsten carbide)

Fig. 4. Metallographic application: detection of defects.

5.4. Camshaft manipulation

The purpose of the application is to grab by a robot a set of camshafts placed in a bin. This is the typical complex application as there are some lighting problems, some precision difficulties to locate the edges, and then I/O problems to move the robot which will grab one camshaft after another.

Moreover, the last difficulty is that a new image has to be acquired after each grabbing as the remaining camshaft in the bin may move after one is taken. The algorithm will involve the following image transformations:

- Image acquisition (Fig. 5a)
- Median 3×3 filter to clean the image
- Sobel edge detector (Fig. 5b)
- Suppression of the non-local maxima of the Sobel

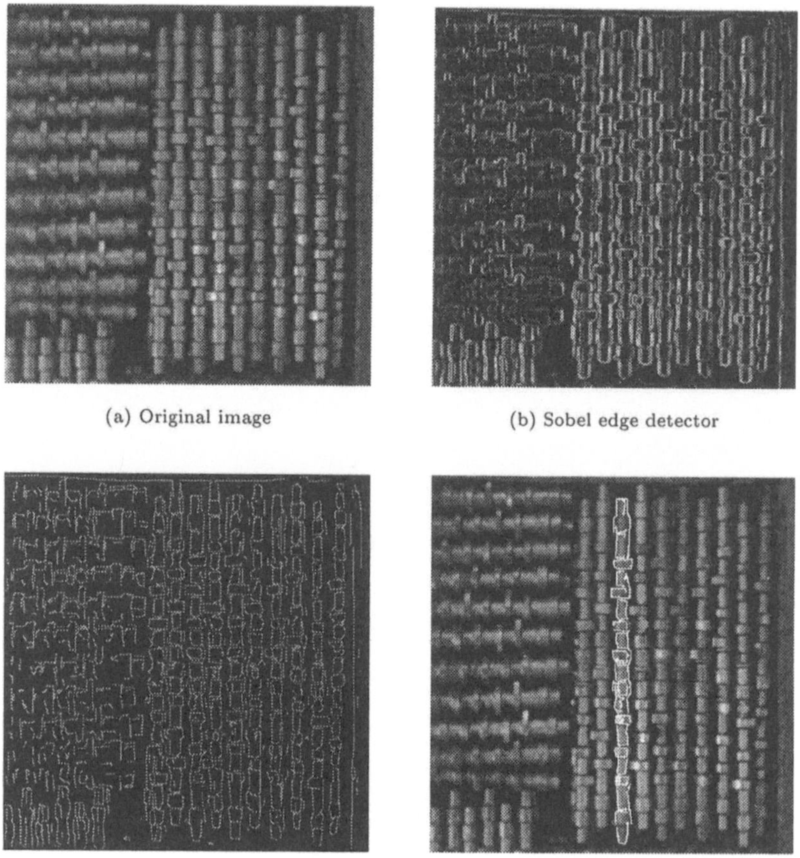

(a) Original image (b) Sobel edge detector

(c) Polygonal approximation (d) Result

Fig. 5. Camshaft detection

- Hysteresis thresholding
- Chain linking and polygonal approximation of the edges (Figs. 5 c and d)

The last stage of the algorithm, which is only running in software on a fast CPU is based on a definition of a database with only two possible parts: the camshaft is at 0 and 90 degrees directions, and the matching between the current edges and the ones in the database. The method developed at the INRIA by N. AYACHE, is built around the prediction and verification of hypothesis, which means that two segments are matched, one from the database and one from the scene.

The first part of the algorithm is running in 200 ms on the DMA machine (Depth and Motion Analysis) developed within the Esprit Project P940.

Finally, the location of the edges is given to a robot which is able to grab in about one second each camshaft.

6. Detection of defects on small mechanical parts

This application has been developed for a small company providing very specialized mechanical parts for the automatic industry.

This company is making a set of metallic parts using the technique of "cold pressing". A small iron segment of defined section is placed into a matrix whose shape is the negative shape of the object and receives an important pressure of few hundreds tons to give it its final shape. Precision of cold pressing systems is such that the parts obtained have the same quality than bright parts.

One of the piece we analyze is a small cross shape part used for producing camshafts (Fig. 6a). The defect types we look for are:

- Strange defects on the boundary, usually performed by the break of the pressing tool (Fig. 6b).
- Random, small and unusual defects looking like small grooves.

Before the use of image processing, strange defects were detected by manual control, and small objects were not detected.

Due to heavy competition in this industry, customers now reject all parts which are not 100% correct.

The vision system NOESIS developed is based upon a very efficient sensor allowing the detection of very small defects, and a user friendly software to be used by any technician.

The system is currently working 24 hrs a day, has been adapted to the current available conveyor system, and can analyze up to 40 pieces per minute (Fig. 6c).

The algorithm involves the study of the edges, by using linear edge detectors, and an approximation by line segments, and morphological transformations to detect small grooves.

7. 3D Neuron Reconstruction

Despite this last application is not an industrial one, it is very interesting as it involves a lot of processing power, and is helping the researcher in a boresome task which used to take several monthes before the introduction of a vision system.

The following system has been developed for the Center for Health Sciences at Ben Gurion University, Israel. The main goal of the system is to provide an environment for reconstructing and analyzing neurons.

Analysis of neurons whose 3-dimensional geometry is often complex can be made much easier by the use of numerical techniques, among which is a 3D reconstruction algorithm.

Typical data consist of a set of cross sections of mouse cerebral nerve cells obtained from a Transmission Electron Microscope (TEM).

Usual series consist of 200 to 300 sections evenly spaced (80 nanometers). Images are digitized at a resolution of 512 square pixels.

Cross sections of nerve cells result in two-dimensional structures within each section which may be difficult to identify for non-specialists. Directions of dendritic shafts may vary, which means that the same dentrite may look pseudo-circular or very elongated depending on the sections.

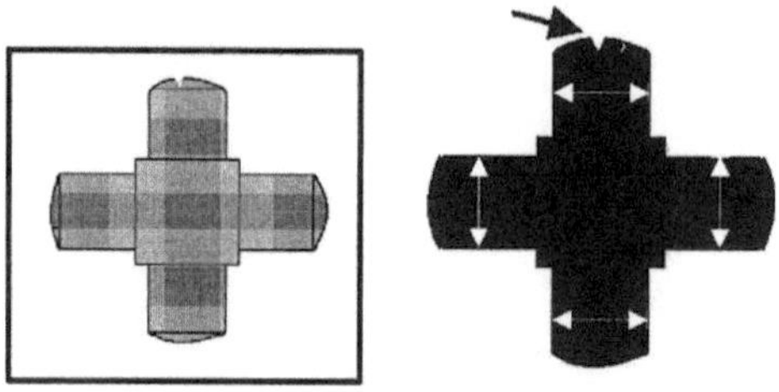

(a) Part to be analysed (b) Measures

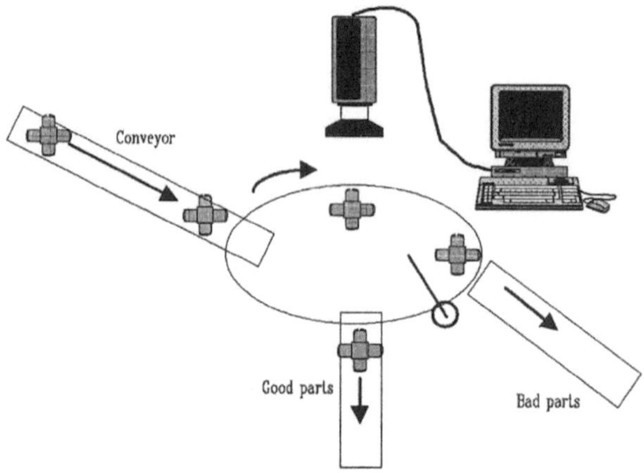

(c) Conveyor set-up

Fig. 6. Cold pressing application.

As sections provided by the TEM are not aligned, images need to be registered to find a coordinate system common to all sections. The technique used here for registering a pair of images relies on a fairly simple principle: one of the image is moved in translation and rotation over the other until a maximum number of matches between feature common to both images is found.

The technique described above requires a sample of edge points of the cell of interest in each section. These contours are rather difficult to detect using standard image processing techniques, however an aided-edge detector based upon watershed techniques is used. Later, an edge editor is provided to let the user interactively modify points on the edges which are not correctly set at the correct location. The result of the edge editor is sent to an automaton which approximates edges by closed polygonal lines. These points are used as input data to the triangulation algorithm.

From the set of 2D contours, one may then obtain a 3D object using the Delaunay triangulation technique, derived from the Voronoï tessellation, which is represented as a partition into tetrahedra.

One of the main function needed by neurobiologists is then the ability to find the axis of reconstructed dendrites, which may exhibit several branches, arising from neuronal branching process. The detection of the median axis is very similar to the computation of the skeleton using Mathematical Morphology techniques.

Figure 7 shows a perspective view of a reconstructed dendrite, the main body is the dendritic shaft and the spines are pointing outwards. The objects include more than 200 sections. This reconstruction required a few hours of work to obtain the 3 objects, from which 3D data can be measured, to be compared with several months with the previous approaches.

8. Conclusion

The progress made in the performance of standard computers, and the emergence of multi-processing systems enabling real-time operations, allow us to solve very complex vision applications involving high-level image transformations such as morphological functions or recursive edge detectors.

References

Boissonnat, J.-D. (1984), 'Geometric structures for three-dimensional shaper representation', **3**(4), 266–286.

Faugeras, O. (1993), *Three dimensional computer vision: a geometric view point*, The MIT Press, Cambridge, MA.

Serra, J. (1982), *Image analysis and mathematical morphology*, Academic Press, London.

White, E. *et al.* (1994), 'A comparison of synapses onto the somata of intrinsically bursting and regular spiking neurons in layer V of rat cortex', *The Journal of Comparative Neurology* **342**, 1–14.

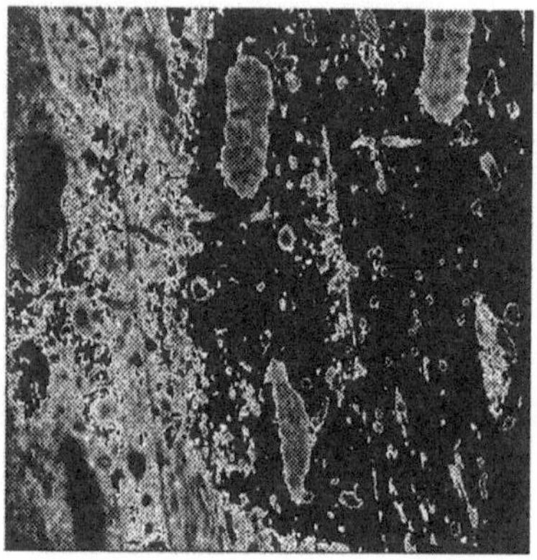

(a) Cross section of the cellular body

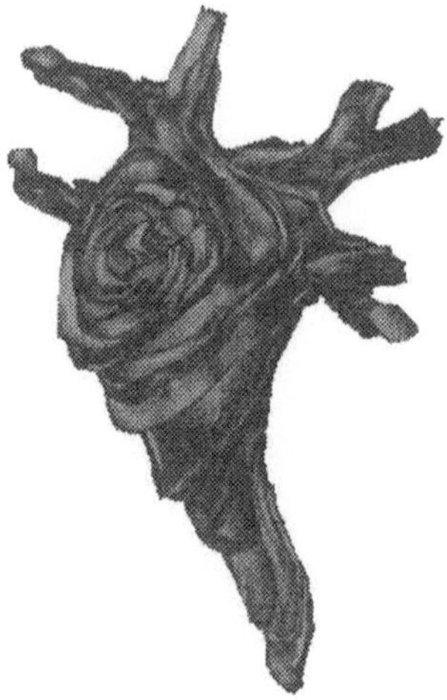

(b) Neuron

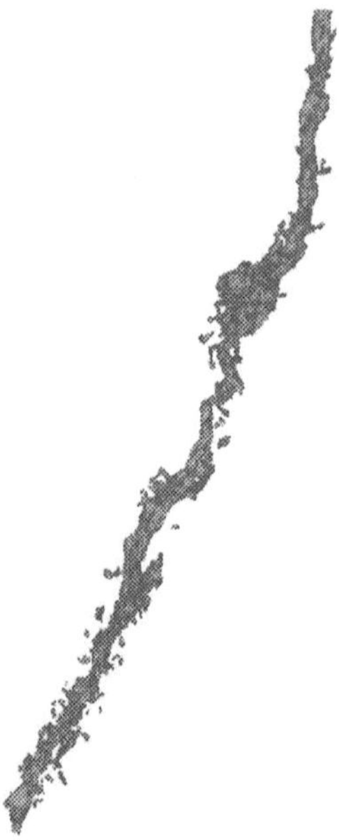

(c) Dendrite

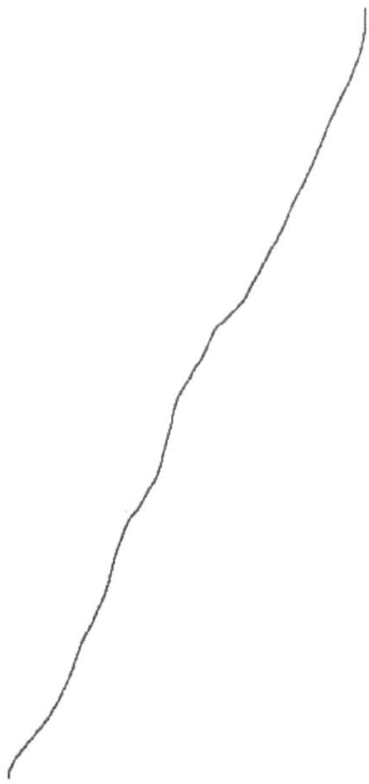

(d) 3-D skeleton of the dendrite

Fig. 7. 3–D reconstruction of a neurone from successive cross sections

RADAR IMAGE ANALYSIS USING MORPHOLOGICAL FILTERS

Application to geological mapping

C. MERING* and J.-F. PARROT†
Département de Géotectonique, UPMC PARIS VI
4, place Jussieu F-75252 Paris Cedex 05, France

Abstract. The speckle noise is one severe obstacle for automatic mapping from radar images. For geological mapping, the connectivity of structures has to be restored. New filters for speckle reduction are presented here and compared to already known ones according to an index of connectivity.

Key words: Radar images, Speckle removal, Morphological filtering, Geological mapping

1. Introduction

On radar images, topographic variations are enhanced by high contrasts of reflectivity. This property is very useful for geological structural mapping based on the recognition of geomorphological objects such as faults, versant orientations, thalwegs or crest lines. The speckle makes although difficult the contrast feature extraction by classical techniques (Mering *et al.*, 1993). We present here a panel of filters having the property of reducing the speckle while preserving the radiometrical and the spatial resolution of the initial image. Two classes of methods have been already developed: (a) statistical methods where the existence of an additive or multiplicative noise is assumed (Lee, 1981). (b) morphological methods which achieve the smoothing of the grey-tone images thanks to the properties of the morphological transformations (Safa and Flouzat, 1989). We propose here other filters belonging to both classes.

The tested area is located in western Spitsbergen, centered on the Broggerhalvoya peninsula. It presents a mountainous topography due to the glacier activity. This area has been previously studied by using ERS-1 imagery (Parrot *et al.*, 1993). The main structural features correspond to sharp crest lines and rock-glacier boundaries. On the other hand, the front of the active glaciers is underlined by morainic accumulations.

---

* Affiliated to ORSTOM, Paris (France)
† Affiliated to ORSTOM, Paris (France)

J.Serra and P. Soille (eds.), Mathematical Morphology and Its Applications to Image Processing, 353-360

2. Statistical Filters and Rank Operators

2.1. Lee filter

The statistical methods of noise removal are based on the minimization of the error between the noiseless image and its estimates, given a model describing the nature of the noise (multiplicative or additive). We have tested this approach by applying to the original image the Lee filter (1981). The principle is the following:

$$z_{i,j} = x_{i,j} + \omega_{i,j},$$

where $z_{i,j}$ is the value of the pixel (i,j), $x_{i,j}$ the value of the pixel before degradation and $\omega_{i,j}$ the additive noise with zero mean and σ^2 variance. It is assumed that the theoretical mean and variance ($\bar{x}_{i,j}$ and $Q_{i,j}$) are approximated by the local mean variance of all pixels in the neighborhood surrounding $z_{i,j}$. The estimate $\hat{x}_{i,j}$ is given by:

$$\hat{x}_{i,j} = \bar{x}_{i,j} + k_{i,j}(z_{i,j} - \bar{x}_{i,j}),$$

where

$$k_{i,j} = \frac{Q_{i,j}}{Q_{i,j} + \sigma^2}.$$

In this version of the Lee filter, the neighborhood is chosen in order to preserve the edges.

2.2. Punctual filter

A similar approach consists in sorting the values of the pixels within a given neighborhood. The median filter is one of the more frequently used for image smoothing. Considering that the speckle corresponds to punctual anomalies, it would be more pertinent to eliminate them. It is done by replacing the isolated values of reflectivity by a statistical estimator (median or mean) computed within 3×3 square neighborhood. The algorithm is the following: the absolute value of the difference between the central pixel and each surrounding pixel is computed. The value of the central pixel is considered as unique when all these absolute values are greater than a given threshold. In this case, the value of the central pixel is replaced on the resulting image by the mean value of the height surrounding pixels; else, the value on the resulting image remains unchanged.

3. Morphological Filters

Morphological Filters are not based on any probabilist model of the grey-tone distribution. They are based on Morphological Openings and Closings with a given structuring element. If utilized alone, a Morphological Opening (resp. Closing) smoothes only white (resp. dark) details. But on a grey-tone image like the radar ones, the noise may be composed both of dark or white details. Classical smoothing filters such as the median filter acts the same manner on high and low values. Many Morphological Filters have been proposed for image smoothing. They are the result of a determined composition of Openings and Closings. We have applied here two Morphological Filters designed for smoothing noisy grey-tone images: the Center filter and the Comparative filter. A third one is proposed which is a Connected filter.

3.1. Comparative filter

Safa and Flouzat (1989) have proposed morphological filters to remove speckle on radar imagery and especially one called the Comparative filter. This filter is built from local transformations which are defined as algebraic Openings and Closings. The structuring elements used in these transformations are not convex. In their definition, the center of the structuring element is omitted. The two basic transformations utilized in the comparative filter are:

$$\varphi_B f(x) = \max(f(x), \min_{B^*(x)} f),$$

$$\gamma_B f(x) = \min(f(x), \max_{B^*(x)} f),$$

where $B^* = B(x) - \{x\}$. The operator φ_B suppresses the "isolated" minima with respect to B and γ_B acts on the minima in the same way. The actual implementation is more complex. It is based on two operators ψ and ψ' and on a family of structuring elements of increasing radii $B_1, \ldots, B_n$. They are defined in the following way:

$$\psi_{B_1,\ldots,B_n} f(x) = \max(f(x), \min_{B_1^*} f, \ldots, \min_{B_n^*} f),$$

$$\psi'_{B_1,\ldots,B_n} f(x) = \min(f(x), \max_{B_1^*} f, \ldots, \max_{B_n^*} f).$$

We used the following step of the filter:

$$m_\lambda = \gamma_{B_\lambda} \varphi_{B_\lambda} = (\psi'_{B_\lambda})^k (\psi_{B_\lambda})^k,$$

where $k = 3$ and B_λ is composed by three circles surrounding the origin and having increasing radii defined from the square grid.

3.2. Center filter

Self duality is one of the property required for grey-tone image smoothing. In this perspective, Serra noticed that the median filter is self-dual but not idempotent and showed are to build filters having both properties from morphological filters (Serra, 1988). In the general case of complete lattices P, the centre β between a *vee*–filter f and a *wedge*–filter g is given by the general formula:

$$\beta = (I \wedge f) \vee g = (I \vee g) \wedge f,$$

where I denotes the identity transform. Given a Morphological Opening γ with a convex structural element B and the dual Morphological Closing ϕ, the centre b is constructed with $f = \phi\gamma\phi$ and $g = \gamma\phi\gamma$. We used here a Morphological Opening (resp. Closing) with a square structural element of size 1.

3.3. Centre connected filter

It has been said that, for geological mapping from radar imagery, thin white structures have to be preserved or even restored. It has been now frequently shown, that connected filters on grey-tone images product grey-tone flat zones. Moreover, filters resulting from a composition of connected Openings and Closings have the same algebraic properties than the equivalent ones made of morphological filters (Crespo *et al.*, 1993). Given the two filters γ_c and ϕ_c which are respectively an Opening and a Closing by reconstruction, we applied to the original radar image (Fig. 1a) a filter which is the centre β_c between f_c and g_c defined as follows:

$$\beta_c = (I \wedge f_c) \vee g_c,$$

where $f_c = \phi_c \gamma_c \phi_c$ and $g_c = \gamma_c \phi_c \gamma_c$. One can see on the Fig. 1b that the speckle has been partially removed and that the contours of the structures have been restored.

4. Comparison and valuation of the filters

The results of the various filters may be visually compared. But visual estimation of the quality of the grey-tone images obtained by filtering is difficult to objectively carry out. Therefore we have compared binary images resulting from an automatic thresholding (Fig. 2). Moreover, a quantitative index based on geodesic parameters is defined here to valuate binary images obtained by this thresholding. This quantitative index, called here connectivity index, is based on the definition of the geodesic length of connected components on binary images (Lantuéjoul and Maisonneuve, 1984). For each connected component of the binary image, we compute the geodesic length according to the algorithm of the geodesic Euclidean distance function proposed by Soille (1992). The connectivity index I_c is defined as follows:

$$I_c = \sum_{i=1}^{N} \frac{l_g(X_i)}{N},$$

where $l_g(X_i)$ is the geodesic length of the component X_i, and N is the number of connected components. A normalized connectivity index NI_c can be defined as:

$$NI_c = \frac{I_c}{l_{gmax}},$$

where l_{gmax} is the maximal geodesic length on the binary image. These two indexes have been used to compare the results of the filtering.

4.1. Connexity index on filtered images

Assuming that the connectivity of white structures, in the case of geological structural mapping, is an index of quality, we thresholded the first decile of the grey-tone distribution of the original image and the five filters formerly described (see Fig. 2). The results presented on Table I show clearly that the use of the connected filters enhance the structural features. On the other hand, the use of structuring elements with a central hole (cf. punctual and comparative filters) seems to improve the speckle removal.

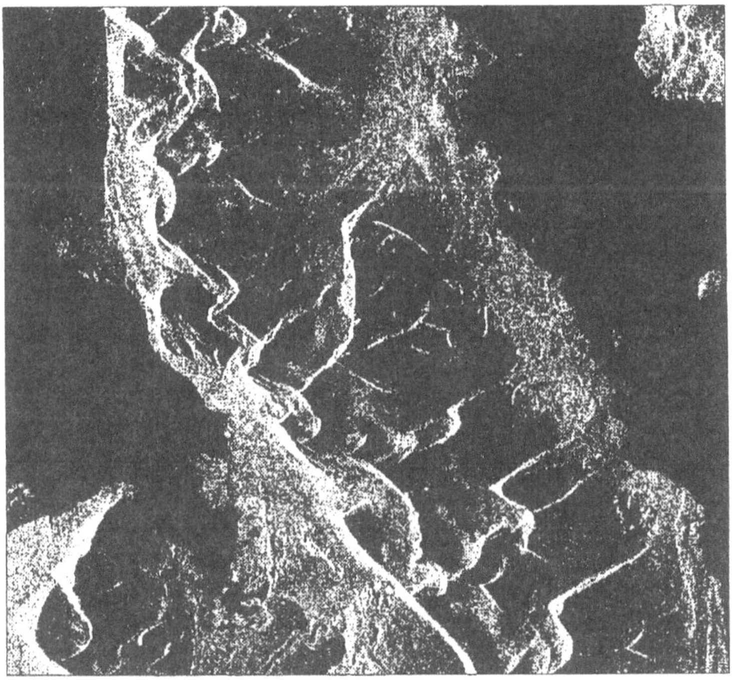

Fig. 1A. Original radar image

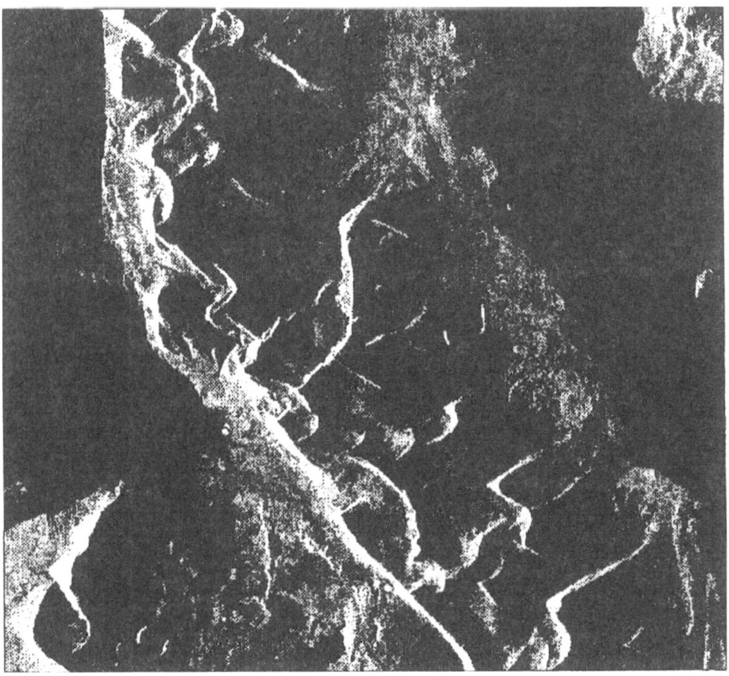

Fig. 1B. Connected Center Filter

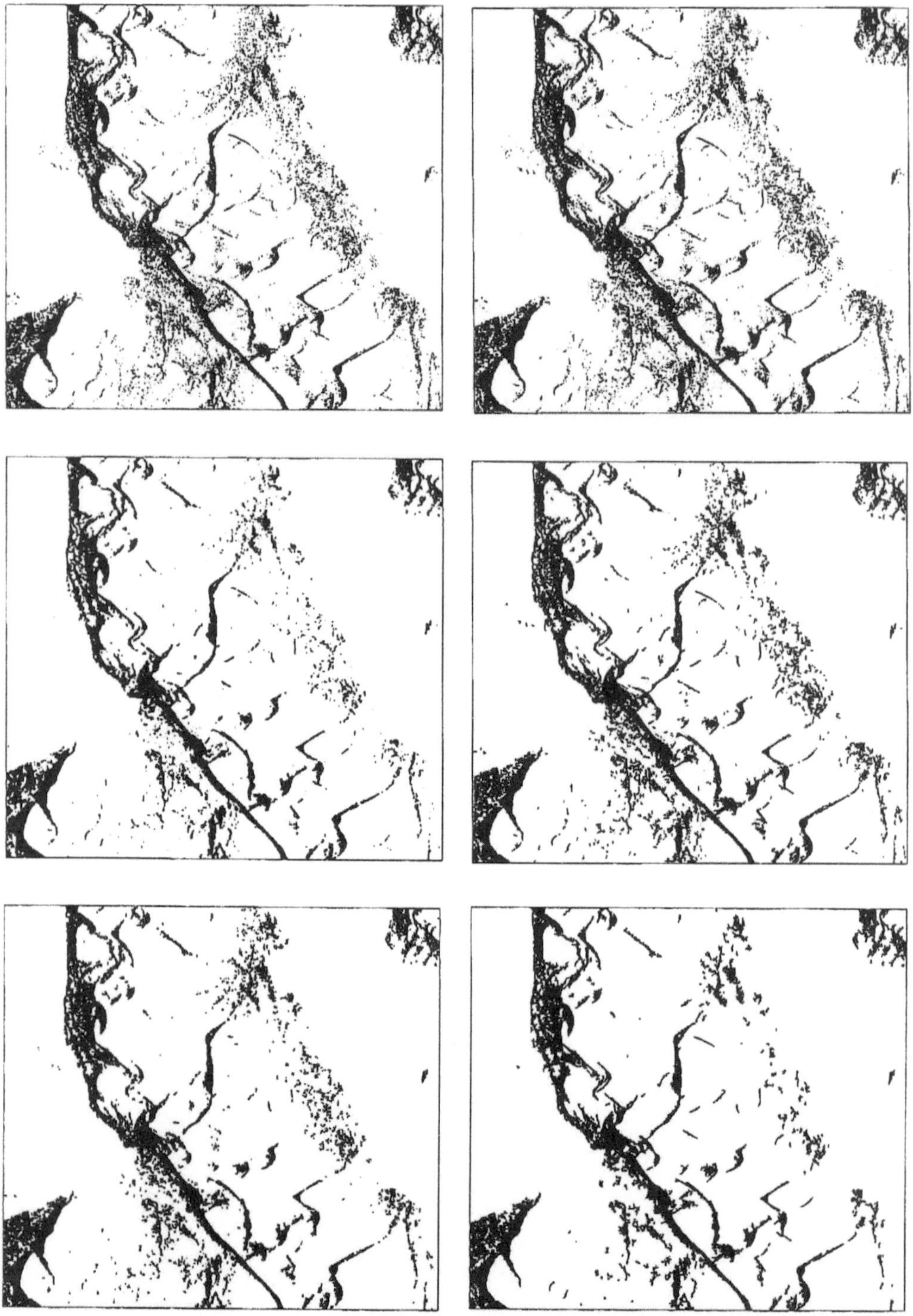

Fig. 2. Thresholding on filtered images: A. Original radar image; B. Lee filter; C. Punctual Filter; D. Comparative Filter; E. Center Filter; F. Connected Center Filter

TABLE I
Connexity index on filters

Filters	connexity index	normalized index
unfiltered image	5.18	0.0050
Lee filter	5.21	0.0051
punctual filter	13.6	0.0101
comparative filter	12.7	0.0112
center filter	9.82	0.0084
connected center filter	59.2	0.0312

4.2. Connexity index on the residual filtered images

Previously, features have been extracted only by thresholding. The contrast feature extraction by means of a White Top Hat transformation has been also experimented on the filtered images. In order to simplify the residual images which are quite noisy and to enhance the contrasts, a κ^2 morphological contrast filter (Meyer and Serra, 1989) has been applied on White Top Hat images. Before the computation of the two connectivity indexes, the thresholding previously described has been used. Table II shows that the valuation of the filters based on their morphological residues is quite different than the one presented formerly on Table I. In particular, it is not surprising that the β_c gets low values of index. Actually, if the use of connected filters improves the aspect of noisy images better than classical morphological filters, this is not any more true for their residues.

TABLE II
Connexity index on residues

Filters	connexity index	normalized index
unfiltered image	5.931	0.0068
Lee filter	5.938	0.0068
punctual filter	6.430	0.0212
comparative filter	9.114	0.0133
center filter	8.783	0.0170
connected center filter	8.059	0.0158

5. Conclusion

Space radar images are very useful for geological purpose if one can reduce the speckle while preserving the fine structures. A solution of filtering is proposed here based on connected filters. The valuation of this solution led us to define an index of global connectivity. In this study we compared filters reducing the noise and minimizing the loss of information about fine details. In the general prospect of removing the speckle for image segmentation at larger resolutions, the use of Alternate Sequential Filters should demonstrate good results.

References

Crespo, J., Serra, J. & Schafer, R. (1993), Image segmentation using connected filters, *in* J. Serra & P. Salembier, eds, 'Mathematical morphology and its applications to signal processing', Universitat Politècnica de Catalunya, Barcelona, Spain, pp. 52–57.

Lantuéjoul, C. & Maisonneuve, F. (1984), 'Geodesic methods in image analysis', *Pattern Recognition* **17**(2), 177–187.

Lee, J.-S. (1981), 'Refined filtering of image noise using local statistics', *Computer Graphics and Image Processing* **15**(4), 380–389.

Mering, C., Callot, Y. & Chorowicz, J. (1993), An application of mathematical morphology to geomorphology and structural geology, *in* J. Serra & P. Salembier, eds, 'Mathematical morphology and its applications to signal processing', Universitat Politècnica de Catalunya, Barcelona, Spain, pp. 204–209.

Meyer, F. & Serra, J. (1989), 'Contrasts and activity lattice', *Signal Processing* **16**, 303–317.

Parrot, J.-F., Lefauconnier, B., Mering, C., Lyberis, N., Taud, H., Chorowicz, J. & Rudant, J.-P. (1993), Etudes des glaciers subpolaires du Spitsberg à l'aide des données SPOT, ers-1 et hypsométriques : résultats et perspectives, *in* 'Colloque SPOT ERS-1'.

Safa, F. & Flouzat, G. (1989), 'Speckle removal on radar imagery based on mathematical morphology', *Signal Processing* **16**, 319–333.

Serra, J., ed. (1988), *Image analysis and mathematical morphology. Volume 2: theoretical advances*, Academic Press, London.

Soille, P. (1992), Morphologie mathématique : du relief à la dimensionalité—Algorithmes et méthodes—, PhD thesis, Université Catholique de Louvain, Louvain-la-Neuve, Belgium.

APPLICATION OF MORPHOLOGICAL OPERATORS TO SUPERVISED MULTIDIMENSIONAL DATA CLASSIFICATION

FERNANDO MUGE and PEDRO PINA
CVRM, Instituto Superior Técnico,
Av. Rovisco Pais, 1096 Lisboa Codex, Portugal

Abstract

In this paper the use of mathematical morphology (MM) operators in the several steps of supervised multidimensional data classification methods is discussed. In a first step, that can be called low-level feature extraction, morphological operators are usually applied with filtering purposes but can also be applied to extract topological features that can be used to generate extra information enhancing the phenomena representation. In a second step, MM operators can also be used to to improve pixel based classification algorithms in the following phases : i) modelling of clusters hulls training samples, ii) definition of criteria for processing overlapping clusters hulls and iii) 2D pattern space partition and distance function definition. Finally, in a third and last step of the classification procedure, low-level generalization algorithms can be used to perform the spatial arrangement of primitive image objects, giving a smoother, more simplified view of the classified image. Two examples of the application of this methodology to supervised classification are presented. The first one concerns the interpretation of geochemical data in a region in the south of Portugal, while the second one concerns the identification and mapping of the areas occupied by different forest cover types.

Keywords: Supervised multidimensional classification, ASF filters, cluster hull, distance function

1. Introduction

The several supervised classification algorithms can be roughly subdivided in three main groups. A brief description of each one is given next:

i) Minimum-Distance classifiers - These algorithms are based on the definition of an euclidean distance to the centroid or barycentre of each object (class) presented in the images. The set of training samples are used to calculate the centroid coordinates (into nD space) of each one of the k objects (classes). Each pixel x is then classified according to the value taken by an euclidean distance function $d(x,k)$ defined in relation to each k class centroid. Each pixel is affected to the least *distant* class according to the mentioned euclidean metrics. These algorithms do not take into account the shape of the nD clouds of training pixels. The occurrence of higher concentration zones (clusters) of pixels is therefore disregarded. The only aspect of this important features retained by these methods lies on the averages calculated for the centroids definition.

ii) Parallelepiped classifiers - These methods are similar to the preceding ones in the sense that they also need a centroid definition of each class, but they intend to model the shape of each training nD cloud by defining nD parallelepiped centered at each class centroid. The modelling of the nD training cloud performed by these methods is rather poor, do not taking into consideration irregular and complex shapes and also the occurrence of disjoint clusters of pixels belonging to the same class. Overlapping between parallelepipeds belonging to different classes can occur as a consequence of the chosen rather simple shape

J.Serra and P. Soille (eds.), Mathematical Morphology and Its Applications to Image Processing, 361-368

model and of the overlapping between training clouds.

iii) Statistical classifiers - Many multidimensional data classification methods make an explicit statistical hypothesis about the sample distribution of each class. The commonly used maximum likelihood classifier assumes for each class a multigaussian distribution. As the preceding methods, this kind of statistical classifiers, do not take into account irregular and complex shapes of the training clouds. Overlapping can frequently occur but is not dealt directly by those methods. Usually classification of pixels belonging to overlapping ellipsoids is complementary achieved by using minimum distance classifiers (*i*).

Due to the rather poor modelling of the shapes of the training clouds when they present irregular and complex shapes, another approach is needed to improve the classification procedure.

2. The use of morphological operators in the several steps of supervised multidimensional classification methods

Mathematical morphology operators can be used in the several steps of supervised multidimensional data classification. They can be grouped in a set of three steps and consist on a low-level feature extraction, morphological enhancement of classification and low-level generalization algorithms.

2.1. Low-level feature extraction

The alternating sequential filters (ASF) have been defined (Serra, 1988) as families of openings (γ_λ) and closings (φ_λ) parametrized by a positive number λ (the size of the structuring element). The family of ASF used in this work can be defined as:

$$M_\lambda(f(x)) = m_\lambda\, m_{\lambda-1} \cdots m_1\, f((x)) \qquad \lambda > 1 \tag{1}$$

where:

$$m_\lambda = \varphi_\lambda\, \gamma_\lambda\, (f(x)) \tag{2}$$

This ASF is a sequence of products of openings (γ_λ) and closings (φ_λ) of increasing size (from 1 to λ).

The proposed ASF acts alternatively and sequentially upon the peaks (through the opening) and the valleys (through the closing) of increasing length. Each opening of size λ, suppresses the peaks of lengths $\leq \lambda$ and each closing of size λ, fills the valleys of lengths $\leq \lambda$.

2.2. Morphological enhancement of classification algorithms

In this classification step MM operators can play an important role in the enhancement of pixel based methods. Indeed, as Madier *et al* (1986) points out, *many multidimensional data classification methods make an explicit or implicit statistical hypothesis about samples distribution of each class. This type appears unadapted when the training samples produce clusters with complex shape.* Thus, at this stage, MM operators can be applied in the following three phases:

i) Modelling of clusters hulls of training samples: it consists on a morphological closing for reconnecting close points, followed by a geodesic opening - erosion followed by a reconstruction - to eliminate small unconnected points;

ii) Definition of criteria for processing overlapping regions: it is composed by a morphological filtering of the non-overlapping parts of the clusters hulls followed by the geodesical SKIZ of the disjoint parts, conditioned by the union of all clusters hulls;

iii) 2D pattern space partition and distance function definition: determination of the influence zones of the set of cluster hulls obtained in ii) by an *internal distance function* for each cluster hull made of successive elementary erosions till the ultimate erosion and by an *external distance function* for each zone of influence made of successive elementary erosions of the respective cluster hull.

2.3. Low-level generalization algorithms

Finally, in the last step of the classification procedure, low-level generalization algorithms can be used to perform the spatial rearrangement of primitive image objects, giving a smoother, more simplified, view of the classified image. The simplified image should, however obey certains constraints. The most important constraint is the local area accuracy, *i.e.*, there must be a correct local representation of the areas of the different classes. This can be achieved by using a local estimation of areas occupied by each class (using, for example a kriging estimator based on local information). These area statistics are then used to drive the generalization process. The approach used combines morphological filtering in order to suppress small unconnected pixels and agglomerate close pixels, with growing (conditional dilation) in the class domain in order to ensure a correct areal balance between the classes.

3. Application of the proposed methodology. Two case studies.

3.1. A case study in the Moura-Ficalho region (Alentejo, Portugal)

The methodology presented above is tested in the Moura-Ficalho region located in Alentejo, Portugal. The information available for this case study is constituted by geochemical data (kriged and topological maps) and by satellite data (Landsat TM images).

Physiographically this region is a peneplain with some NW-SE oriented residual rugged hills of low relief some of tectonic origin. Numerous economic concentrations are found in the zone. The most characteristics are polymetallic sulphides of Pb, Zn and Cu occurring spatially linked with Cambrian dolomites. The oxidation of some sulphide deposits has led to significant gossan development during which enrichment reached economic values (Preguiça, Vila Ruiva). A detailed description of the geology of this area can be found in Oliveira and Piçarra (1986). The geological map of this region is presented in figure 1.

The geochemical data used in this study consists on grades of copper (Cu) and zinc (Zn) in soils, obtained in exploration surveys over Moura-Ficalho area. The samples were taken over a regular grid of 200m x 200m in an area of 13.6 x 17.8 km^2. Using the sampling points, the values of both variables were estimated in a regular grid of 30m x 30m using geostatistical methods (kriging). A detailed description of this procedure can be found in Vairinho *et al* (1990).The resulting kriged values in each point were converted into grey level values (0-255) using an histogram equalization (each grey level class has the same frequency). Images of Cu and Zn were produced this way having a spatial resolution of 30 metres per pixel.

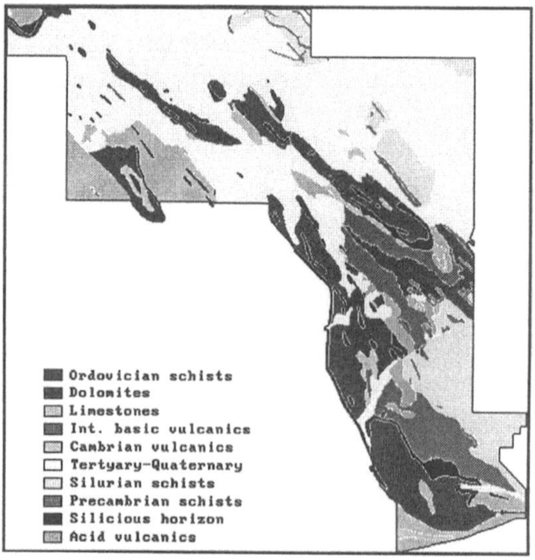

Figure 1 - Geological map of Moura-Ficalho area, Portugal (Oliveira and Piçarra, 1986)

The topological behaviour of both variables can be used as *extra* information in the classification procedure of the lithological formations. Maps enhancing these features were built by means of ASF filters (Muge and Pina, 1993).

Remote sensing data comes from Landsat TM spectral bands. The six digital images with a spatial resolution of 30 metres per pixel, have been previously submitted to radiometric and geometric corrections (Sousa *et al*, 1993). The radiometric correction was applied to correct some wrong information given by a malfunction of the sensors (periodic stripping in the images) and to attenuate the atmospheric effects. The geometric correction gives a geographical referential to the satellite images.

The available data consisted on the following : 2 geochemical (Cu and Zn), 6 topological (3 for Cu (sizes 2, 8 and 19) and 3 for Zn sizes (2, 8 and 15)) and 6 satellite images (bands TM 1, 2, 3, 4, 5 and 7). This information was then reduced to a 2D pattern space, by retaining the images corresponding to the first two axes of a PCA.

Classification tests were done in a subzone of the study area. The results obtained by the morphological approach method are compared with the ones obtained by applying the classical methods: minimum distance, minimum weighted distance and maximum likelihood. Figures 2 shows the classified image for this method, while the results of the classification procedures are presented in table I, and correspond to the main diagonals of each confusion matrix. The results obtained show that the morphological method is, in general, the best one, leading to an improvement in the classification. For the 10 lithological classes, 6 are best classified using the morphological approach, 2 using the minimum distance, and 1 each using the other two methods.

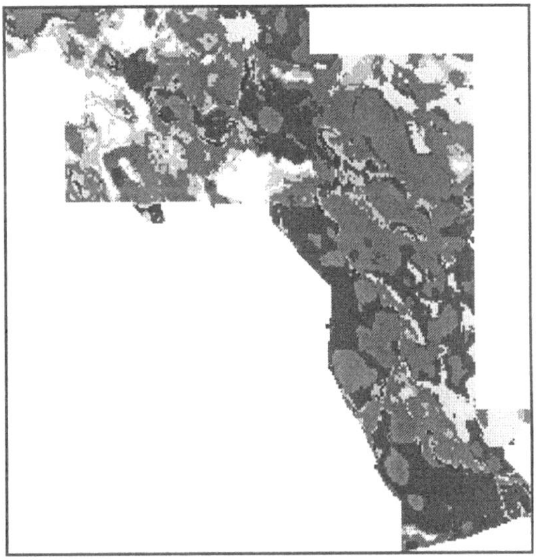

Figure 2 - Map produced using the morphological classifier (Moura-Ficalho case study)

CLASSIFICATION RESULTS (%)				
Lithologies	**Minimum distance**	**Minimum weighted distance**	**Maximum likelihood**	**Morphological**
Ordovician Schists	12.58	10.11	8.75	11.95
Dolomite	50.12	45.46	51.91	48.74
Limestones	13.00	13.42	13.19	20.82
Inter. Basic Vulcanics	8.09	6.58	7.15	11.89
Cambrian Vulcanics	2.45	2.73	2.84	3.39
Tertiary-Quaternary	71.65	77.88	79.37	86.29
Silurian Schists	45.04	42.64	40.50	35.03
Precambrian Schists	0.57	0.96	1.20	1.96
Silicious Horizon	6.05	7.86	6.82	7.25
Acid Vulcanics	2.14	2.51	2.69	4.61

Table I - Confusion matrix results (Moura-Ficalho case study)

The definition of a distance function (normalized or not) in the space of the variables (figure 3) allows the construction of images according to its degree of classification given by its distance to the points of the ultimate erosion of each class. Being the minimum value of the distance function the maximum grey level allowable (255) and the maximum value of the distance function the minimum+1 grey level available (1), it is possible to know immediately, by a simple thresholding operation, what are the points classified in certain domains. For instance the Tertyary-Quaternary lithologie has a global classification accuracy of 86.29%. If only the points *belonging* to the internal distance function are retained the classification accuracy increases to 94.90%.

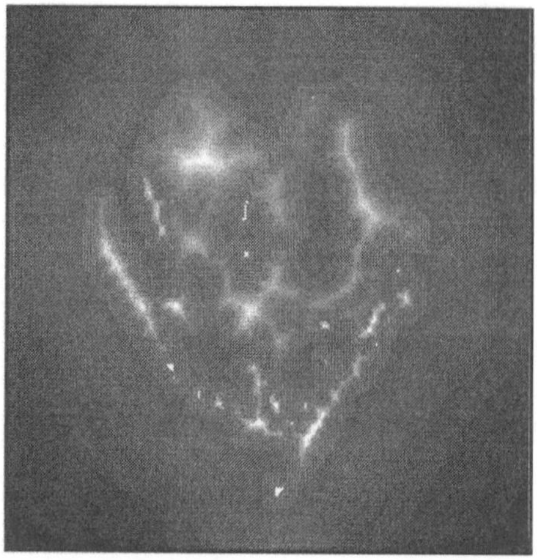

Figure 3- 2D pattern space partition: normalized distance function

3.2. Case study on forest imagery (aerial photographs)

The second example, at a different scale, concerns the application of supervised classification methods to identify and to map areas occupied by different forest cover types based on colour infrared aerial photographs.

In this case study only the second and third steps of the proposed methodology were applied, *i.e.*, the morphological enhancement of the classification and the low-level generalization algorithms. The average value of each forest cover area for each aerial photograph was obtained by two different ways: estimation by kriging using the information given by a dot grid superimposed to a sampled subset of aerial photos and delimitation of the area of each forest cover type by an expert.

The images used in the classification procedure were taken from the three components RGB (red, green and blue) of a colour image. In figure 3 is presented an image of a study area located in a region of Portugal. The classification was performed using the same methods applied in 3.1, giving the morphological one the best results. The thematic map produced for 5 different forest cover type classes (here simply named A, B, C, D and E) can be seen in figure 4, being the classification accuracy given by the respective confusion matrix in table II. In that table are presented the results obtained before and after the low-level generalization step (LLG).

The classification of four of the five forest cover types improves after the low-level generalization step: only class A decreases its level of classification accuracy.

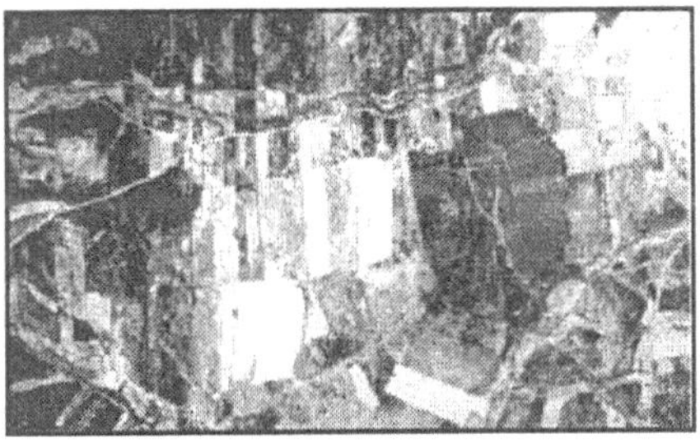

Fig. 3 - Aerial photograph of a region occupied by different forest cover types

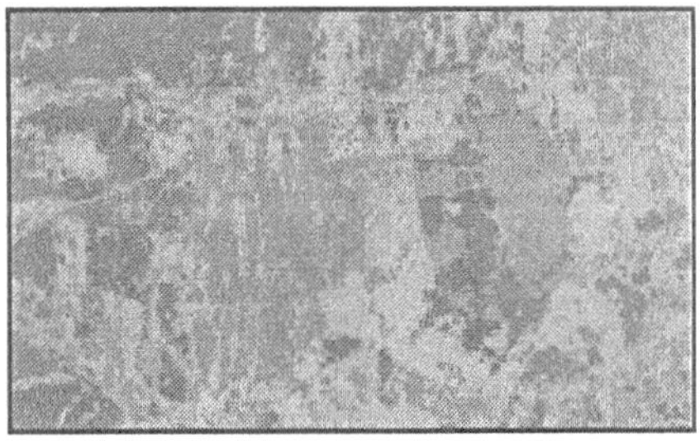

Figure 4 - Map classified using the morphological classifier (forest imagery case study)

CLASSIFICATION RESULTS (%)		
Forest cover types	Before LLG step	After LLG step
A	47.46	44.62
B	50.26	58.45
C	62.69	65.13
D	37.15	39.85
E	26.60	27.80

Table II - Confusion matrix results (forest imagery case study)

4. Conclusions

The several phases of the classification procedure where the morphological operators are introduced and that are presented in this paper do not need any statistical hypothesis on sampling distribution and can be applied to irregular complex shapes of training clouds. To conclude, the results obtained show the interest of using this morphological operators to supervised multidimensional data classification.

Acknowledgements

The case study presented in this paper related to the Moura-Ficalho region is partially included in a research project between CVRM/IST and IGM - Instituto Geológico Mineiro.

References

Madier J.P., Flouzat G. & Jourlin M. (1986), A Non-Parametric Supervised Multispectral Classification Method Using Binary Morphological Operators, *IGARSS'86, ESA-SP-254*, Zurich, Switzerland, vol.1, pp.547-552.

Muge F. & Pina P. (1993), Some Applications of Mathematical Morphology based Image Analysis Techniques to Remote Sensing, *Proceedings of Recpad'93 - 5th Portuguese Conference on Pattern Recognition*, Porto, Portugal, pp.287-294.

Oliveira V. & Piçarra (1986), Litoestatigrafia do Anticlinório de Moura-Ficalho (Zona de Ossa-Morena), *Bol. Inf. Soc. Geol. Port.*, **2**, 13.

Serra J. (1988), *Image Analysis and Mathematical Morphology vol.2: Theoretical Advances*, Academic Press, London.

Sousa A.J., Pina P., Muge F., Vairinho M. & Mariano A.C. (1993), Improvement of Geostatistical Treatment of Geochemical Data by Inclusion of Remote Sensing Information, poster presented at 25th IAMG Meet., Prague, Czech Rep., Oct.93 (to be published).

Vairinho M., Sousa A.J., Oliveira V., Guerreiro L. & Gonçalves A. (1990) - Tratamento Geomatemático e Cartografia de Dados da Prospecção Geoquímica da Região de Moura-Ficalho, *Geociências*, Vol.6,fasc.1-2, pp.145-159.

Vairinho M., Pina P., Sousa A.J., Muge F. & Oliveira V. (1993), Geostatistics and Image Analysis in the Interpretation of Geochemical Data, presented in *3rd CODATA Conference on Geostatistics and Geomathematics*, Enschede, The Netherlands, June 1993 (to be published in *Sciences de la Terre*).

APPENDIX A

THE "CENTRE DE MORPHOLOGIE MATHÉMATIQUE": AN OVERVIEW

(Welcoming Speech to the Second International Conference on Mathematical Morphology and its Applications to Image Processing, Fontainebleau, 5–9 September 1994)

JEAN SERRA
Ecole des Mines de Paris, Centre de Morphologie Mathématique, 35, rue Saint-Honoré, F-77305 Fontainebleau Cedex, France

Since the present workshop enables our gathering here at Fontainebleau, at the very place where mathematical morphology has expanded, let me introduce you briefly, in this welcoming speech, the "Centre de Morphologie Mathematique" and its history.

The Sixties

For a long time, Mathematical Morphology had seemed to confine itself to a small coterie. Was it because its first publication had been a patent, in 1965? or because it had originated outside from any academic context? Its birth took place thirty years ago exactly. G. Matheron supervised my PhD thesis, a work devoted to ore reserve estimation, for the iron deposit of Lorraine. The quality of ore was more related to its ability to be enriched, after appropriate milling than to the iron grade. Transposing the tools of geostatistics, I decided to compute variograms on ore thin sections, and in order to do so, to construct a digital device. Thanks to this first "Texture Analyser", developed in cooperation with J.-C. Klein, I understood that such different operations as covariance, chord length distribution, perimeter measurement, or particle counting were particular cases of a unique concept, which I called Hit or Miss Transform (Serra, 1965*b*; Serra, 1967; Haas, Matheron & Serra, 1967).

In the meantime, on a more theoretical level, G. Matheron had undertaken the study of permeability for porous media in relation with their geometry (or their 'texture'). When we look, today, at the publication he made following this first work (Matheron, 1967), the morphological aspect clearly prevails over the hydrodynamics part. For the first time, the notion of a morphological opening was introduced and associated with the convexity of the structuring element, leading to granulometry. In parallel, a random approach was explored, via the Boolean and

J.Serra and P. Soille (eds.), Mathematical Morphology and Its Applications to Image Processing, 369-374

the semi-Markov models, which also appeared for the first time.

Three years after the publication of *Eléments pour une théorie des milieux poreux*, we realized that our nonlinear approach was in line with Integral Geometry, and that G. Matheron had rediscovered Steiner formula and Minkowski functionals: the history of ideas is nonlinear either.

Finally, this first period yielded, besides a first set of result, a certain sketch for the future, namely:

- the wish to develop theory from actual (physical) issues,
- the primacy given to 'hit or miss' type relationships,
- the cross-fertilization between deterministic and random approaches,
- the symbiosis between method development and system design.

Also, one evening of winter 1966, in a pub of Nancy, following a full-day lecture on probabilities, and perhaps a few pints of beer, G. Matheron, Ph. Formery and I, decided to call "Mathematical Morphology" the foreseen method.

The seventies

An institutional basis was provided by the Ecole des Mines de Paris. They had received substantial funds from the government, in order to create centres of applied research, and the city of Fontainebleau had offered room for these scientific activities. Our application was accepted, and the Centre de Morphologie Mathématique was born in April 1968, in the building it still occupies today. We were ten people (including staff and the first four PhD students), under the direction of G. Matheron.

This was the anchoring point. Very soon, it turned out that the chaining of successive hit or miss transforms actually generated new operations such as particle reconstruction. This resulted in a second patent in 1970 (Serra, 1970), and in the Texture Analysis System of the German company Leitz. This system has probably been one of the most important ones in image processing, if we consider the turnover (30 to 50 million dollars), and surely a long life record (12 years).

On the theoretical level, the seventies were marked by G. Matheron's work: topological foundations, random sets, increasing mappings, convexity, several models of random sets, etc. Part of this material became the subject of a second book (Matheron, 1975). On the level of operators, it can be said that the core of the morphological tool box was discovered during this period (except for morphological filtering). Based on iterative processing, binary thinning, skiz, ultimate erosion, conditional bisector and their geodesic framework were introduced. Meanwhile, the initial set-oriented approach was extended to numerical functions, giving birth to morphological gradient, top hat transform and watershed, in particular. The main actors of this development were S. Beucher, H. Digabel, D. Jeulin, J-C. Klein, Ch. Lantuéjoul, F. Meyer and J. Serra (a list of the first papers covering each topic is given in the references).

Although, the centre was already known in the field of geometrical probability (see the proceedings of Buffon's symposium (Serra, 1977)) our work was practically not known to the community of signal (or image) processing. This is perhaps because the Leitz-TAS, in spite of its success, reached mainly the world of users, and often of naturalists. A contrario, this demonstrates that the scientists who adopted morphology at the beginning of the seventies (G.S. Watson, R.M. Haralick, M. Coster, J.-L. Chermant, J.-C. Binet, among others) denoted a real independent mind.

The eighties

Four events marked this decade, namely

- the opening to the outside world, and especially to the United States,
- the setting up of Mathematical Morphology in the convenient mathematical framework of lattices,
- algorithmic developments and
- the renewal of random processes.

The opening to the outside world was produced by both a book and a man. The first volume of *Image Analysis and Mathematical Morphology* reflected the state of the art in 1980 at Fontainebleau (40% of the book had not been published before, another 40% came from Fontainebleau school but was not well known, the rest came from other sources). The person was S.R. Sternberg. He liked the way of thinking in Mathematical Morphology, adopted it, and organized a number of courses on the subject at Ann Arbor (1980-1985). I also co-organized three of those courses with him, and participated in two others.

This sudden broadening came as new fields opened to apply Mathematical Morphology. The oil crisis had resulted in the development of automated visual inspection, and the method could obviously provide means to solve part of such tasks. At Fontainebleau, in 1984 and 1986, two opportunities to create companies occurred. They led to launch MorphoSystems (finger print recognition, 200 people in 1994) and Noesis (image processing, 25 people in 1994). As another consequence of this broadening, about ten research centres were created in Europe, America and Australia. For the first time, substantial developments in morphology stemmed from other sources than Fontainebleau.

The second typical feature of the eighties was the setting of the method (at least of its deterministic aspect) in the mathematical framework of complete lattices. The variety of applications brought us back to theoretical reflection. Although the initial operators were set oriented and translation invariant. They were now transposed to other situations and to other objects (graphs, numerical functions), where translation might influence the process (geodesy, edge conditions) or even not exist (graphs). Finally, the core of essential axioms could be reduced to the complete lattice structure.

In 1986, I worked out a new formulation of Mathematical Morphology on this basis, and tried to figure the additional assumptions necessary for some particular notions. For example, the concept of a connectivity needed a lattice of $\mathcal{P}(E)$ type, but no additional requirement. It is this reorganization that led G. Matheron and myself to the theory of morphological filtering. A contributed book (Serra ed., 1988) gathered these advances. interpreters to renew stochastic approaches appeared in the late seventies through the works of D. Jeulin and J. Serra on Boolean functions. During the nineties, it continued on both levels of theory and applications (D. Schmitt, F. Prêteux), while D. Jeulin explored new models, (conditional) simulation, and lattice gas approaches.

The third characteristic of the eighties concerned the emphasis put on algorithmics. It has its root in the relative growth of morphological software packages, versus dedicated processors. They concerned elementary operations, such as binary dilation, or sophisticated ones such as watershed. The classical data flow was conveniently replaced by edge tracking, (hierarchical) queues, arrow propagation and rewriting. At the Centre, this activity was mainly associated with the names of S. Beucher, F. Meyer, M. Schmitt and L. Vincent. They benefited from the extraordinary improvements in computation and processing speed, during the decade. But, paradoxically, this acceleration urged them to speed up even more.

The nineties

We do not have the required distance to step back and evaluate the present time. However, two major trends can be discerned at Fontainebleau Centre. First, the predominant role devoted to motion analysis: it concerns both encoding and description of moving scenes. Second, the permanent symbiosis between algorithms and hardware architectures has continued (J-C. Klein, M. Bilodeau, R. Peyrard, Ch. Gratin), as well as the design of operators for numerical functions (M. Grimaud, L. Vincent, P. Soille).

Conclusion

The future of a theory and a praxis generally escapes their founders (fortunately so!). As a method for artificial vision, Mathematical Morphology will be, and already is, trapped by its inability to catch the universe of meanings and the symbolic representations of the human mind. If it turns out to be, sometimes, more efficient than other approaches in pattern recognition, this comes from a better hold on the geometry of the scenes under study, but nothing more.

On the other hand, physics, or biology, offer situations where the method may be fruitful. An example is given by the lattice gas, which combines morphological operators and digital substitutes for partial derivative equations in a very subtle way. Another example is given by the current trends to give differential expressions to Minkowski operations. More basically, there are so many natural phenomena that are managed by sup/inf type relationships (possibly combined with other laws) that one can hope Mathematical Morphology will continue to be useful.

Last word: although this overview has, on purpose, focused on the contributions of Fontainebleau School, and on the first appearances of the concepts, it is clear that Mathematical Morphology is not reduced, today, to this particular group. The amount of publications in the field, and the recent books from Dougherty (1993), Schmitt & Matioli (1994), or Heijmans (1994) attest it. But the proof of this dynamism will be given during these three days: it is the workshop itself.

References

Beucher, S. (1982), Watersheds of functions and picture segmentation, *in* 'IEEE Int. Conf. on Acoustics, Speech and Signal Processing', Paris, pp. 1928–1931. [Examples, and use of watershed on gradients].

Beucher, S. (1990), Segmentation d'images et morphologie mathématique, PhD thesis, Ecole des Mines de Paris. [First apparition of the combination of connected operators and watersheds, in a hierarchical way, constitutes a compendium of watershed performances and applications].

Beucher, S. & Bilodeau, M. (1992), 'Road tracking, lane segmentation and obstacles recognition by mathematical morphology', *Proc. of Intelligent Vehicles '92, IEEE.*

Beucher, S. & Lantuéjoul, C. (1979), Use of watershed in contour detection, Rennes, France. [First publication of the watershed for numerical functions].

Bilodeau, M. (1992), Architecture logicielle pour processeur de morphologie mathématique, PhD thesis, Ecole des Mines de Paris.

Digabel, H. & Lantuéjoul, C. (1978), Iterative algorithms, *in* J.-L. Chermant, ed., 'Sonderbände der Praktischen Metallographie', Dr. Riederer-Verlag GmbH, Stuttgart, pp. 85–99. [First publication of the Skiz and of the watershed, the later presented as a set oriented notion].

Dougherty, E., ed. (1993), *Mathematical morphology in image processing*, Marcel Dekker.

Gratin, C. (1993), De la représentation des images au traitement morphologique des images tridimensionnelles, PhD thesis, Ecole des Mines de Paris.

Grimaud, M. (1992), New measure of contrast: dynamics, *in* P. Gader, E. Dougherty & J. Serra, eds, 'Image algebra and morphological image processing III', Vol. SPIE-1769, pp. 292–305. [First publication, in English, of the notion of the dynamics].

Haas, A., Matheron, G. & Serra, J. (1967), 'Morphologie mathématique et granulométries en place', *Annales des Mines* **11 and 12**, 736–753 and 768–782. [First publication of the connectivity numbers and of linear opening].

Heijmans, H. (1994), *Morphological image operators*, Advances in Electronics and Electron Physics, Academic Press.

Jeulin, D. (1989), 'Morphological modelling of images by sequential random functions', *Signal Processing* **16**, 401–431. [First publication in English of sequential random functions].

Jeulin, D., Vincent, L. & Serpe, G. (1992), 'Propagation algorithms on graphs for physical applications', *Journal of Visual Communication and Image Representation* **3**(2), 161–181.

Klein, J. C. (1976), Conception et réalisation d'une unité logique pour l'analyse quantitative d'images, PhD thesis, Université de Nancy. [First publication of geodesic methods].

Lantuéjoul, C. (1978), La squelettisation et son application aux mesures topologiques des mosaïques polycristallines, PhD thesis, Ecole des Mines de Paris. [First theory of the Skiz].

Lantuéjoul, C. & Beucher, S. (1981), 'On the use of the geodesic metric in image analysis', *Journal of Microscopy* **121**, 39–49. [First theory of the geodesy].

Matheron, G. (1967), *Eléments pour une théorie des milieux poreux*, Masson, Paris.

Matheron, G. (1975), *Random sets and integral geometry*, Wiley.

Meyer, F. (1978), Contrast feature extraction, *in* J.-L. Chermant, ed., 'Sonderbände der Praktischen Metallographie', Vol. 8, Dr. Riederer-Verlag GmbH, Stuttgart, pp. 374–380. [First publication of the top hat transform and of gradient by erosion].

Meyer, F. (1979), Cytologie quantitative et morphologie mathématique, PhD thesis, Ecole des Mines de Paris. [Various notions applied to cytology, first publication of conditional bisector].

Meyer, F. & Beucher, S. (1990), 'Morphological segmentation', *Journal of Visual Communication and Image Representation* **1**(1), 21–46.

Meyer, F. & Serra, J. (1989), 'Contrasts and activity lattice', *Signal Processing* **16**, 303–317. [First publication of idempotent contrast operators].

Prêteux, F. (1987), Description et interprétation des images par la morphologie mathémathique. Application à l'imagerie médicale, PhD thesis, Université de Paris 6.

Salembier, P. & Serra, J. (1992), Morphological multiscale image segmentation, *in* 'SPIE Visual Communications and Image Processing 92', Boston, USA, pp. 620–631. [First apparition of the combination of connected operators and watersheds, in a hierarchical approach].

Schmitt, M. (1989), Des algorithmes morphologiques à l'intelligence artificielle, PhD thesis, Ecole des Mines de Paris. [First publication of the chain and loop algorithms for binary dilation and for artificial intelligence in mathematical morphology].

Schmitt, M. & Matioli, J. (1994), *Morphologie mathématique*, Masson, Paris.

Serra, J. (1965*a*), 'Automatic scanning device for analyzing textures'. [Inventor, granted to IRSID. Priority date: July 2, 1965, France. Patented in: Belgium, Canada, Great-Britain, Japan, Sweden, USA].

Serra, J. (1965*b*), L'analyse des textures par la géometrie aléatoire, Technical report, Comptes-rendus du Comité Scientifique de l'IRSID.

Serra, J. (1967), Remarques sur une lame mince de minerai lorrain, Technical Report N6, Bulletin du B.R.G.M.

Serra, J. (1970), 'Device for the logical analysis for textures'. [Inventor, granted to ARMINES and J. Serra. Priority date: June 10, 1970 (70/21 322), France. Patented in: Austria, Canada, France, Germany, Great-Britain, Japan, USA].

Serra, J. (1975), Les fonctions à peu près en tout ou rien, Technical Report CMM-N-406, Ecole des Mines de Paris. [First publication of morphology for grey tone functions].

Serra, J. (1977), 'Geometrical probabilities and biological structures', *Buffon's 200th Anniversary*.

Serra, J. (1982), *Image analysis and mathematical morphology*, Academic Press, London. [Number of new notions, in particular first theory of mathematical morphology for grey tone functions: models, increasing transformations, stack operators, homotopy, etc].

Serra, J. (1986), Eléments pour une théorie de l'optique morphologique, PhD thesis, Mathématique univ. PM Curie. [First publication of mathematical morphology for complete lattices, first theory of alternating sequential filters].

Serra, J., ed. (1988), *Image analysis and mathematical morphology. Volume 2: theoretical advances*, Academic Press, London. [First publication of the theory of morphological filtering, and of number of notions: connected operators, activity lattice, properties of the skeleton, symmetries on convex sets, advances in Boolean functions].

Soille, P. (1991), 'Spatial distributions from contour lines: an efficient methodology based on distance transformations', *Journal of Visual Communication and Image Representation* **2**(2), 138–150. [First publication on interpolations and on geodesy].

Soille, P. & Vincent, L. (1990), Determining watersheds in digital pictures via flooding simulations, *in* M. Kunt, ed., 'Visual Communications and Image Processing'90', Vol. SPIE-1360, Lausanne, pp. 240–250. [First publication in English of a watershed implementation based on queue algorithms].

Vincent, L. (1989), 'Graphs and mathematical morphology', *Signal Processing* **16**, 365–388. [First comprehensive publication for the morphological processing of graphs].

Vincent, L. (1990), Algorithmes morphologiques à base de files d'attente et de lacets. Extension aux graphes, PhD thesis, Ecole des Mines de Paris. [Basic book in morphological algorithmics, first publication for queue algorithms].

APPENDIX B

LIST OF POSTER CONTRIBUTIONS PRESENTED AT ISMM'94

The following contributions have been accepted for a poster presentation at the second international conference on 'Mathematical Morphology and its Applications to Image Processing', Fontainebleau, September 1994. They are published by and available from the *Centre de Morphologie Mathématique de l'Ecole des Mines de Paris* 35, rue Saint-Honoré, F–77305 Fontainebleau Cedex, France (email: ismm@cmm.ensmp.fr). Each contribution consists of a 2 page paper:

Representations

- *Centro-normal function and basic mathematical morphology using splines*, J. Becker, I. Fillere, M. Jourlin, ICPI-CPE Lyon, France; M. Laboure, Universityé Jean Monnet, Saint-Etienne, France
- *Morphological signal decomposition in digital image compression*, D. Coltuc and I. Pitas, Aristotle University of Thessaloniki, Greece
- *Symmetries of mathematical morphology transformations on complete lattices*, A. Tuzikov and P. Zalesskii, Academy of Sciences of Republic Belarus, Minsk, Belarus
- *Polymorphism, an extension of binary opening*, M. Van Droogenbroeck, Belgacom, Brussels, Belgium

Applications

- *Automatic assessment of skeletal maturity by digital image processing methods*, Y. Jiang and C.V. Howard, The university of Liverpool, U.K.
- *Automated texture segmentation in images of the human cerebellum*, K. Sutherland, D. Rutovitz, J.E. Bell, and J.W. Ironside, Western General Hospital, Edinburgh, U.K.
- *Use of geodesic dilations for analysis of hematological images*, C. Souchier, M. Benchaib, R. Delorme, Université Claude Benard, Lyon, France; A. Manel, Université Claude Benard and Hôpital Debrousse, Lyon, France; N. Shen, Institut Pasteur, Lyon, France; J. Tigaut, Hôpital ED Herriot, Lyon, France; P.A. Bryon, Université Claude Benard and Hôpital ED Herriot, Lyon, France
- *Morphological characterisation and modeling of polymer blends filled with carbon black*, S. Blacher, F. Gubbels, F. Vecoven, F. Brouers, J. Destiné, and R. Jérôme, Université de Liège, Belgium

J.Serra and P. Soille (eds.), Mathematical Morphology and Its Applications to Image Processing, 375-376

- *Automatic process for image segmentation: application to plastic deformation localisation,* N. Ben Amar, A. Beghdadi, and P. Viaris de Lesegno, Université Paris Nord, France
- *Directional mathematical morphology for the textural segmentation of urbain images,* S. Loumi and B. Sansal, U.S.T.H.B., Alger, Algérie
- *A mixed morphological and spectral procedure to improve the accuracy of the built area classification from multisensor satellite data,* M. Pesaresi, Venice University, Italy
- *Real-time morphological processing: an application for automated navigation,* A. Broggi and S. Bertè, Università di Parma, Italy
- *Road segmentation using a fast watershed algorithm,* S. Beucher and M. Bilodeau, Ecole des Mines de Paris, France

Segmentation

- *Hypergraph and image processing,* A. Bretto and B. Laget, Laboratoire de traitement du signal et instrumentation URA 842, Saint Etienne, France
- *Binary and multivalued morphological analysis of a multidimensional data set for pattern classification,* C. Botte–Lecocq and J.-G. Postaire, Université des Sciences et Techniques de Lille, France
- *A dynamic hierarchical segmentation algorithm,* L. Najman and M. Schmitt, Thomson-CSF, Orsay, France
- *Image segmentation in morphological scale–space,* R. van den Boomgaard, A. Smeulders, and J. Schavemaker, University of Amsterdam, The Netherlands
- *An improved split-and-merge watershed algorithm,* B.P. Dobrin, T. Viero, and M. Gabbouj, Tampere University of Technology, Finland

Fractals

- *Mathematical morphology and fractal theory: a new concept to characterize fractal objects,* I. Terol Villalobos, Centro de Invest. En Electroq. del Edo de Qro., Sanfandila-Pedro Escobedo, Mexico
- *On the robustness of fractal dimension measurements in image analysis,* P. Soille, Ecole des Mines de Paris, France; J.-F. Rivest, University of Ottawa, Canada

Author Index

Subject Index

Computational Imaging and Vision

1. B.M. ter Haar Romeny (ed.): *Geometry-Driven Diffusion in Computer Vision.* 1994 ISBN 0-7923-3087-0
2. J. Serra and P. Soille (eds.): *Mathematical Morphology and Its Applications to Image Processing.* 1994 ISBN 0-7923-3093-5

Kluwer Academic Publishers – Dordrecht / Boston / London

MIX
Papier aus verantwortungsvollen Quellen
Paper from responsible sources
FSC® C105338

If you have any concerns about our products,
you can contact us on
ProductSafety@springernature.com

In case Publisher is established outside the EU,
the EU authorized representative is:
Springer Nature Customer Service Center GmbH
Europaplatz 3, 69115 Heidelberg, Germany

Printed by Libri Plureos GmbH
in Hamburg, Germany